UNDERSTANDING THE POLITICS OF PANDEMIC EMERGENCIES IN THE TIME OF COVID-19

This book reviews the political significance of COVID-19 in the context of earlier pandemic encounters and scares to understand the ways in which it challenges the existing individual health, domestic order, international health governance actors, and, more fundamentally, the circulation-based modus operandi of the present world order.

It argues that contagious diseases should be regarded as complex open-ended phenomena with various features and are not reducible merely to biology and epidemiology. They are, as such, fundamentally politosomatic, namely that they disrupt, agitate, and trigger large-scale processes because individual somatic-level anxieties stem from individuals' sensing immediate danger through the networks of their local and global connectedness. The author further argues that pandemics have somatic effects in political expressions that transform the epidemic into national security dramas which should not, for the sake of efficient health governance, be treated as aspects extraneous to the disease itself. The book highlights that when a serious infectious disease spreads, a 'threat' is very often externalized into a culturally meaningful 'foreign' entity. Pandemics tend to be territorialized, nationalized, ethnicized, and racialized.

This book will be of key interest to scholars and students of global health and governance, pandemic security, epidemics, history of medicine, geopolitics, international relations, and general readers interested in the COVID-19 pandemic.

Mika Aaltola is Director of the Finnish Institute of International Affairs, Finland; Full Professor of International Relations and European Studies at Tallinn University, Estonia; and docent of International Relations at the University of Tampere, Finland.

The Politics of Pandemics

Understanding the Politics of Pandemic Emergencies in the Time of COVID-19
An Introduction to Global Politosomatics
Mika Aaltola

UNDERSTANDING THE POLITICS OF PANDEMIC EMERGENCIES IN THE TIME OF COVID-19

An Introduction to Global Politosomatics

Mika Aaltola

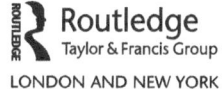

Routledge
Taylor & Francis Group

LONDON AND NEW YORK

First published 2022
by Routledge
4 Park Square, Milton Park, Abingdon, Oxon OX14 4RN

and by Routledge
605 Third Avenue, New York, NY 10158

Routledge is an imprint of the Taylor & Francis Group, an informa business

British Library Cataloguing-in-Publication Data
A catalogue record for this book is available from the British Library

Library of Congress Cataloging-in-Publication Data
Names: Aaltola, Mika, author.
Title: Understanding the politics of pandemic emergencies in the time of
    COVID-19 : an introduction to global politosomatics / Mika Aaltola.
Description: Milton Park, Abingdon, Oxon ; New York, NY : Routledge, 2022. |
    Series: The politics of pandemics | Includes bibliographical references and index.
Identifiers: LCCN 2021051860 (print) | LCCN 2021051861 (ebook) |
    ISBN 9780367769666 (hardback) | ISBN 9780367769659 (paperback) |
    ISBN 9781003169147 (ebook)
Subjects: LCSH: COVID-19 (Disease) | COVID-19 (Disease)—Political aspects.
Classification: LCC RA644.C67 A22 2022 (print) | LCC RA644.C67 (ebook) |
    DDC 616.2/414—dc23/eng/20211123
LC record available at https://lccn.loc.gov/2021051860
LC ebook record available at https://lccn.loc.gov/2021051861

ISBN: 978-0-367-76966-6 (hbk)
ISBN: 978-0-367-76965-9 (pbk)
ISBN: 978-1-003-16914-7 (ebk)

DOI: 10.4324/9781003169147

Typeset in Bembo
by Apex CoVantage, LLC

CONTENTS

PREFACE

Pandemics are now acutely felt. COVID-19 has ripped through human, societal, economic, and global dimensions. When I published an extensive study on the topic of plague and people in 2012, 'Understanding the Politics of Pandemic Scares: An Introduction to Global Politosomatics', I was focusing on the long history of plague encounters. I wanted to show how extensive and consequential the outbreaks and waves of them have been in the past and how they still impact us. This new book reworks the more lasting themes and materials of the 2012 book. It expands to cover the (geo)politics of COVID-19 from a perspective that I coined 'politosomatics'. The basic premise is that individual somatic anxieties and fear of global regressive currents catapult pandemic emergencies to a class of their own and catalyse the lasting cross-cutting consequences. Moreover, the intellectual history of plagues and people points to the tendency that violent outbreaks do not happen in isolation and vacuum. They are indicative of failures of the human political space, the ability to control and govern wars, violence, and the accidental nature of human surroundings. Pandemics are bad omens of weakening, weak, and non-existing global governance.

1
INTRODUCTION

Diseases desperate grown
By desperate appliances are relieved,
Or not at all.

—Shakespeare, *Hamlet*

It struck the city of Athens suddenly.
People in the Piraeus caught it first,
and so, since there were not yet any fountains there,
they actually alleged that the Peloponnesians had put poison in the wells.
—Thucydides, *The History of the Peloponnesian War*

As evidenced by COVID-19 (coronavirus disease), deadly contagious diseases have the potential to catalyse societal havoc, heighten enmity between political actors and different levels of governance, and set out unforeseen, cascading negative chains of events. The crucial driver is the pandemic's ability to disrupt not only complex societal, economic, and political systems but also, most fundamentally, people's individual lives and to elicit somatic fears and catalyse projections of anxieties to the political situation around them. The pandemic is translated into fear at both political and individual levels, producing combinations of the two. The resulting politosomatic nexus is expressed in streets, in social media, and in geopolitics election booths. By no means trivial and insignificant, this is largely unacknowledged, but extremely consequential politosomatic relationship is the key topic of this work (Aaltola 2012a).

In our modern times, body politics and globalized individual bodies are uniquely exposed to pathogens spreading through the arteries of global interdependence, in particular through modernity's air-travel vector. Antibiotic resistance is looming on

DOI: 10.4324/9781003169147-1

the horizon in a way that accentuates worries about the re-emergence of older pestilences. Pandemics and fears of them embody our global way of life in a regressive way. Instead of economic growth and increasingly efficient value chains, pandemic scenarios introduce dystopian fears of contagious interdependence between differentially exposed individuals. The source of global power, status, and wealth—the globalized world order's key modes—turns into channels of potential political and somatic regression. The growing dis-ease—the nexus between political order and somatic anxiety—morphs a diversity of characteristics into one scenario where the sentiments of containment, severing connections, and enmity are more pervasive than high reliance and optimism concerning integrated regions or a seamless global sky. Under this regressive scenario, any anticipation of an epidemic becomes newsworthy but also symptomatic of the perceived underlying unsustainability of the global order and the hostile relationship with the mutating natural surroundings. Hyperbole, politicizations, misinformation, and rumours interact with each other and trigger deep anxieties concerning the sustainability of the way of life of a particular hegemonic order and global epoch.

The dreams of the post–Cold War world were crystallized in ideas of integrated mobility infrastructures and a seamless sky standing in sharp contrast to the dividing territorial political borders of the past. The flows of disease agents can illustrate, signify, and embody the regression of the global vision and governance as well as reveal the lack of solidarity and trust if (re)-emerging diseases interact with human polities in waves one after another. They disempower the citizens of the increasingly exposed globality, highlighting the international and intra-communal borders, and reveal the injustices of a differential spread of vulnerability and production of immunity. Pandemic fears can ultimately undermine the trust placed in states as the Hobbesian reality of a life, which is dis-eased, short, nasty, and brutish, becomes acutely felt inside many states. The key is to understand that micro-level contagions go hand in hand with a heightened sense of macro-level enmities, and one pattern of enmity translates into and readily combines with the other. For example, COVID-19 translated almost effortlessly into a catalyst of great power rivalry between the United States of America (the US) and Russia China, and inside states, it fed existing stereotypical patterns of suspicion and prejudice.

As COVID-19 has demonstrated, a pandemic outbreak can show how suddenly, and swiftly, the world can be brought to its knees driven by somatic fear and anxiety. It seems that the major players of the rule-based world order and global governance, ranging from the major political powers to global health institutions, cannot be fully trusted to fulfil their responsibilities. Moreover, the pandemic itself seems like a worrying portent of more governance regressions to come. This can further undermine the trust and legitimacy needed for regional and global order.

In pandemic security emergency situations, the likely global sentiment yearning for leadership is not one of mobilized global empathy, humanitarian solidarity, or desperation for a timely cure for everyone. Instead, we recoil and sever connections. We try to instinctively secure the borders of our immediate communities. This is the antithesis of the humanitarian impulse usually connected with localized human suffering due to natural disasters. The sight of a starving child in places of misgovernance may lead to a sense of compassion and the need to rush in to intervene on behalf of this distant sufferer (e.g. Aaltola 2009). Highly rehearsed donor behaviour and rescue efforts are likely to follow. The international community tries to move fast to ameliorate conditions in places of misery. Yet the sight of the dead and suffering swine flu victims in Mexico in the spring of 2009 led to a sudden global jolt of aversion and fear. Similarly, fear of COVID-19 started to spread soon after the containment failure in Wuhan in late 2019. The immediate global reflex—a reaction similar to the emergence of those infected by other perceived pandemics—was that of distancing and severing contact with the site of the unfamiliar and deadly disease outbreak. The momentum of pandemic emergencies is aimed at disengagement with the suffering distant other and taking care of one's own community, where one feels more securely embodied. The rush is towards proximate containment rather than the compassionate crossing of distances. In this sense, a pandemic's affective flows are unlike other global emergencies—they are seemingly non-compassionate rushes towards withdrawal and to contain the disease in a certain place, spot, or 'zone'. If there is altruism, it is towards the people living close by or towards the 'general public', conceived of in terms of national or regional bubbles. As a sentiment, containment sets a scene for paranoid governance whereby rational and conspiratorial content mixes, and any attempt to help is treated with suspicion and is likely to be merely pandemic diplomacy or vaccine statecraft. Legitimate global power tends to disappear, accentuating cold calculations, motivations of self-interest, and sentiments towards decoupling from the global contacts. When the wave of a new variant recedes, connections are restored with hesitation. However, the element of distrust is bound to linger, setting the scene for a political long COVID as the earlier value placed on rule-based or liberal order has lost its momentum.

The acute global relationships of anxious containment shed light on the power-related dynamics of pandemic emergencies. In this work, I will use the term 'politosomatics' in reference to how lived-life, individual, somatic-level anxieties couple with the hierarchical interconnectedness of the global polity. Politosomatic relationships interlink the global hierarchy's differential spread of risk—the inequalities in the disease burden together with the associated imbalances of wealth and power—with individuals' expectations and fears of bodily harm.[1] The world order translates into a configuration of differentially exposed individual and political bodies, which, in turn, causes anxiety and leads to political reactions, market panics, consumer reactions, a race to develop vaccines, fear of public spaces, wearing of masks, changing social expressions, and other types of disease-related expressive behaviour. Moreover, the containment sentiment also finds its expression in catalysing existing and emerging geopolitical, cultural, moral, ethnic, and sexual cleavages and enmities.

The more encompassing political 'bodies', such as states, the world order, and humanity itself, can also be felt as being under pressure and duress. Dis-order and dis-ease at those levels can directly link with somatic-level pains, a sense of being exposed, and individual-level anxiety. It is hardly surprising that after several millennia of this interaction, people often sense their wider surroundings and their world as embodiments with which they identify in varying ways and on behalf of which they worry. They feel and react to the community's or world's pains, and, as a result, these wider embodiments may turn into bodies in pain. And, it can be suggested, these political or world-related pains have long cultural histories, memories, and expressive practices that also condition our contemporary sensitivities, for example, when it comes to regressive processes or 'fatal blows' delivered by lethal epidemic diseases. These imageries of regressive circulations and flows cannot be anything but intense. Their judders lead to expectations of corresponding pain in other less expansive but far more intimate bodies such as individual bodies. In this way, actual and feared political pain may become somatized and vice versa, with the result that it is possible to speak about politosomatic disorders in much the same way as it is possible to discuss psychosomatic or socio-somatic disorders.[2]

Politosomatics builds an overview in which people's bodily fears are contextualized in both narrower and wide political embodiments and the power relations therein. Similar tendencies have prevailed in social sciences for decades ranging from psychosomatic to socio-somatic approaches. Psychosomatics developed based on the need to bridge a dichotomy inherent in the term and to understand how the mind and body are interrelated—how somatic symptoms lead to mental outcomes, disturbances, and vice versa. The field challenged the clear-cut division between thought and the material body's physical mechanisms. Due to the incommensurable nature of the two elements bridged, mind and body, the field has suffered from conceptual issues (Hitzer and Leon-Sanz 2016: 67). However, despite the inherent complexity, clear tangible interrelations can be seen. Socio-somatics, similarly, contains an attempt towards a more comprehensive understanding of the place of the mind and body in social interactions and communities. A social setting with its norms, practices, and interpretations affects the way in which communities and individuals give meaning to somatic processes such as diseases (e.g. Kleinman 1986). The body does not exist in a vacuum but is psychologically and socially embedded, thus opening up complex yet conventionally bound interrelations.

It is clear that contagious diseases exist, flourish, and die in wider than physical environments, as they adapt to local memories, practices, and cultures, as also to patterns of political order, governance, and power. For example, the communal responses to avian flu were commonly based on the practical logic developed on the basis of existing stereotypes, media representations, government information campaigns, and popular rumours (Padmawati and Nichter 2008: 31). Moreover, diseases are embedded in and readily react with the fabric of political power. In this process of mutual adaptation, the responses to diseases inevitably turn into signifiers of the underlying patterns of power. For example, in the early 1980s, the Soviet authorities insisted that HIV was the outcome of an American military experiment that had gone wrong (Nelkin and Gilman 1991: 39). The purpose could have been to point out that the US was a vicious and underhanded superpower that should not be trusted. Moreover, for the Soviet Union, the HIV and

AIDS epidemic offered an opportunity to point out that it was AIDS free because it had no 'degenerate' and 'corrupted' homosexual elements. However, HIV and AIDS never became a very potent propaganda weapon, partly because it could be externalized into 'undesirable' and long stigmatized internal elements such as homosexuals, prostitutes, and recreational drug users. In other words, many people in the West connected the disease with what was back then the 'unnatural' gay community, rather than with the general 'corruptness' of Western societies. HIV and AIDS were also used effectively by the American neo-conservative movement in the beginning of the 1980s to promote its own message about family values and the need for religious revival in the US (Aaltola 2008: 67). It may be further argued that the public meaning of suffering from HIV and AIDS changed the expressive pain behaviour of those who had the syndrome. Their suffering was stigmatized and used for purposes related to political power. Thus, the syndrome became politosomatized. The fact that the suffering became more silent was in itself a politosomatic phenomenon. HIV and AIDS, like many pandemic diseases before and after, reacted with the prevailing perceptions of power, hostility, and enmity. COVID-19 revealed similar patterns. It became a sign of the worsening great power relations, and it was translated into the language of enmity. In the US, there were discussions that featured the expressive term 'China virus', while China declared that the disease had not originated in China but could have had its origins in the US. In the paranoid atmosphere of a pandemic, misinformation and disinformation are norms that reflect underlying power-political cleavages. People, communities, and states tend to decipher the state of the world through contagions, and the world, with its power patterns, tends to give meaning to diseases. Pandemics seem to forcefully register the world of hostility as well as the world's hostility (Tuan 1979: 87).

In the case of pandemics, the power-political embeddings are increasingly global. In most studies on lethal epidemic diseases before the COVID-19 outbreak, this macro-level political aspect is missing or only implicitly recognized. There are a few notable studies that have focused on the power aspect of pandemics and researched how public health has interacted with conquest and governance (McNeill 1976; Panisset 2000; Price-Smith 2009). Going against this tendency of overlooking power and politics, I will chart pandemic diseases and their scares as being inherently power related (Aaltola 1999, 2005a, 2012a, 2012b). I will use the term 'politosomatics' to describe how the constitution and interaction of different embodiments—ranging from the wider political embodiments to the somatic ones—are shaped by political and power-related processes. Political imageries can be deeply integrated into understanding and awareness of the body. The direct impact of the political context on the various kinds of disease experience and on the practices of pain-expressing behaviour is to be expected. Disease, as a socially interpreted physical and physiological process, is fundamentally shaped by prevailing political culture and practices. In this way, pandemic scares can be identified as polysemous, yet forceful, idioms of distress and anxiety. By using politosomatics as an analytical concept, I will explore how these disease-related hyperbolic and widespread experiences of fear are linked to global power structures, which differentially expose bodies to various risk factors. While the prevailing and underlying political anxieties may be projected into interpretations of pandemic diseases, the opposite is equally likely: the emergence of acute pandemic emergencies reinforces the corresponding imageries of both declining and reviving political power. I will draw from disease-related memories and histories to show how these politosomatic interactions are supported by traditions of political theory and thought that are still under-researched.

It can be argued that the recent pandemic scares may be regarded as 'politosomatic disorders' or 'dis-eases'. It has been widely recognized in psychosomatics and socio-somatics that 'disease behaviour'—or how people express their fear of diseases—is influenced by factors other than physiological ones. For example, different people react differently to pain and death, in a way that reflects their 'learning history, socialization, and cultural predisposition to behave in certain ways in particular circumstances' (Chapman and Wyckoff 1981: 35).[3] Moreover, this relationship is often perceived as complex and entangled with 'cultural, psychological, and physiological factors' (Bever 2000: 581). However, the aim here is to highlight how expressed pain behaviour calls for a deeper appreciation of our political embodiments, their wider interrelatedness, and the associated grammars of politically expressible pain. The politics of bodily suffering, pain, and death has two main dimensions. First, physical suffering and fear of it are a highly iconic and readable part of disease as well as of different forms of political violence. Second, there exists a long tradition in which political bodies—such as societies, communities, empires, states, nations, and humanity—have been seen as 'subjects' of suffering. In the case of pandemic diseases, which often provoke the image of much hyped 'blows against civilization', both the somatic and political embodiments can be seen as suffering, and the expressive language of such suffering can be connected. Politosomatics is a bridging concept in discerning the nexus between the different forms of 'bodily' pain.

Susan Sontag (1988) can be read as having captured the underlying dynamic. She notes that all attention-catching diseases were always ideally comprehensible entities in their own time. They serve and are co-opted to crystallize an epoch's hegemonic individual and political fears. I will use this insight to claim that the reason pandemic emergencies become so urgently anxiety-provoking also stems from the prevailing declinist imageries—how political affairs and external power positions are in decline—and from other historically conditioned political sensibilities, insecurities, and vulnerabilities. The declinist interpretations lead to calls for reform to find shelter in some perceived form of politics and civil religion free of dangerous contact and 'unnatural' habits. The present pandemic scares and, very importantly, the silence of pandemics that do not catch public attention are intimately connected with the contemporary construction of crises and threats in global politics. The politosomatic perspective links the recent pandemic outbreaks—from Ebola to COVID-19—to the imageries of political decline and regression of the prevailing globalized world order as a hegemonic embodiment. The central theme in these imageries is that the interaction between different perceived crisis factors and dynamics—for example, global warming, collapsing public health, weakening democracies, political polarization, economic turbulence and changing demographics—will further induce the expectations and likelihoods of eruptions of perceived emergencies and catastrophes. The related uncanny anxiety creates a political context pregnant with anticipation of different imageries of coming bodily discomfort. Such declinist crisis imageries also make the time ripe for perceptions of pandemic emergencies. Furthermore, the appearance of other forms of emergency, especially large-scale wars, heightens still further the expectation of pandemic emergencies and their spectacles. From this perspective, pandemic emergencies and scares can be seen as symptomatic of the underlying political power worries. Thus, they embody many fears that stem from visible stress on the existing world order, anxiety concerning the order that turns into deep disease. This world order has been able to provide specific forms of bodily comfort. The blow by a pandemic plague is a major way of imagining and embodying the possible unmaking of the bodily comfort embedded in the globalized order. Thus, the added value of the politosomatic approach stems from the ability to understand the nexus between macro-level political processes, one's place in the hierarchy of empowerment, and personal-level disease fears.

Before they become ideally comprehensible, sudden and rampant contagious diseases transform their epoch and can accentuate already pronounced social and political trends. They function as triggers for contemporaneous interpretations in ways that may be, to a degree, unrelated to their biology in the human body but change the way in which the bodily processes are politically understood and acted upon. However, as showcased by SARS (severe acute respiratory syndrome) and COVID-19, they are made to fit the prevailing vulnerabilities inherent in the social, economic, and political fabric: 'Epidemic diseases are not random events that afflict societies capriciously and without warning. On the contrary, every society produces its own specific vulnerabilities. To study them is to understand that society's structure, its standard of living, and its political priorities' (Snowden 2020).[4] The more serious the pandemic, the better the fit between it and the vulnerabilities in the global system. The global mobility and circulation-based order were the vectors for the spread of COVID-19, and as such, it can catalyse and trigger underlying challenges and pressures in the highly mobile global order. These 'comprehensibles' were also made to rhyme with the rise of China and the decline of the other main stakeholder, the US, with the heightening power-political competition among the major powers, as exemplified by the Russia's geopolitical moves in Europe during the Spring of 2022, and the sustainability of present-day institutions such as the World Health Organization (WHO), which are founded on the existing global order.

The world order, as a hierarchical hegemonic political embodiment, causes incongruence with the more or less peripheral local, national, and state embodiments. These conflicts and contestations reflect, in turn, on the individual bodies caught in the middle. All this finds an expression in the ritualistic nuances and entanglements of pandemic situations. Outside of the West, many just suffer, expressing their misery through their local iconic pain language, which does not come under the global public gaze if there is no sense of an uncontained contagion. In other words, pandemics, as embodiments of feared 'dis-eases', are reflective of the underlying power flows and circulations in the prevailing human polity. In this sense, the specific forms of pandemic scares reveal the underlying political dynamics. Figuratively speaking, lethal epidemic diseases provide an X-ray of their embeddings (Herdt 1992: 8). This resonates well with Sontag's notion that all attention-catching diseases are always ideally comprehensible entities in their own time: they fit and are made to encapsulate their political surroundings, as their alarming nature is constructed from the prevailing declinist fears (Ungar 1998: 37).

This book examines the overall politosomatic dynamics of pandemic scares. What are their common tendencies? What do they reveal, and how is that linked to their production and staging? How do political concerns shape the emergence of lethal epidemic diseases? The answers to these questions are based on rediscovering some of the central proto-political scenarios and characteristics as well as on illustrating how they still shape present-day pandemic emergencies. The phenomenon of politosomatics allows for a more comprehensive and critical evaluation of how pandemic scares are much more substantive parts of the global experience than would first appear. Pandemic emergencies are regarded as politosomatic disorders that link individual-level stresses, strains, and fears with global circulations of power and with the global and local polity's production of legitimacy. While examining their underlying dynamics, this book provides an overview and history of recent politosomatic pandemic emergencies and scares.

Before COVID-19 shook the world, the precursor pandemics (Ebola, bovine spongiform encephalopathy (BSE), SARS, Middle East respiratory syndrome (MERS), avian flu, and swine flu) were seen more like duds—scares with fewer than feared deaths—than feared plague blows. However, they were both spectacular and hyperbolic when it came to eliciting fears and being comprehensible expressions of their epochs. They are in themselves worthy of critical examination, especially because they shaped the laggard response to COVID-19, but also because they rehearsed and brought to our epoch the old imaginaries of coming plagues. The present-day pandemic imagery is so interwoven with the fabric of global politics that by studying the precursor epidemics and pandemics, crucial knowledge can be gained concerning how power and legitimacy are created through somatic fears and threats. It should be noted that power-embedded politosomatic pains and anxieties can lead to a sense of relief and restored normalcy. Furthermore, past scares are also relevant because they reveal how the sentiments of fear, anxiety, and scare are converted into opportunities for legitimizing power spectacles branded as 'effective health governance' till the hyped devastating blow is once again averted and the scare subsides. They have been useful in painting an image of prepared and resilient communities, thereby creating a sense of sheltered citizens.

The focus of this book is on the politosomatic dynamics of recent pandemic emergencies, which 'suddenly burst forth in a catastrophic manner' (Kilbourne 2009: 218). The diseases in themselves, as physical and epidemiological phenomena, fall largely outside the scope of this work. The emphasis is on how diseases are interpreted and co-opted in their social and political contexts and how these interpretative constructs interact with sudden pandemic emergencies. On the one hand, pandemics emergencies are often defined by hyperbolic attention, which, in hindsight, can appear to be 'grossly disproportional in relation to its low mortality rate' (Caballero 2005: 483). However, the status of recent pandemic emergencies as 'scares' does not detract from their political significance. On the contrary, pandemic scares are highly significant situations that highlight the ways in which global politics is inherently glued on to individual bodily fears and anxieties. On the other hand, pandemics can truly shake the world, going much beyond the scale of being scares, as demonstrated by COVID-19. They suddenly bring the global reaches closer to human bodies and change the way in which people express their fears in politics. The underlying medicalized geographies of power turn into concrete political manifestations. Fears and anxieties connected with the circulation of disease agents are always non-abstract but acute and consequential. They are deeply felt. People sense their globalized surroundings, thereby creating points of attachment for relevant understanding of their own 'locatedness' in the interconnected global embeddings. Waking up to a world that is experiencing a pandemic instantiates a relationship of worry that is bound to have a more than fleeting influence. Through them, people re-remember the high personal stakes involved in the global polity and enact deeply seated historical memories of interactions between plague and people.

The politosomatic interface allows for highly comprehensible re-enactments of power, which are seen as highly pertinent to the present circumstances faced by differentially situated individuals. Because these connections to a part have been instantiated just then, they appear to be still murky and ill-defined. They are explicated at the level of abstract public health knowledge. Yet, at the same time, the themes involved—that of plague and people—are ancient. Only the scale has changed, and much of the old 'disease frame' has been forgotten because of the triumphant claims in the mid-twentieth century that the era of major lethal epidemics was over. The recent pandemic scares and emergencies reactivate and rearticulate the older and almost instinctive registers of rendering relevant the interconnectedness and inter-locality of people. The use of the term 'politosomatics' involves an effort to explicate the silent knowledge involved in the disease-politics nexus. Examples are many from propaganda to status and blame games. Politosomatics changes people's voting behaviour and galvanizes the political expressions in social media and on the streets. It also finds its expression in global politics and great power competition.

This work is fundamentally about bodily pain, fear of it, and the pain-conducting links between differently embodied kinds of suffering. Besides being abstract, the study of politics can be seen as embodied. Its main subject has been the various political bodies—yours, mine, and ours. It has also strived to understand more encompassing embodiments such as community, state, world, and, now, globality. Often, without being aware of it, the corpus of political knowledge has charted the nuanced entanglements through which these bodies interact and feel each other. The central conceptual configurations have tried to understand the violence between the bodies as well as to come to terms with the internal violent conflicts of contesting and failing bodies. Many of modernist research energies have focused on the way in which political bodies are constituted and governed—that is, on progressive narratives. At the same time, the shadow of the intense regressive processes of decomposition still looms large over the ways in which the world is sensed. Against the background of the unravelling of the modernist progressive paradigm, the central research interest is on how the narrower and larger of our political bodies can become entangled in mutual regressions or downward-sloping slides of less order and governance. Politosomatics entails an awareness of the interrelated nature of embodiments. The pulses of political shivers, pains, and convulsions of a feverishly globalized life travel through the different political fabrics, which echo worries over the dangers of interrelatedness.

Thus, politosomatic intimacy involves sensing the world's pains on one's body. The two most distant embodiments—individual bodies and world order—come into direct contact in pandemics and their scares. As a child growing up during the 1980s, I remember when the worst-case scenario consisted of a nuclear holocaust. Posner (2004: 71) aptly states that 'during the half century of the cold war . . ., the catastrophic risk that attracted the most attention was that of a nuclear and a thermonuclear war'. Imagining what a nuclear holocaust would mean sent shivers down the spine of the young boy that I was. It was felt bodily in sweating and nightmares. My reaction was politosomatic. The worst-case scenarios of more recent times have focused on pandemic diseases. Many people, young and old, feel them. Pandemic scenarios have become more ideally comprehensible about our times than scenes of nuclear war. It is also noteworthy that pandemic anxieties co-exist with anxiety scenarios of rampant global warming. Pandemics fit their political power surroundings, and their alarming nature is sculpted from the prevailing sensibilities concerning what might go wrong. These bodily felt world-order anxieties are also involved in the recent pandemic diseases enabled by the ancient sediments of memories written in the language of bodily disfigurement and suffering. An individual nested in and enabled by the world must have a near instinctual sense of the power dynamics which can also catalyse large-scale disasters.

Turning to the theoretical framework of this book, I remember reading with keen interest Elaine Scarry's 1987 book, *The Body in Pain*, while lecturing at the University of Minnesota on the nexus between lethal epidemic diseases and world politics during the spring of 2008. In it, I saw many bridgeheads to the politics of pain. As one can imagine, Scarry's work was full of morbidity: the text and many visuals in the book described a world of contorted and convulsing human bodies, vivid images of agony, and a masterful account of the unmaking of bodies through the processes of torture and war. The intensity of the pain language brought to my mind the classical account of war, Thucydides' *History of the Peloponnesian War*. For Thucydides (*c.* 460–395 BC), the deepening and widening vortex of macro-level war induced pulses and co-currents. These emerging sub-currents occurred in the vicinity of the war's rhythmic expression of regressive energy. The increasingly violent circular motions meant that intervals in extreme pain production became progressively shorter: violence kept coming back, cutting across and within bodies in increasingly intense spirals, circling round and back, again and again. The drama that Thucydides describes spreads from the inter-poleis level to local slaughters and to that unforgettable sub-current of war, the Plague of Athens. The comprehensive nature of Thucydides' overview, which covers the macro, local, and individual levels, might be better understood through a comparison with how he might have approached contemporary times: the wars fought by the hegemonic power, such as the US—in Iraq and Afghanistan—open a context in which individuals' disease-related fears—those of SARS, avian flu, and swine flu—can be interpreted as sub-manifestations of the overall dynamics of terror and war in our world. Thucydides' model is also felt to be relevant for the subsequent phase of the hegemonic struggle, the rise of China, and the US attempts to contain its power (e.g. Allison 2017). Thucydides would not have been surprised by the sudden emergence of COVID-19 in the middle of this geopolitical heat. Things are interrelated: the regressive tensions at the macro level lead to the weakening of overall governance and governability. The human space—the space that allows for control over the power-political jungle and over the accidental randomness of nature—gets narrower and more exposed to war and pestilence. 'Pestilences' are more likely and tend to come together if the human governability weakens, he seems to be saying. One regression increases the likelihood of the other. Vulnerability to crises, disasters, and diseases can spill over and result in complex entanglements, the true nature of which cannot be discerned with the customary disciplinary bracketing.

Thucydides' influential narrative of the Plague of Athens may be read as a story of how disease causes a political community to regress in the same way as external and internal wars. Moreover, Thucydides' analysis contextualizes the plague in the wider dynamics of the hegemonic war. He seems to hint that disease is an expected part of a wider, violent power struggle. The widening and deepening vortexes of hegemonic contestation are a dynamic that engulfs individual polities through extreme communal violence and individual bodies through plagues and famines. This nexus between wars and diseases also leads to corresponding expectations and fears for one in the presence of the other. This is a powerful associative tradition.

I will examine plague and people interactions and proto-theories in the first two chapters of the book to give an overview of the modern pandemic scenarios and content to the politosomatic hypothesis. Chapter 2 examines the intellectual and conceptual histories of the containment based on the 'nearest is dearest' logic and contrasts it with the politics of compassion for the distant other underlying humanitarian governance. In Chapter 3, 'Understanding Grand Vortexes: The Classical Model for Politics and Plagues', I will further develop a politosomatics reading based on Thucydides' classical account and its more modern interpretations. As said before, politosomatics has a deep and influential cultural and intellectual history. For example, it is often said that before World War I, more people died because of disease in the context of war than because of actual fighting, although this statement is likely to be inaccurate since the Spanish Influenza killed millions during and after the war. The war provided a ripe context for the Spanish Flu through large-scale troop movements. However, besides providing the physical context for a disease, the war heightened the sense of an especially serious disease. To a degree, it was because of the war that the disease was seen as significant from a highly (geo)political angle. It heightened the sense that political enmities were so deep that they produced a disease, thereby feeding the enemy images and propaganda and conspiracy theories. This link can be seen in the use of the disease in the war propaganda of the time.

After reviewing the proto-theoretical aspects, I will move to specific pandemic cases. In Chapter 4, 'Global Mobility-Based Order: The Disruptions of SARS and COVID-19', I will examine more closely the present global order and how its vulnerabilities surfaced during the recent serious pandemic outbreaks. Chapter 5 takes a closer look at these two global outbreaks to see how historical patterns were rehearsed in our contemporary geopolitics and geo-economy. Chapter 6 examines the political vortexes of COVID-19 in more detail focusing on the historical patterns and how the pandemic is creating political distancing as one of its major enmity-promoting outcomes. Chapter 7 is a detailed study of the local consequences of an epidemic outbreak. It charts the dynamics of the Haiti cholera outbreak in the wake of the devastating 2010 earthquake there. The domestic reactions are descriptive of how the level of trust between international actors and local actors can suffer in the long term, as the cause of the disease was 'internationalized' to the United Nations (UN). This internationalization can be contrasted with the pattern of localization which has been a major way for locals to try to come to terms with a disease outbreak. The second part of Chapter 7 examines these two tendencies, localization/nationalization versus internationalization, in the case of the mad cow disease (or BSE). The focus is on how communities react politically to disease by heightening acrimony between different local, state, and international interfaces. The work concludes by providing critical insights into how the modern pandemic scenarios are constructed in an attempt to strip down some of the anxious hyperbole associated with pandemics that allows for its (geo)politicization.

Scarry's multidimensional argument was about the unmaking of an individual's world. For Scarry, the painful unmaking refers to a flow of events in which the supporting constructions of everyday life become radically undone.[5] Her central notion was that fears of pain and anxiety motivate the making of things in a process of world-making. These supporting constructs and architectures become, so to speak, 'pain relievers' and 'pain killers'. They ease the burden of pain by containing some of the burden and moving it onto external supporting and comforting 'objects'. Thus, troubled by gravity, human beings have created technologies and governance institutions to support their bodies' freedom from the likelihood of pain. Hobbes, who translated Thucydides' work, used similar motivations for the need to build state-level governance to free people from a life that is 'nasty, brutish, and short'. Troubled by subsistence, they have created organized communities. Troubled by war, famine, and disease, they have built states and international bodies such as the WHO. These supporting constructions, in their turn, reinvent what being a human means with inherent liberties and constraints. In this way, relieving pain becomes an important political motivation: a reason for any political archi-tecture is partly to remove discomfort, to relieve pain, and to produce security and the absence of 'dis-ease'. In other words, a state or international organization can be regarded as objects, political architectures, aimed at relieving particular types of aches and pains stemming from violence, famine, and disease. The state, as a made artefact, becomes dependent on the underlying bodily discomfort it aims to relieve. Extending beyond the state, any political order legitimizes its existence through the absence of a particular type of bodily harm, for example, terrorism, torture, or disease. From such a perspective, the state relieves more territorially bound discom-forts, whereas global governance structures relieve other more de-territorial types of pains, such as pandemics, which have notably been constructed as mutating and penetrating political borders.

At the same time, embedded in such a pain-relieving context, the absence of bodily pain gets its second-order dynamics. Individual bodies become inher-ently linked with and integrated into wider social and political embodiments. Any movements in these embodiments are directly translated into the underlying anxi-eties concerning bodily pain. In the same way as the anxious awareness that one is lacking a vital medicine creates ominous expectations and fears, the perception that global structures are lacking can lead to fears at the level of somatic security. An argument can be made that this dynamic of worry is fundamental to the recent spectacles that have been termed 'pandemic scares'. Imageries of political disorder are implicated when it comes to the perceived sources of bodily harm. Bodily comfort becomes identified with the existence of political structures and political bodies. Moreover, the 'suffering' of these pain-relieving bodies becomes synony-mous with the acute possibility of somatic physical suffering. This offers one way of understanding the political function of recurring pandemic scares. They create a demand for particular types of governance systems seemingly able to match the challenge of a mutating disease agent, which is able to penetrate natural and politi-cal boundaries. In a way, pandemics may have their uses because they address basic bodily needs. The dramatic form of a pandemic scare might offer ways of connect-ing with people's fears in answering key questions: 'What and how pain means, how such meaning can be embodied, how such embodiment can be dramatized, and how such dramatizations can be put to use and made meaningful in a variety of contexts' (Allard and Mathew 2009).

Theoretical Approach

The politosomatic perspective draws from a nexus between felt and interpreted somatic sensations and power structures. It is clear that this framework has to draw theoretical and methodological support from models that take into account the embodied aspect of knowledge (e.g. Ignatow 2007; Marlin-Bennett 2013; Hutch-ison 2018). In order to understand how the different modalities of knowledge link together, the recent 're-challenge' of the mechanistic and simplified assump-tions concerning the primacy of the characteristics of abstract knowledge in social theory scenarios offers a useful bridgehead (Zerubavel 1997; DiMaggio 2002; Ignatow 2007). The critique has led into studies of modalities of knowing such as emotional, motor, and sensory qualities (Barsalou 1999). The key driver of this turn in approaches has focused on taking into account more embodied characteristics such as emotions, visuality, and kinaesthetics. The emphasis is not on knowing something only abstractly and intellectually but on seeing, feeling, and sensing the world. In this way, the abstract topologies—such as systems, grids, diagrams, knowledge trees, and hub, and spoke models—are embedded in other more felt and sensed modalities such as power, emotions, movements, and flows. What has emerged are embodied intermediaries that fuse abstract thinking with perceptual motor and sensory experiences, for example, in the so-called cultural models (Ignatow 2007: 124). These more encompassing and overviewing intermediate scenarios capture the core relationships between the key objects and contain 'image schemas' of the possible interactions between the primary objects of a particular situated scenario (D'Andrade 1987; Lakoff and Kovecses 1987).

Thus, 'disease' and its derivative, 'pandemic', can be seen as providing an overall embodied scenario, a disease object world. Its processes of contagion and spread provide for the understanding of the kinaesthetic, motion-based interactions between the key objects: 'I' extends to 'we', and both stand in opposition to 'them', 'a foreign element' and 'disease agent', through a sense of spread, contagion, and possibilities of containment, cure, and immunity. The object world of a contagious disease is part of our embodied DNA because it has been experienced in some way by all, and historical encounters of such diseases are read about in schoolbooks and rehearsed by popular culture. These embodied scenarios of disease involve deeply personal struggles while being inflicted by a serious illness. Most know how diseases limit personal agency within economic, social, and political embeddings, which set the possibilities and limits as people struggle to manage their daily lives while sick. The conflicted disease subjectivities and the vicissitudes of their adaptive strategies are felt deeply as people react to renegotiate their positions within their surroundings. They might rally round their local and national leaders, turn to the streets, express their anxieties in voting booths, or turn to conspiratorial content and answers. The modalities of disease scenarios are thus anything but just abstract. This is sensed even in the middle of the emergency by outside actors who use their resources of personal protective equipment (PPE) or vaccinations to turn loyalties towards them. The citizens of the polities of the sick and exposed are restless and open to stimulation. Bodily fevers are manifested in increasingly feverish polities.

Emotions of pain and anxiety colour—and fuse with—the underlying cognitions and cultural beliefs. The expressed pain behaviour becomes a register of self- and other knowledge as one navigates the course of an illness (Parish 2008). Often, at one point or another, a person becomes dependent on their social safety nets; on local, national, and global authorities; and on the medical world. In this way, the object world of disease contains the emotions of comfort, compassion, and containment as well as fears of exclusion, isolation, and aloneness. These emotions are tightly connected with the reconstruction of one's sense of the underlying fabric of social interaction. How sheltering is it? How exposed to the disease can it be? Through a disease, one becomes aware of the complexities of individuality, family, society, economy, medicine, and politics in ways that are hard to express in terms of simple amodal abstractness or the usual patterns of producing authority and expertise that are empty of the tempos and rhythms of disease waves and emotional insecurities.

It can be argued that the highly embodied and deeply felt disease sentiments are readily projectable onto the more encompassing spatio-temporal understandings concerning the wider surroundings, ranging from the immediate to encompassing notions such as 'world', 'global', and 'humanity'. In this way, the world can become embodied through it starting to exhibit disease characteristics. This projection provides the framework for the 'enactualization' of global politosomatics when deeply personal disease experiences blend with the 'disease' seen as affecting or stemming from these wider conceptual 'bodies'. In this connection, it is important to note the power of the disease object world—that is, the disease proposition schemas—to contain visually and emotionally charged 'pictures' of the dynamic interactions between the key objects (Lakoff and Kovecses 1987). Pandemic diseases, as a scenario with multiple characteristics, provide a core relational structure. This structure allows for the embodied interpreting of events in more abstract domains by importing them by analogy from a tangibly concrete realm (Boroditsky 2000: 3). Such projected disease scenarios of situated knowledge contain kinaesthetic meanings—that is, spread, tempo, speed, directionality, tempos of waves, and modes of contagion—associated with the dynamically changing relationships between key embodied objects. Who are those around me possibly endangering me or to whom I might give the disease? How does it feel to get an infection? How would others interpret my illness? Should I use a mask? Can I touch door handles or press elevator buttons? Must I stay home? Can I shake hands? Should I hide my sneezing? The mental projections of this lived life object world into different scenarios existing in the physical, social, and political realms are what are at stake in embodied knowledge. The projections of the disease object world's dynamics have been omnipresent in the times of COVID-19. However, the contagion scenario extends to world politics and world economy. We speak about contagions of violence, for example, in terms of rioting or terrorism. We fear economic contagions from one region to other, in terms of market panics. Why? Because the underlying scenario is tangible, embodied, and easy to understand. In a way, it is proto-politics and deep-seated to a degree that its common uses might be unnoticeable. Without probably intending to, Skillen (2001) provides an unusually explicit example of how the disease object world can guide the understanding of political-level developments:

> The purpose of surgery on cancerous cells is to remove danger to an otherwise healthy body. However, many political bodies around the world, including those in Afghanistan and a number of other countries, are not healthy. The terrorist cells feed on those unhealthy political bodies. A sharply focused

campaign to rid the world of terrorist cells will not by itself help to create or strengthen the healthy states that are needed.

That said, the projection of diseases onto the world also changes the way in which diseases are felt in private and public life. The severity, for example, of contagion is continuously being reimagined and reinvented when it is seen as afflicting different social and political bodies. With COVID-19 hitting the globality, many of the expanded ideas of what a lethal contagion means are being enactualized, and the underlying situated scenario is transforming into an even wider scenario with even more dynamically interacting characteristics such as great power rivalry and vaccine nationalism.

The object world of diseases has often been used in politics. The kinaesthetic processes involved in the disease object world are used in making sense of things that are contagious, getting out of control, containment, and decelerations of spread, the coming and going of waves. The dynamic kinaesthetics and its 'comprehensibles' are central to the understanding of power-political processes and flows. Broadly speaking, the term 'contagion' is used in reference to the idea that political violence—for example, external or internal wars—in one region or state influences the possibility of violence in another region or state (Li and Thompson 1975: 63). Political violence and its sub-categories, such as war and terrorism, are often treated in terms of a disease (Spilerman 1970; Zartman 1995: 9). There are numerous examples equating different forms of extreme political violence with disease as a regressive process. Most and Starr (1980) refer to 'war disease' when they discuss the spread of war. Hamilton and Hamilton (1983: 41) state that the main paradigm in terrorism studies holds that 'terrorist incidents may encourage further violence through a process of imitation or diffusion, giving rise to a dynamics of terrorism analogous to that observed in the spread of a contagious disease'. These widely used contagion models in politics arguably have their roots in politosomatics. The path is historically well trodden. It is here that Thucydides' points concerning war and plague become relevant. They both belong to the underlying scenario of combined regressions feeding each other. Contagions are seen as mutually reinforcing in a causally non-linear way influencing the likelihood of each other.

Besides allowing for a culturally deeply entrenched way of understanding violent political processes, the disease object world highlights fundamental tensions. Susan Sontag (1978) referred to the ability of the disease metaphor to crystallize the enmities inherent in the world: 'Feelings about evil are projected onto a disease. And the disease (so enriched by meanings) is projected onto the world'. In a politosomatic way, political enemies turn into potential sources of regressive contagion. The talk about superspreaders/events and diseases carries additional embodied ways of picturing rogue and inherently hostile elements. Political enemies are treated as diseasing, and diseases are seen through the lens of political enmities. Enemies within and without are perceived as sources of potentially dangerous physical maladies. In this way, the association of COVID-19 and SARS with China allowed for a strengthening of China's otherness as well as making invisible disease agents more politically comprehensible. In China, reverse imaginaries are used where others unjustifiably blame China because of their deep-seated hostility towards the rise of China. Associating the origin of the pandemics with the perceived Chinese secrecy gave the disease a narrative form that seemed to clarify its nature. There are many such examples. During the BSE (bovine spongiform encephalopathy) scare of 1996, the disease was seen by many commentators as having emerged out of the 'reckless' deregulation policies practised during the Thatcher years in the United Kingdom (UK). Others, especially in the UK, saw the bans on British bovine products as a sign that the European Union (EU) was seriously interfering with British sovereignty. The disease was interpreted through the lens of the political contestations of the time. In the same way, there is a tendency to see the fight against naturally occurring pandemic diseases as 'rehearsals' for the eventuality of a biological terror attack in the context of the War on Terror. This disease frame also offers clues for the present tendency of associating pandemic threats with states that are 'rogue', 'failed', or 'failing'. There might be factual reasons for all of these identifications. However, one hypothesis that can be made is that the inherent usability of the disease object world reinforces such underlying enmity dynamics.

Thus, the sentiment of disease, like enmity, provides an important register for feeling and sensing power in world politics. When real or perceived (e)motions in power-politics favour political enemies, they may also alarm because of the disease-related repercussions of such movements. In her review of the emotional modality of international relations, Neta Crawford traces the origin of the term 'emotion' to 'political or social agitation and popular disturbance' (2000: 124).[6] Against this power-related background of emotionality, it is not a coincidence that the theories of political movements and political mobilizations have been most receptive to giving emotions a central role in their models (Jasper 1998). Research has concentrated on such mobilizing events as moral shocks, frame alignments, and collective identities. The movement itself brings about emotions by stirring up passions and by stimulating people. At the minimum, it stirs the existing patterns of understanding what are positive and negative emotions, what should be expressed and hidden, and what are adequate and inadequate responses (Willer *et al.* 1997: 573). Sentiments ranging from disdain, superiority, hostility, and anger to compassion are equated with the movements and with the changing power relations signalled by the movements. The general idea is that changes in power hierarchies trigger emotions and stimulate participation in further flare-ups of collective feelings. The power status differences are established, challenged, and reinforced by emotions (Lutz and Abu-Lughod 1990: 14). The emotions produced by the in-group or the in-group versus out-group power structures vary from negative to positive, from enmity and containment to compassion (Kemper 1991). It can be argued that the use of the disease analogy influences and directs these power-related emotions. The disease scenario reinforces attributions of deep-seated feelings of enmity and hostility to power shifts that favour actors who have come to be viewed in diseasing terms. For example, globalization as a process of lowering borders is often felt as alarming because it brings places that have been seen as diseased landscapes closer, linking global peripheries with its hubs. It is also possible to speculate that the perceived rise of China is sensed through the lens of a diseasing enmity, thereby making the context ripe for perceiving dangerous processes, such as pandemics, as emanating from China.

Thus, the disease frame can be seen as making some power-related emotional registers more prominent. The perceived global flows of power stimulate their targets according to particular anxieties. These anxieties over the inherent fragility of human beings and humanity during pandemic scares offer insights into how various people sense that they are linked to the world's hierarchical order and how the increased interconnectedness between the global centre and its peripheries results in a heightened sense of worry that gets embodied in pandemics or fears about them. These linkages translate into harm, terror, and horror in more ways than are commonly understood. Anxiety and stress are at their acutest when the 'fevers of the world' physically infect people through the main global arteries—the hub-and-spoke system of air travel. These turn into perceived disease vectors and circuits of contagion and seem to demand spectacles of containment and disengagement to stop their dangerous spread. However, these complex emotional relationships can be further disentangled.

Besides highlighting the dynamics of spread and contagion, there are additional nuances that need to be considered for a fuller grip on how the medico-political heuristic is used to symbolize architectures of global power. The basic disease object world schemata include various kinaesthetic sensations. Among the most important of these is the sense of being diluted or submerged by something negative and overwhelming. It can be argued that the fear of submergence provides a specific hue to disease-related anxieties. Even a quick review of this type of declinist literature reveals a stress on the communal creed—on the moral, religious, and cultural underpinnings, for example, the 'American way of life' or 'Western values' (Huntington 2004). From this perspective, it is often thought that the primary sign of trouble is the sudden disregard of civic virtues and the underlying civil religion. The causes of this are easily associated with foreign disease-like elements: the civil character becomes diluted when the hegemony of the preponderant actor turns into its opposite—into submergence—by excessive assimilation of hostile 'incompatible' elements. It is here that the most common reaction to pandemics becomes relevant. A moral panic to restore the 'healthy' and 'immune' civil religious element can ensue. Questions of who we really are nationally and globally are asked in the middle of the pandemic.

The thoughts that connect world power with constant fear of decline and fall by submergence may be interpreted as a significant cultural stock narrative that dramatizes the contemporary dynamics of global security. The drama of political health is meant to demonstrate that the core element—the top of the power hierarchy—is not going to be dangerously diluted or rendered not vigorous enough to continue to create security and eradicate dis-ease. The associated hierarchical imagery points out the differential place of the various nations, ethnicities, regions, religions, civilizations, and people. Their interconnectedness is interpreted based on the disease frame. In this spirit, it is often argued that the diligent maintenance of hierarchy's divisions—or the new containment boundaries—is the best guarantee against submergence by a wave of anarchy (Kaplan 1994). Robert Kaplan's influential geopolitical imagery is partly composed of 'cities and suburbs in an environment that has been mastered'. He contrasts this with the Third World, from where he sees a wave of dangerous anarchy emanating. His detached aerial view—the first-person account is often based on observations from a cosmopolitan perspective of an airplane—of the ground below seemingly permits him to grasp the politically sig-nificant contrasts and patterns between combinations of scenes. He makes all these relevant as part of an overall emotional scene of fear of the imminent chaos spread-ing from the Third World. This fear of flight—people fleeing and global air flights enabling the fleeing—seems to stem from the expansive reaches of the globalized world's hub-and-spoke infrastructure. It seems that what Kaplan is suggesting as a healthy antidote for the spreading anarchy is the confinement of people to the contours of their territory (Dalby 1996: 472). The confinement of people to their territories and the ranking of people as more compatible and less compatible offer additional substance to contemporary containment dramas. Significantly, Hunting-ton (2004, 2005) identifies foreign immigrants as one major source of decay and reason for worry. According to Huntington (1997: 38), contemporary forms of contact do not cut immigrant umbilical cords in the same way as before. Links and contacts remain, turning people coming from different civilizations into sources of decay and erosion (Huntington 2005: 306). The fear of global contact and intimacy can be seen as an additional consequence of the projections of the disease object world based on a scenario that is highly embodied and contains characteristics that are ideally comprehensive. It blends the declinist modality of submergence with the emotional registers of spread and contagion.

Disease as a crucial embodied object world, or a situated scenario with com-prehensible characteristics, needs further sharpening in order to provide analytical clarity. I will draw from the frame paradigm developed by Erving Goffman (1974) to provide methodological support for the further understanding of present-day pandemics and their inherent politosomatic dynamics. The 'frame' offers a way of gaining insight into health governance composed of politico-cultural perfor-mances—that is, pandemic scares—and supported by the disease as a situated scenario. From a general perspective, the notion of frame refers to an 'organized and bounded social entity most immediate to the individual's experience' (Gonos 1997: 854). Framed public acts involve heightened and engrossing dramas and spectacles. As the recent, approximately 3 years, frequency of pandemic emer-gencies shows, these public events tend to be tense, emotional, theatrical, and spectacular. Pandemic public drama creates a sense of having its own specific type of reality, which suspends and interrupts the way in which events normally take place. The frame produces a sense of realness, comprehensiveness, and enhances its performers with a sense of differentially (dis)empowering solidity. In this sense, any frame offers a clear gallery of figures, which allows the spectators and performers 'to conjure up a desired self-image' (Fine and Manning 2003: 46). These dynamic 'frames' produce suspended circumstances in which the spectators judge things to be dramatically real and critically meaningful. Highlighting this point, Goffman (1997: 150) refers to William James, who argued for a pre- or quasi-cognitive, revelatory status of knowing (James 1985: 352). This type of knowing means that frames are acknowledged, rather than rationally known; authoritative, rather than freely chosen; and emotionally appealing and bodily felt, rather than cognitively satisfactory. Many of the events and reactions to them make sense at the level of proto-theory rather than any explicit analytical model. It can be suggested that a pandemic emergency sets into motion such a frame, or scenario, in which the underlying comprehensibles are being revealed. To an important degree, the question of framed realness becomes a function of specific types of attention, as Goffman (1997: 150) points out, quoting from William James: 'Each world, whilst it is attended to, is real after its own fashion; only the reality lapses with the attention'. The question of realness turns into one of attention: How is attention captured and encapsulated in pandemic spectacles? What is the specific emotional content? How is knowledge revealed, by what figures, and to what audiences? Familiar frames and the shared experiences they contain are fundamentally about fixing the trajectory of acknowledgement and about the production of authority: What is the flow or script of the pandemic spectacle and what can be done with it?

The additional modality of pandemic scares has to do with making the invisible visible. Bruno Latour's (1988, 1993) idea of the 'theatre of proof' offers a history of the medicine-related way of looking at pandemic performances, in which the various protagonists take on their respective roles. The key for them is to demonstrate legitimacy in meeting the challenges posed by the invisible rogue disease elements. Latour's notion draws from a famous 1882 demonstration in which Louis Pasteur revealed the effectiveness of vaccination. The experiment lasted for several days and was the focus of intensive attention by the French media. Twenty-five sheep were vaccinated against anthrax and another 25, which were not vaccinated, were painted with red marks. The success of the demonstration was vividly visible to the onlookers, who witnessed the death of all the animals who were not vaccinated but were visibly marked. This experiment was widely followed and publicized and gave medical research an air of progressive certainty and authority. It offered clear-cut revelatory knowledge about the power of the new health science to tame hard to understand invisible disease agents. Pasteur managed to make the underlying, difficult-to-comprehend, hidden reality visible and controllable. At the level of popular imagination, these laboratory experiments, once transferred into the field, turned into modernity's testing grounds—into theatres of proof. At stake was the legitimacy of modern medicine and the state that had produced it. When the progressive scenario—the theatre of epidemiological might—turns into a sudden regressive encounter with disease agents that cannot be contained, the questions of certainty, legitimacy, authority, and expertise are thrown into the open. A key characteristic of the pandemic scenario as a theatre of 'unproof', when the scenario fails and is not revelatory, is the losing of legitimacy and authority.

This method of demonstration can be argued to still linger. The theatre of proof, as a frame, turned any effective conquering of a disease by public health measures into a power repository, into an opportunity of demonstrating the legitimacy of a particular medicalized ideal of a modern governance structure as an answer to the Hobbesian dilemma of offering refuge from a short, nasty, and brutish life. In this way, pandemic scares offer tools for demonstrating power. The key to understanding them as theatres of proof has to do with clearly identified and visible sources of disease and the protagonist agencies that fight them. Whereas WHO played a prominent role during the swine flu scare, COVID-19 is more challenging for the established authorities. It has left the great powers damaged although the vaccine development and vaccination programmes can restore some of the declinist status worries. Similarly, in the case of SARS in the spring of 2003, the scene was set for the WHO to stop the much-talked-about disease threat. The SARS spectacle managed to convey a sense of security as the disease was contained. However, in the case of swine flu, the theatre failed, partially because of public scepticism that the disease scare had been too hyped up. The controversies over vaccine purchases, effectiveness, and possible side effects demonstrated the limits of the progressive theatre of proof dominated by the key protagonists.

Pandemic spectacles are intense and engrossing scenarios in which the power of modern states and their international health regimes are being tested and demonstrated by diligent—highly visible and dramatic—application of modern health sciences. Moreover, the performer of 'health' is a figure, an embodiment, which objectively and securely meets the external hostile reality. By proxy, the effectiveness of this performance proves the 'true' and 'authentic' foundation of the Western political bodies. In this historically well-rehearsed way, any successful act of the health theatre turns into an empowering foundation for political power. Pandemics are refined into governance exercises that are thought to be beyond politics (Siddiqi 1995: 196; Symonds and Carder 1973: 157).[7] However, a closer examination reveals the close co-optive relationship between the demonstrations of health technologies and hegemonic political power. COVID-19 showed us a failure scenario. Protagonists were largely missing or inefficient. Antagonists gained an upper hand over the supposedly resilient modern way of life. This is going to have repercussions because the comprehensibles are less than ideal and more difficult to fit into any theatre of proof.

Notes

1 The 'root' causes of most violent epidemics can be traced to multilevel political structures and dynamics, which provide the macro-level context for the disease-causing agents (Fassin 2007; Farmer 2004; Joralemon 1997). The local and global circulations of disease agents are largely in accordance with structural imbalances and inequalities in terms of nationality, ethnicity, gender, and wealth. Although recent literature on the anthropology of suffering has highlighted it, this aspect of disease is not a recent revelation. Rather, it can be argued that it has always been encoded in the nuanced quasi-cognitive beliefs about diseases.

2 The theory of socio-somatics is used in reference to those social processes through which patterns of social interaction have an influence on the somatic process, such as heart rate, perspiration, or blood pressure, and vice versa (Kleinman and Becker 1998). These mediating social patterns can refer to various social practices such as humiliation, expressed pain behaviour, and mourning: '[A] person's context . . . influences the severity and type of symptoms experienced' (James and Prilleltensky 2002: 1134).

3 See also Elisabeth Bronfen (1998).

4 See also Frank Snowden (2020).

5 Scarry (1987: 7) uses the term 'radical epistemological doubt' to describe these processes in which violence goes hand in hand with non-acknowledgement of former knowledge and the accompanying unravelling of knowledge/power relationships.

6 Emotion-centred language is omnipresent even in contemporary rational and system-oriented theorizing. Realist ontologies are based on despair over the flaws in human nature and the fragility of human achievement (Clark 1989: 83). This sentiment of despair is paired with constant worry and fear over the unpredictability of events. The more liberalist ontologies build on the possibilities of hope.

7 The medicalized governance language renders the politics of the distant other into a series of rational/technical problem-solving exercises. Although this production of subjects is itself a political act, it is political in a specific sense of the word: it is politically privileged by its appearance of being apolitical. Further light can be shed on this by Barthes' (1980: 45) concept of 'depoliticized speech'. The practice of depoliticized speech is based on rooting the political out of one's actions and turning them into something self-evident and natural.

2

PANDEMIC DRAMAS

Containment Efforts and 'Nearest Is Dearest' Compassions

In the traditional state- and, inevitably, border-centric political thought, physical separation and geographical distance are often equated with security and shelter. When COVID-19 escaped its outbreak zone through global air travel and the global pandemic management system failed to cope, borders went up and an archipelago of state-level containment measures became the new norm. The almost instinctive nature of this reaction provides evidence for the quarantine border qualities associated with national border lines. They can more or less effectively cordon off territorial entities from each other. This health-related function has a long history in the interaction between plagues and people. The identification of borders with security may be seen as a basic conceptualization which has implications beyond the defence- and trade-related functions. Borders can become signifiers of security in an expansive sense. Moreover, the bordered security conceptualizations also lend legitimacy to and catalyse other multifarious political boundaries ranging from cultural, ethnic, and socio-economic to religious and civilizational markers of distinctions, and including the interspecies barrier (Weiss 1997: 457). Pandemics are an open-ended bundle of characteristics that reinforce the comprehensive understanding of borders as communal shelters and, beyond that, as defining characteristics of what a community is as an exclusionary entity and identity.

In contrast to this traditional emphasis on signifiers of separation, the emergence of globality as a process of lowering boundaries, producing seamlessness, and bridging distances is essentially a problematic phenomenon. Pandemics contest the modern paradigm of open spaces. It is in this anxious affective climate of felt global insecurities, stemming from vanishing borders, that pandemic emergencies can become epochally comprehensible and start to carry political, geopolitical, and geo-economic messages that relate to people's need to find shelter from a life that is short, nasty, and brutish. From the politosomatic perspective, the cultural constructions of pandemic diseases are embodied expressions of the underlying

DOI: 10.4324/9781003169147-2

anxieties stemming from such global intimacy between hubs and spokes, centres and peripheries, and one's immediate community and global reaches. It is clear that in the affective rush of a pandemic scenario, these deeply embodied anxieties can be seen as motivating a diversity of multilevel containment activities. The embodied 'object world' of pandemics instantiates strong containment tendencies, instead of a sense of being connected as a compassionate value in itself. The sense of urgency and of things getting out of hand leads to less international coordination and unity as the age-old inward-looking attitude focuses on finding shelter in known and traditional communal spaces.

Thus, it is difficult to conceive of a pandemic emergency's public health dramas without taking into account the value placed on 'containment' and on the sentiment of striving 'to contain'. It is seen as a value aimed at keeping harmful influences under control outside of certain limits, preventing the expansion and spread of a hostile outside element.

Cultural geographer Yi-Fu Tuan, in his book, *Landscapes of Fear* (1979: 6), argues that much of human activity is directed towards securing the freedom of human existence from what he calls chaos: 'In a sense, every human construction whether mental or material is a component in a landscape of fear because it exists to contain chaos'. This is especially pertinent to the conceptual underpinnings of political theory and international thought. Both can be seen as traditions that aim to contain the effects of insecurity, randomness, anarchy, roguishness, and injustice both in and between polities. The idea is to expand the human controllable space between the brute nature of power and the accidental nature of the environment. The usual dynamic of a pandemic scenario can be seen as an expression of this underlying desire to contain and tame disruptive forces. The modern world juxtaposes the disconnectedness of walled-in and contained places—such as states and institutions—and dynamic border-crossing flows of interdependence (Tuan 1995: 229). The balance of these partially contradictory elements is rapidly renegotiated as a lethal contagion is felt to be on the move, crossing distances and closing up. The political emotion of rushing to contain redefines the global order as one of its key recent characteristics, the infrastructure of fast borderless mobility, is limited or even shut down.

The tracing of the affective contours of global containment brings into the limelight its antithesis, the other global public cognition, the mobilizations of compassion, as in humanitarian emergencies. While the sentiment of containment aims to wall off and encircle a community with lockdown restrictions, the emotive flow of mobilized compassion is directed outwards in an attempt to bridge distances: donation campaigns are organized, media is focused on the distant suffering, politicians want to be do-gooders, aid is delivered, and personnel are sent to the disaster areas. In many ways, compassionate activity revolves around the alleviation of global insecurity, lowers the sense of national bordered identities, and includes the idea of humanity and its citizens. In the pandemic scenarios, there is a strong compassionate element. However, as seen with the ineffective and underfunded COVID-19 global vaccination drive, it tends to be undermined if not overwhelmed by self-interested sheltering tendencies. The rational expert-led planning approach struggles to find mobilizing motivations in compassion for the distant other or for humanity as the affective climate of the out-of-control pandemic is rushed and panicky.

In this chapter, I will review practices of compassion in order to contrast them with those of containment and to offer alternative imageries to pandemic scenarios. The idea behind offering these two contrasting views is to map out how pandemic containment, as a scenario, contains tendencies and action sequence directionalities that are unique and different from the humanitarian instincts present in violent conflicts, yet more purely represented in reactions to natural catastrophes. The point is not to suggest that there can be no compassionate, outwardly extended actions during pandemic emergencies but to highlight and characterize the relatively understudied dynamics of pandemic emergencies. After drawing the distinction, the aim is to tie the respective scenarios together schematically to show broad and novel patterns of nuanced similarity and dissimilarity. In this way, further light can be shed on the politosomatic nexus of pandemic diseases by juxtaposing their emotional charges, for example, with the dynamics inherent in the traditions of political compassion.

Political compassions—as expressed in global humanitarianism or in 'nearest is dearest' mobilizations—are often based on action at a distance, for example, when some distant sufferers' plight is relieved through charity, voluntary work, or aid.[1] However, the sentiment of compassion implies global power patterns because such suffering can be seen to be in itself an expression of the world order and global hierarchies (Aaltola 2009). In this way, they are related to the practices of containment, which also accentuate existing power disparities and markers of separation. At the same time, the containment-oriented pandemic security perspective often views humanity as an interlinked whole in that the health of the distant other is intimately linked to the health of everybody. The discourses of global public health often reveal articulations of compassion towards the human polity as a whole. Thus, the panics and scares over pandemic threats may be seen as consisting of a double movement of selective compassion and vigorous containment. In this chapter, I will review how these two essentially nested 'power moves'—compassion and containment—can be used to make sense of underlying pandemic insecurities. The working hypothesis of this chapter is that compassionate worries over public health are entangled with alarm over the general uncontainability of global processes. My aim is to map out the historic complexities involved and thereby shed light on pandemic scares as embodied expressions of this complex entanglement.

This acute global relationship of outward-directed compassion, blended with strongly anxious aversion and containment, provides the Janus-faced template for the understanding of different pandemic emergencies. Such tangible global emotional charges offer insights into how pandemic experiences intertwine with geographies of fear and, moreover, with the dynamics of political power production. I am using the term 'politosomatics' to describe how bodily felt anxiety for shelter couples with the interconnected global landscape in a nexus that, on the one hand, turns the dynamics of power and politics into an embodied and even somatic experience and, on the other hand, gives somatic fears a global extension and offers a framework that gives affective interpretations to global dis-eased politics. The embodied object world of pandemics as a somatic experience opens up in a dynamic relationship between disease agents, methods of infection, and individual bodies. This object world, however, is not only personal, it is also predominantly power related and thus political in that the scenarios of violent diseases have the tendency to embody the underlying patterns of political hierarchy and enmity. That said, it is precisely the personally tangible nature of pandemics that allows them to be used as ways of telling stories of what is at stake in the global order. Taken together, these two juxtaposed object worlds of disease and global order translate into a configuration of differentially exposed bodies which, in turn, give expressive meanings to ritualized pandemic behaviour and relevance to their consequences in political expressions in different political systems. The private and collective sentiments of fear, anxiety, and scare transform into demands and opportunities for calming power spectacles branded as 'effective health governance', the legitimacy of which becomes even more tangible when the devastating blow or wave is averted and fear subsides. If that does not happen and communities are faced with serious wave after wave of disease, the body politic of a community can become restless and authority and loyalty patterns become rearranged.

How the Black Death and Plague Transformed Political Thought

It may be argued that the seminal Western encounters between plagues and people from the perspective of modern imageries took place during the long centuries of plague on the European continent. It took about 400 years for the plague to run its course and disappear, but not without first killing vast numbers of people in different parts of Europe. Between the landmark years of 1346 and 1721, epidemics that killed more than one-third of local populations at a time were more the rule than the exception (McNeill 1976: 10). It was not until after the city of Marseille had been devastated (1720–21) that the deadly shadow of widespread plague epidemics largely withdrew from continental Europe and, much more gradually, if at all, from popular imageries. The plague swept across Europe several times in the form of inexorable tides, leaving behind not only large-scale destruction but also major social, religious, and political changes and sticky memory images.

Thus, the migration of rat species from South Asia to Europe had a disruptive yet also transformational impact on European politics and power. The bacterium, *Yersinia pestis*, is the causative disease agent of plague. This coccobacillus bacterium spreads pneumonic, septicaemic, and bubonic plagues via the oriental rat flea. The pneumonic variant of the disease can also spread through human-to-human transmission. The main reservoir of plague has been several rodent species. A bite of a flea that has fed on a rodent can spread plague. The spread of plague to Europe was originally catalysed by the Roman conquests in the Middle East, which opened up trade routes to the heart of the Roman Empire (McCormick 2003). Thus, a mix of conquest, trade, and rodent migration was the key factor in the introduction of plague epidemics into Europe. The emergence and spread of plague were a symptom of the rise and spread of Roman power and hegemony. Ultimately, it was also a causative agent in the decline and fall the Western Roman Empire.

The Late Roman period came to an end with close to two centuries of the Plague of Justinia (541–750 CE).[2] The key Mediterranean port cities in particular were decimated by the waves of plague that could kill about 50% of the population. It was one of the most devastating and politically consequential epidemics in recorded history. At the same time, research suggests that societies overreact to and hyperbolize sudden epidemic outbreaks and that their consequences are overemphasized later on (Mordechai *et al.* 2019). Yet the opposite might also be true. Although the disease agent itself does not come with a message or function as a direct cause that could be later recognized in research, it can act as a trigger for complex non-linear and lasting cascading effects that can be hard to recognize later on and reduce analytically back to a single cause, an outbreak. In many cases, the expected 'consequential' outcomes of a serious pandemic are the political collapse, instability, and other regressions—for example, war and famine—that are associated with it. Thus, an epidemic, to be consequential, has to cause a regression in the political and social order and be accompanied by and happen in tandem with war and upheavals. Historically speaking, 'plagues' and wars do coincide. However, the causal linkages are hard to disentangle. This methodological challenge should not lead to the conclusion that serious epidemics do not matter. It is suggested that a more comprehensive approach be adopted.

As the role of *Yersinia pestis* as the cause of plague via rats and fleas remained unknown for centuries, people thought of plague as a terrifying and unusual fever that was intimately connected with filth and foul-smelling miasma and ultimately tied in with various ideas of broken 'sacred' communal boundaries and with different embodiments of foreignness (Palmer 1982: 358). Very often, it was assumed that the ultimate reason for plague had to do with communal irreligiousness or God's divine and mysterious providence. The communal quilt-related beliefs were strengthened by the inability of alternative perspectives to satisfactorily explain the connection between the people who died of plague as other than their own sins or God's will. In the plague years, people were generally more accustomed to the different pestilences that caused pain, suffering, poverty, desolation, and death as compared to the modern day. Even in this disease-saturated context, plague was a case apart because of its lethality, bodily manifestations, mysterious pattern of spread, lack of perspicuity, and staying power. Its extraordinary and ominous character led to anxiety and fear of a kind that was unparalleled in European history and during the emergence of key modern-day political institutions and ideas such as 'state' and 'borders'.

Despite the distinctiveness of plague, many fail to appreciate its effects on the political and intellectual development of modern political thought. This disregard is one reason why it is fairly common to think that the ramifications of plague were not dramatic or long lasting. However, plague did leave its marks because it contained powerful, persuasive, and constraining narrative charges that were able to create lasting associations even when any causal relations had become too entangled and imperceptible to distinguish. These analogical influences are consequential because everyday routines and discourses absorb them effortlessly, extending their impact beyond causal attributions. These profuse complexities were synonymous with plague as a social and political phenomenon.

In studies and popular culture products, people of the plague years are cast more often than not into passive suffering roles. However, occasionally, plague offered more possibilities for conceptual control and political agency. For example, it allowed localities, city-states, and states to demonstrate their own status or point to the weak status of outside actors. In other words, the way in which plague's contemporaries perceived it contained combinatorial possibilities with religious and political understandings such as enemy images: witches were burnt, minorities were killed, and enmities were reinforced as churches were built and alms were given. Reactions were many and context dependent; however, civil religious purity and strictness was usually one significant consequence. Moreover, a related political embodiment that was emerging in the plague-saturated context was that of a bordered state as a concept. Thus, judging by some relevant perspectives, pestilence, and politics first collided, then tangled, and finally combined, actualizing, moulding, and reinforcing one another as changed entities. This interacting nexus between state and plague included important points of affinity such as border, threat, enemy, shelter, and survival. Thus, it can be suggested that the state involved scenarios of knowledge and practices that matured and became deeply ingrained in a context permeated by plague.

During the early modern period, the fight against plague assumed an increasingly secular and physical form as the attempts made to check its spread were formalized in various quarantine and *cordon sanitaire* regulations. The use of soldiers and medical police in upholding the numerous regulations and restrictions, together with occasional violence, gave an increasingly military and political character to the battle against plague, with the result that it began to resemble, metaphorically, a defence against an invading army. The tempting nature of the enemy analogy was reinforced in the Christian tradition, which includes numerous references to plague in connection with war, defeat, and invasion. The analogy between political practices—state, border, and war—and plague became even more pronounced when large-scale troop movements and plague were usually simultaneous and accompanying events. Troop mobility increased contact and the likelihood of spread. These associations were also highlighted in narratives that often drew strong causal inferences between long-distance activities—such as commerce and travel—and plague. The figures of the soldier, sailor, and vagabond were inherently dubbed as dubious in the plague context. The general perception was that foreign influences were framed as plaguing. Thus, it may be hypothesized that plague formed easy-to-tread combinatorial paths that did not limit its effects to a few common points of attachment. Rather, it resonated with other scenarios. These mutually accentuating and reinforcing object worlds or scenarios influenced and legitimated the maturing of the central political practices and the meanings of their use.

Plague outbreaks were considered causes of significant embarrassment both individually and locally because they were thought to be a mark of the sinful, indecent, and unconfined life of a political community. In this context, the threat of plague easily became or was made analogous with exogenous enemies and foreign sources, as in the form of rival city-states. Enemies of Christendom, foreign elements in general, and domestic minorities—mainly Jews and perceived heretics such as witches—were often thought to be well poisoners and plague spreaders during the long plague years (e.g. Dols 1974). These rudimentary yet influential analogies were further supported by the conclusion that the spread of plague, with the resulting economic losses and societal paralysis, was clearly in the interest of rival communities and states. It was often thought that what these outside forces could not achieve by honest means, such as political, economic, and strategic competition, were being attained with the help of plague. Although it often became necessary eventually, it was harder for the proud citizens of city-states to imagine that the deaths were due to their own moral corruption. Thus, the general argument pointed to the immorality and sins of outside forces or to one's internal minorities, who were deemed to be wickedly and deceptively spreading the plague to the more morally upright individuals and communities. In this way, the pattern of plague, which was in reality quite random, reinforced existing and emerging imageries of hierarchies and boundaries.

The placing of blame on foreign entities or unwanted internal minorities could justify their harsh and violent treatment and turn public attention away from the authorities' inability to maintain public safety and order. For example, it was not uncommon that the hospitals set up for the containment of quarantined people were also used to imprison politically unwanted elements (Carmichael 1986). The references to a foreign threat in connection with plague were not limited to the elements of foreignness within the borders of a city-state but offered possibilities from the point of view of intercommunal competition. It should be noted that the policies and actions based on taking advantage of the disease were less dishonest and sinister than they may sound at first because of the mysterious and puzzling way in which plague spread. Plague manifested itself in a paranoid context filled with supernatural, inexplicable, and dangerous forces. It is, therefore, quite possible that the officials of city-states and the clergy could believe that their explanations and allegations were true, independent of their own political motives. Thus, purposefulness and ignorance often combined dangerously in explosive and unpredictable mixtures. Hidden motives, deception, and secrecy, together with well-intended but misguided actions, were a prominent part of the internal and external policies when plague struck.

During the plague years, the more or less arbitrary effectiveness of quarantines as a preferred disease control method manifested itself from time to time in a frightful way and added weight to views critical of them. In hindsight, quarantines offered only a relatively weak protective barrier against diseases that spread via and from animals (plague and yellow fever) or through water (cholera). On the other hand, experience seemed to suggest that diseases were somewhat contagious. In other words, there existed much scepticism towards the idea that climatic, hygienic, or geographical features caused diseases, as the miasmic theory claimed. Practical knowledge dictated that diseases spread through contact and proximity and that containment sometimes worked against the spread of diseases (e.g. Zuckerman 2004: 273). Yet, although quarantines did not always work against the plague-bearing black rat, the conceptualizations behind quarantines were somewhat logical and persuasive at the time. Moreover, quarantines gave the political authorities the means to do something that could be used as proof of their effectiveness in containing the plague. For example, it gave states a means to prevent people from escaping their plagued communities and protected the property of the fleeing upper class. Thus, the survival and viability of a state as a political entity under the dramatic conditions of plague required drastic political measures. On the other hand, citizens often associated quarantines with the very thing that quarantine measures were supposed to protect them against. Hence, it was often not the epidemics that caused political disturbances but the authorities' actions such as quarantines (Evans 1992; Pullan 1992). From the perspective of sceptics and authorities alike, it can be said that quarantines had an important political existence; saving individual lives was often of secondary importance.

Despite the mixed success record of the quarantine and *cordon sanitaire* regulations, their widespread use can be contextualized in connection with the emergence of centralized states and encircling state boundaries. As said, state boundaries offer a major conceptual connection between politics and epidemic diseases: 'European states adopted and implemented national quarantine measures in an effort to keep diseases from entering their territories from foreign lands' (Fidler 2004: 27). Several writers have seen the Peace of Westphalia as a turning point in the history of diseases. Eckert (2000: 25) perceives a direct link between the establishment of state boundaries and a major decline in plague outbreaks.[3] Before the late seventeenth century, the enforcement of quarantine systems was mainly the responsibility of city-states. Local quarantines encircling a city or village were the most significant plague control policy. The coming of the state system changed all this. Thereafter, state interventions efficiently utilized their administrations and large armies. Surveillance also became much more organized. Like natural barriers such as mountain ranges, rivers, or oceans, increasingly, effective political borders too provided a formidable obstacle to the spread of epidemic diseases. Human-made borders clearly affected epidemics and changed the appearance of randomness by influencing which places were devastated and which were spared by diseases. Through efficient and well-maintained political borders, it was possible to convey a sense of the legitimizing quality of political order. The modality of health started to occupy an even more prominent role in the scenarios of political power. The growing legitimacy of borders and the practice of developing border controls changed the nature of communities. In reference to the emerging well-contained communities, Ehrenberg (1960: 7) writes that '[t]he narrow space, admitting of little variation, produced a marked unification of the civic type and a very distinct political consciousness'. Every time an epidemic struck somewhere else, the state's legitimacy as a secure, privileged, inimitable, and exemplary entity, predestined and chosen for glory, was reinforced. In many ways, thus, it seems that the need to combat diseases may have intertwined with and complemented the efforts of state-building.

Pandemic Containment Scenarios

It can be suggested that containment-related tendencies are also present in the more altruistic compassionate strategies that target the maintenance of national, regional, and global pandemic security. The containment strategies focus on containing an emerging disease at the site of its outbreak and, if that fails, at different global hubs and, ultimately, at national and sub-national borders. As evidenced by the lost days in the initial stages of the COVID-19 outbreak, the clock was ticking fast and national authorities were expected to notify the WHO in time and also allow immediate access to the hot zone. The idea is that the containment of a disease in the limited area of its initial occurrence is in practical terms the only effective option. After this, the bets are on recognizing the disease carriers in the global airport hubs. This is much trickier if the contagious people do not show symptoms for days or if the symptoms are relatively unnoticeable, such as a low fever or headache, as in the case of COVID-19.

Once a pandemic disease has broken out, efforts have to concentrate on ways of reducing mortality and morbidity and on mitigating other consequences. Even if a pandemic outbreak cannot be totally contained, efforts to do so might serve to delay an all-out pandemic and provide time for the preparation of other actions:

> The international containment strategy is based on studies suggesting that efforts centred on using antiviral drugs to prevent infection as well as treat cases might contain a pandemic at the site of the outbreak or at least slow its international spread, thus gaining time to put emergency measures in place and develop vaccines.
>
> *(Crosse and Gootnick 2007: 16)*

Containment is based on the geographical notion of a 'containment zone'. A containment zone is large enough to circumscribe all the known cases and those in close interaction with them. Movement of people across the limits of this zone needs to be restricted.

One way to understand a lethal epidemic disease as a contagious process with geography is also to embed it in a political landscape. The evolving disease language becomes a vital part of this political landscape. Political borders between and inside states have played an important role in the history of disease. The practice of quarantine offers a case in point of borders in connection with diseases. Quarantine refers to the isolation of known and possible sources of contamination, whether humans, animals, commodities, or things. Quarantine practices started to take shape at the end of the fourteenth century in the context of freely spreading plague epidemics. In its most basic form, a quarantine consisted of keeping a ship docked outside of the harbour for 40 days (Kilwein 1995). Inland quarantines isolated those actually or probably infected with plague to their homes or to lazarettos. On a wider scale, it was common practice to set up roadblocks to city gates or along roads to stop dangerous contact and to stop commerce. For example, during the Great Plague of 1664, King Charles II moved his court to Oxford. The city gates were closely guarded, and most traffic was stopped. Plague carriers were moved outside the city to specially made huts. The range of quarantine methods used has also included large-scale military *cordon sanitaire* practices involving the isolation of localities, cities, and villages in siege-like arrangements (Slack 1991). As stated previously, evidently, borders, diseases, immunity, and cures are intimately connected from the historical perspective.

Modern pandemic-related containment measures are coordinated by the WHO.[4] However, there are states that have declared that efficient worldwide pandemic control measures are also in their national interest. The inclusion of pandemic threats in national security strategies anticipates more forceful public health interventions in case of an alarming outbreak. The WHO's World Health Assembly of 2005 started a process to reform the global protocol for rapid response and containment in the eventuality of an epidemic breakout called the International Health Regulation (IHR). In March 2006, WHO held a global technical meeting to finalize the early containment protocols for pandemic influenza. The draft protocol (WHO 2006a) highlighted the unpredictable nature of pandemic influenza:

> [G]iven the unpredictable behaviour of influenza viruses, no one can know in advance whether the start of a pandemic will begin gradually, following the emergence of a virus not yet fully adapted to humans, or be announced by a sudden explosion of cases, thereby precluding any attempt at containment.

In cases where containment was possible, the protocol stated that the mass administration of antiviral drugs must begin within 21 days following the initial detection. This placed much importance on the early detection, notification, investigation, and reporting of influenza symptoms. The protocol made it clear that local government cooperation was vital for any efficient response. The immediate control measures included the following:

> 1. Isolation of clinical cases of moderate-to-severe respiratory disease and other patients under investigation in respiratory isolation rooms or single rooms. 2. Identification and voluntary home quarantine of asymptomatic close contacts and daily monitoring for symptom onset. 3. Administration of antiviral drugs for the treatment of cases and, if domestic supplies permit, for the targeted prophylaxis of close contact. 4. Strict infection control and the use of PPE in health-care facilities caring for cases during the delivery of health care. 5. Intensive promotion of hand and cough hygiene. 6. Domestic

cleaning, using household cleaning products, to reduce transmission via fomites (infectious respiratory secretions on surfaces).

(WHO 2006a)

The exceptional measures, when the situation worsened, included quarantine:

> The SARS experience suggests that quarantine, applied on a voluntary basis only, is preferable to enforced quarantines and may be equally effective. . . . At the same time, however, national, sub-national, and local governments should be legally prepared to enforce individual and community-based containment measures if warranted.

The protocol also recommends methods of 'social distancing', which 'might increase the likelihood of successful containment'. Social distancing methods can include the closing of schools and workplaces, cancellation of mass gatherings and public transportation, community-based confinement within homes, and border controls. The term 'extraordinary public health action' is used by national and international public health authorities to refer to rapid containment procedures to stop the spread of a pandemic.

The WHO faces the challenge of deciding whether evidence suggests that a localized outbreak may have global effects and start a pandemic. The declaration of various states of emergency is tied to the legislations of multiple countries as triggers of national pandemic preparedness plans. The extraordinary measures fall in the hands of national and local authorities who are provided extensive international assistance with the expectation of efficient sharing of information and communication. Under such measures, people interaction is restricted in the containment zone: the current version of the WHO protocol

> takes a geographically based approach where the initial area of outbreak becomes the main target—the containment zone—in which actions are taken to stamp out the infection and prevent its spread. Within the containment zone and in an area around it called buffer zone, surveillance and community mobilization will check and maintain containment. In the buffer zone, any 'breakthrough' cases are quickly detected and isolated.

(Dutta 2008: 15–16)

Perimeter controls are enforced on the boundaries of the containment zone. Around the buffer zone, there are no perimeter control measures. The protocols are based on the assumption that the state first affected will be willing to accept the interventions, 'which will be intrusive and could be viewed as infringing on national sovereignty' (Eurosurveillance 2006). Although the WHO lacks reinforcement mechanisms to force affected states to participate in the containment strategy, it is clear that other countries would be willing to enforce such policies. For example, the US 2010 and 2015 National Security Strategies categorize pandemics with terrorism, natural disasters, and large-scale cyber-attacks. As evidenced by the 2014–15 US reaction to the Ebola outbreak in West Africa and the Obama administration's decision to send medically trained American troops to the outbreak area, pandemics can lead to US intervention 'as we do everything within our power to prevent these dangers' (NSS 2010). The US 2015 National Security Strategy puts the onus on 'shared spaces' defined as high seas, airspace, space, and cyber space. The US has a commanding position in these realms as well as ready access. This is related to the pandemic—air traffic nexus. It is therefore significant that the regulation concerning access to international air travel has been a policy much emphasized since 9/11. Access to the shared space of international air travel was filtered and restricted during the 2014 Ebola outbreak to stop its intercontinental spread. The Trump administration's 2017 National Security Strategy makes pandemic threats explicitly national security concerns—what is at stake is not only public health but US security as more traditionally understood:

> Naturally emerging outbreaks of viruses such as Ebola and SARS, as well as the deliberate 2001 anthrax attacks in the United States, demonstrated the impact of biological threats on national security by taking lives, generating economic losses, and contributing to a loss of confidence in government institutions.[5]

Although left unsaid by the WHO, it is clear that the military and the police are the only institutions in most states that are able to organize, implement, and maintain containment and buffer zones. National security becomes at least one key characteristic of the pandemic security scenario alongside the welfare and public health characteristics. The imageries of the worst-case scenarios do not offer much time for effective action, which has to be implemented in the absence of extensive knowledge of the fundamental nature of the (re)emerging pestilence. Because there is much uncertainty, the most probable reaction to a perceived pandemic outbreak is likely to be to mix the expert approach with national security safeguards and culturally important stereotypical reactions to violent epidemic diseases.

Before proceeding to a more detailed analysis of public health practices of containment, it is useful to touch upon the meaning of containment in the nexus between politics and plagues. The link between foreign policy containment and pandemic control has been noted in research literature (e.g. Annas 1999: 37). So it seems useful to review the practices of containment in the general international relations discourse, where containment is explicitly about sculpting the contours of power. I want to point out the parallelism between power-political containment and public health containment, instead of claiming that political containment is primary. On the contrary, there is much truth in Ellis' (2001: 106) point about the power of disease to 'order spatial information' and to distinguish between safe and unsafe areas. It is clear that the age-old general disease scenarios still heavily influence our perceptions of political enmities, as was pointed out in Chapter 1. The connection between diseases and enmities has a long cultural history. This history may be read to comprise a proto-theory of politics and plague, which still stimulates contemporary disease imageries. Moreover, the way in which this proto-theory dynamically embodies the object world of disease puts containment in the centre of the narrative. Generally speaking, the perceived effect of diseases on communities can be seen to be about imagined broken and transgressed boundaries, whereas the act of healing is often made to stand for the restoration of proper boundaries and for the virtuous nature of acts of such containment.

In order to further triangulate the political meaning of containment dramas, it is useful to see how they have been used in international relations thought. The strategy of containment is commonly linked with expansive strategies by some actors as in the case of the US containment of the Soviet Union after World War II.

In his Long Telegram of 22 February 1946, George Kennan famously spelt out the malignant dangers of Soviet expansionism, which worked by sowing internal cleavages within the West through networks of collaborators and fifth columnists: 'World communism is like [a] malignant parasite which feeds only on diseased tissue'. Contagious disease became the embodied scenario through which to understand a superpower clash (Aaltola 2020: 4). From a more theoretical standpoint, according to Hans Morgenthau (1955), the fundamental aim of expansive actions is to dispose of a prevailing status quo so as to advantage one's own power position and bring about a more favourable resolution. To establish this kind of an advantageous relationship, Morgenthau (1955: 54) maintains that states use three different types of techniques or methods: military, economic, and cultural imperialism. The practice of imperialistic policies on the part of some state(s) requires reciprocal actions on the part of other state(s) to resist (containment) or allow (appeasement) changes to the status quo.[6] In the traditional realist understanding of major power foreign policy, the policy of containment refers to restraining, restricting, and confining the expansion of other state(s) within certain limits that are spelt out in forceful and uncompromising terms. The various reciprocal actions to expansive moves include confinement of an instigator inside some economic, military, and cultural limits so as to make the attempts to change the status quo futile:

> The policy of containment erects a wall, either a real one, such as the Great Wall of China or the French Maginot Line, or an imaginary one, such as the line of demarcation drawn in 1945 between the Soviet orbit and the Western world.
>
> *(Morgenthau 1955: 59)*

The strategy of containment is often seen as the preferred option in world politics. It establishes firm limits to a particular world order and renders the actions of different actors legitimate by demarcating a common frame and grammar for interpretation. The language making containment a normatively sanctioned option in power-politics is deeply entrenched. Such thinking can become important in the nexus between politics and plagues because it reinforces containment-oriented cultural forms.

Examples of the influential overlap between medical and political views are many. Diseases interact with power in that they can be read as signs of illegitimating weakness or as demonstrations of unimaginable strength. The production of health has often been framed as a powerful demonstration of the legitimacy of political rule, and the absence of health suggests the existence of fundamental injustice and transgressions, not only at the physical level, but in the way political power is upheld. The corresponding mythologies of this link are rich. For instance, when Sophocles' Oedipus 'intellectually' kills the Sphinx which had plagued the city of Thebes by answering the riddle it poses to him correctly, he gets the crown and the power. The Sphinx, a hybrid creature, half-lion, half-human—in itself an embodiment of transgressed boundaries—poses a riddle for those trying to save the city: 'What has one voice and is four footed, two footed and three footed?' According to the story, anyone who could solve the riddle would save the city from a ravaging plague, but the ones that failed would be eaten by the Sphinx. Oedipus, who is later to kill his father, unwittingly marry his mother, and, as a result, tear his own eyes out of his head, answered: 'Man'. The Sphinx then annihilates herself by throwing herself off the cliff. The correct answer to the Sphinx's question restores health in the city of Thebes and brings it new legitimate rule. It is a very commonsensical answer, which lacks any of the pomp and splendour that might have been expected of something that would save a huge number of lives. It can be taken to symbolize the restoration of civic virtue and common sense within a now better bordered city, which, according to the story, was beset not only by plague but, more fundamentally, by the supposedly moral transgression of homosexuality. Oedipus' answer restored the 'commonsense' morality of the community, although it is not very self-reflective, which bears upon the later tragic consequences in the story. Oedipus himself, as his name, Oedipus the 'swollen-footed one', suggests, used a stick while walking as a youth. The answer he gives is the right answer from the general perspective, although the 'man' in the answer does not include Oedipus himself. By producing such a self-alienating answer, he manages to restore the city's health but, at the same time, breaks the sacred boundaries by committing incest and, as a result, excludes himself from that community and is banished from it. The mythologies of plague and immunity are full of warnings against hybridity, border-crossing, and transgressions. The proto-theory—an ancient synthesis of tacit and non-tacit interrelated characteristics—concerning plagues and politics is composed of these characteristics.

In order to gain better appreciation of disease mythology, it is useful to examine for a moment artistic dramatizations of disease containment dramas. I have already pointed out the plague depiction in the frontispiece of Thomas Hobbes' *Leviathan*. Next, I will turn to a few other pandemic emergency visualizations to illustrate still relevant proto-theoretical models of politosomatics. The famous painting, *St George and the Dragon*, by the great Renaissance painter and architect Raphael (1483–1520), painted between 1504 and 1506, offers a case in point. The scene of the painting is set on the outskirts of a community, the epicentre of which is depicted by the church tower in the horizon. There are three main figures in the dynamic movement of the painting: the dragon emerging from a cave, the armoured St George riding on a white house, and the praying maiden. The hybrid figure of a dragon is a largely unrecognizable creature to the contemporary imagination. The figure of the dragon was used until the early modern times as an allegory for pestilence, which was itself a symbol of sin and evil. In a more embodied everyday sense, the figure of the dragon referred to encounters with violent epidemic diseases (Horden 1992: 20; Chiu 2017: 143). The fiery and burning breath of the dragon referred to the equally blistering effect and 'burns' of plague on human bodies. This should be read against the miasmatic conceptualization of disease causation, which stated that the cause of diseases was the bad, polluted, and stale air that contaminated communities. Disease did not spread through contact but through bad air. In this way, the painful symptoms of the plague were caused by stagnant, and thereby polluted, air, which spread the disease like fire. The fieriness of the dragon was an expression of this conceptualization, which emphasized the 'mal', or bad, air in the atmosphere. Bad air took over the political community in a process emphasizing diseases as moral, religious, and political complexes.

The painting captures much of the proto-theory. For a modern viewer, it is a static image. However, when one understands it as a depiction of pandemic emergencies complete with drama and lessons learnt, it comes alive and the figures become more identifiable as signifiers of our own pandemic times. Plague was part of everyday life for Raphael and his contemporaries. Before his untimely death caused perhaps by plague or syphilis, Raphael painted another pandemic emergency scene, the *Plague in Crete* (1515–16) based on the story in Virgil's *Aeneid*. The relevant quote from Virgil conveys the sense of emergency: 'Men were losing the lives they loved or dragging around their sickly bodies'. Restoration of health meant finding the true telos of the community, restoring the common sense and civil religious virtues.

Raphael's iconic painting is about a community in a terrible crisis, the cause of which is embodied in the figure of the dragon. The epicentre of the scene— the confrontation with the dragon—is located at the margins of the community. The limit of its power—its *potential*—is a presumed circular perimeter emanating from the centre of the community. This power is being contested by the plaguing dragon, who is being fought by the patron saint of the community, whose relic is kept in the church. The object world of the painting comprises the dragon, the saint, the pious sacrificial maiden, and the community. The painting may be read to capture the dynamic containment-related narrative between these objects. The embodiment of the plague—the dragon—has emerged at the limits of the community. Its existence poses an imminent threat to the existence of the community. To discern the movement within the painting, one should remember the close connection between diseases and the religious conceptualization of morality. The moral content of the painting is signified by the patron saint of the community, which has been reanimated, and the praying figure in the right-hand corner. The praying figure represents the role of piety in protecting against dangerous hybridity, besides being a potential sacrifice or victim. The expression of piety by the members of the community enables the elimination and banishment of the source of contamination. The saintly figure symbolizes the civil religion, unity, and cohesion of the community in the spirit of St Augustine's conceptualizations. Only this embodiment has the power to confront and defeat the hybrid creature, whose confusing hybridity stands for broken, transgressed boundaries. The figure of the saint radiates a higher order over the physical place and the people living inside it. This characteristic quality of saints to radiate 'potentia' could exist only if the community maintained the rituals of remembrance enacting what the saint stood for. The 'proper' remembering and the civil religious rites associated with it represented the cohesion of the community and consolidated its members around a sense of the community standing for something higher (Brown 1980: 96).

Raphael's painting contains dynamic movement between its key objects. Many of the animating elements have been forgotten by contemporary audiences. The painting has become static for the contemporary viewer—there is no sense of immediacy or alarm. Discerning the movement in it would require memory concerning disease symbolism that many no longer possess. The painting can be seen as a restaging of a pandemic-related genre of politosomatic painting. It may be argued that this genre contains an influential proto-political theory concerning the nature of the political community. The key to this genre is to perceive it as expressions of alarm, worry, and anxiety over secure borders and common sense within the secure parameters.

Moving to more modern-day containment dramas, there are numerous other examples of this proto-theoretical genre of imagining. These re-enactments are meant to arouse general compassion and point to the dangers of uncontained civil irreligion. They also provide an expression of remedy; acts of containment restoring the communal external and internal boundaries can stop decline and the eventual fall. Arnold Böcklin's (1827–1901) painting, *Der Krieg* (1896), represents the same dynamics as Raphael's work. The walled community at the bottom of the painting is being ravaged by pestilences represented by the four horsemen of the apocalypse flying above the community: Death, War, Famine and Plague. The situation is even more serious than the scene in Raphael's painting. The image is focused on the four horsemen. The community below is burning. Its walls are collapsing, and the gates are wide open. It seems that the vortex of violent chaos has entered through the open gates and engulfed the community. The horsemen are hurrying away from the collapsed city to its neighbouring ones, symbolizing the spreading nature of violent political regressions. Böcklin's bleak painting lacks the triumphant revivalism of the curative action in Raphael's painting. The armies of violence are on the march. The grand movement is convulsing the civic nature of the *civitas terrana*. In Böcklin, this genre has acquired a deeply melancholic declinist form where plague-like regression can prevail over hope.

During the Middle Ages, the iconic plague figure turned from the classical hybrids into the Christian symbols of godly thunder, arrows, and equally fiery dragons, which exhaled poisonous vapours (Horden 1992: 47; Chiu 2017: 139–181). The dragon that lurked at the city gate ready to kill its inhabitants was a completely inhuman hybrid, an unreal blend of reptiles and birds. In the case of the Greek myths, the elimination of the problem required rhetorical healing words to restore common sense and political friendship, a task that was much more physical in the case of the disease-spreading dragons. However, the thematic emphasizing the healing power of common sense remained at the centre of containment dramas. In the language of plagues and people, the curing, containing action is often directed at the therapy of the political bodies. Entralgo (1970: 177), in his book concerning the classical notions about 'healing speech', compares the fundamental aim of political rhetoric to the mission of medicine in that

> the mission of rhetoric is . . . not to persuade but to discover the persuasive element that there may be in each case, just as the mission of medicine is not to cure . . . but to ascertain how and in what measure each patient is curable.

Every successful act of political rhetoric is based on there being a resonating board of shared ways of interpretation, which the speech act further reinforces and restages. The central insight is the equation of the establishment of the shared area of persuasion with the establishment of the general curability as a realm of deliberate politico-medical action. In Entralgo's nuanced study of classical thought, the realms of rhetoric and Hippocratic medicine were highly interchangeable in that the existence of a realm of persuasive and convincing political rhetoric created the conditions that were conducive for the successful therapy of the political body. The locus of 'health' becomes a reusable chalkboard for the articulation of various visions for creating and maintaining political communities. In this way, the tangible curing of somatic bodies creeps into politics, as the proto-theories of health also address how to form self-contained constitutive elements for different political communities. The embodiment of a legitimate political actor is conceived of in terms of its ability to exert a cure or containing influence on the community, whereby the community's persuasive element is given additional staying power.

The intertwined themes of breaking of boundaries and liminality are present in this genre of containment drama. The external boundary of the community is broken, or at least there is an acute danger that a source of contamination might be getting into the community. The affliction of the community is connected not just to external forces. Far more importantly, the source of the danger is inside the community, in the form of moral corruption, fifth columnists, plague spreaders, and other dangerous forms of disobedience. In the genre, diseases are 'reactive complexes' stemming from and further inducing broken multidimensional boundaries. Even today, many diseases are readily read as signs of the dubious moral nature of the disease carrier embodiments. For example, HIV and AIDS explicated for some a stereotypical image of 'wrong' sexual contact between members of the same sex, thereby signifying the breaking of old and strict boundaries. It is no wonder that the disease was distorted to mean the 'gay plague' when it first appeared in the US in the early 1980s (e.g. Dowsett 2003: 121). In a way, HIV and AIDS, as many other diseases with strong moral and political overtones, have been equated with crossed limits and are represented by supposed liminal or peripheral creatures—the African orphan who is wasting away, the Indian prostitute, or long-haul truck driver, the Western homosexual, or the injecting drug user. It seems that at the level of the collective memory, much is still remembered and re-enacted when it comes to the genre of containment drama.

The dramaturgy of the containment scenes visualized by Sophocles, Raphael, and Böcklin seems to highlight the link between bodily suffering and communal regression. The co-instantaneous nature of war and plague is made understandable by linking them both to an underlying regressive process or flow whereby community constitutive sacred boundaries have become loose and uncontained: 'As a disease besetting a whole town, province or area, [the plague] threatened the cohesion of the social bond and called for action and containment upon a mass scale, involving socio-medico-political, and therefore also ethical, decisions' (Cooke 2009: 2). What happens tangibly in the soma of a disease sufferer and what more metaphorically happens to a political community is interlinked in the embodiments of political maladies, which cause the decomposition of the perceived underlying essence of together-mindedness. The importance of the communal staying power is made visual and tangible in the bodily suffering caused by the hybrid monster of war and disease. And the field of expectations conditioned by this dramatic visual language and its narrative logic is saturated by the looming anxiety of more disease and war. Judged from this perspective, the double movements of compassion and containment start to overlap and become partially just one overall movement. The compassion is felt towards the communal ethos, and the curative practice is one of strict containment—of re-establishing, renewing, and putting together the boundaries of rule accordance in the community.

Thus, the aforementioned disease imageries are indicative of a powerful cultural construct. The suffering inflicted by both violence and diseases is seen as consequences of an overall communal regression. Construed in such a way, the object world contains a normative directionality. The compassionate curative action is one of restoration or reform of the presumably broken communal element. Furthermore, although the curative action deals with the somatic suffering, it is often seen as secondary and as a by-product of the curative action at the level of more encompassing and wider political bodies. These bodies have traditionally involved nested and layered embodiments ranging from the local and state-level communities to the hegemonic, imperial, and global communities. In this language, the compassionate containment has different implications, depending on how the primary object of the curative action is construed.

It can be suggested that the central legacy of the proto-politics of disease causation has been the sense of communal threat associated with the transgressions of a community's perceived sacred boundaries. The perceived transboundary intermixtures easily signify and start to embody diseasing political regressions. To address this dynamic, public rites are often directed against illegitimate trans-border contacts for they contain the constant possibility of contamination. Unsafe contacts, especially those taking place at a great distance, have often been viewed with suspicion.

Lee (1998) offers a fascinating example in her essay on English poet Samuel Taylor Coleridge's attitude towards the slave trade. During colonial times, yellow fever spread around the world. The common conception was that it did not affect 'black' people although it had very severe consequences for the 'whites'.[7] Because of this unequal effect of the fever, in many parts of the world, it was called 'strangers' fever'. Lee cites the literature of the time to point out that the wickedness associated with the slave trade was thought to spread through the social body like a disease. Some thought that the consumers who enjoyed the fruits of the slave trade shared this disease of guilt and were thus inviting the physical malady.[8] The nature of the dangerous transgression connected with yellow fever was twofold. First, the disease contained a sense of the inhuman treatment of the 'blacks'. On the other hand, the chain running from the 'blacks' to slave owners, to the producers, and finally to the consumers was in a sense a chain of contagion. The sharing of the guilt also contained the breakdown of the normal barriers between localities and, thereby, between people.

> [I]t was the geographical movement of this disease that determined its interpretive implications. Because these early medical studies nearly always referred to yellow fever as a Caribbean disease, and since the Caribbean was synonymous with the slave trade and colonial slavery, yellow fever itself became intimately tied to the physical and philosophical effects of slavery. Together, the medical study of yellow fever and the debate on the abolition of the slave trade and of slavery kindled a series of specific concerns . . . about what happened when 'foreign' matter, or 'foreigners', became part of the physical or political body.
>
> *(Lee 1998: 675)*

The debate concerning yellow fever illuminates the geopolitical imagery that epidemic diseases have inevitably had.

From a general perspective, an uneven distribution of the disease burden offered culturally accessible ways of embodying and explaining it. This fact alone instantiates politosomatic explanations: the disease often turns into a sign of 'unnatural' imperial long-distance contact. Second, a disease tends to become a signifier of an unnatural and perverse contact between a foreign, racially different community, which was brought into misery, and the European consumers. The uneven distribution of epidemic diseases turns into a sign of the corrupting effects of a contact between two far apart localities and into a symptom of imperial decline germinating from its peripheries.[9] The logic of an emerging medical topography during the early modern times contained a sense of geographical demarcation and difference. Besides highlighting the differences between faraway localities, racial distinctions were brought up to 'understand' the physical and moral aspects of diseases. The ability of the Western colonial powers to subdue most of the world directly or indirectly led to a pronounced sense of racial superiority. Whereas most of the associated distinctions conveyed a legitimizing sense of the white man's burden, the distinctions based on disease topographies showed the other side of the coin. Thus, the power to dominate brought along unimaginable vulnerability (Harrison 1996: 70).

Plagues and the Proto-Conceptualizations of International Politics

Plague imageries may have had important ramifications when it came to the understanding of states as contained, unitary, and bounded entities. However, the cultural history of plague also had a pronounced influence on the development of the imagined antithesis of the state. Plague gave substance to the discourse that later came to be framed as 'international anarchy'. The conceptualizations concerning the state of nature were made vivid and striking by memorable associations with plague. In the atmosphere of plague, statements such as Hobbes' definition of life in the absence of state as short, nasty, and brutish must have been more persuasive. As said, it is important to note that both the concept of state and the practices constituting the state system developed in a context permeated by large-scale plague epidemics in Europe. This connection between politics and plague can be dismissed as a mere historical coincidence, but there is some evidence to the contrary. I will next provide a general account of the commonalities between the discursive practices of plague and anarchy. My intent is to show that the inherent discursive connection can provide insights into shared discursive dynamics and into even present-day pandemic scenarios. Plagues have a place in the ways in which interstate power is said to have been traditionally imagined and embodied. This connection provides vital substance to the politosomatic phenomenon. I will argue that pandemic plagues have not been and are still not encountered in a historical vacuum. The response patterns are not only 'non-linear' and 'catalysing', but some of them are well trodden and clearly repetitive. It can be argued that the cultural history of the construction of modern-day pandemics draws from the powerful past associations between plague and political conceptualizations. It is possible to entertain the thought that the embodied plague scenario may have an often unrecognized place in the established imageries of international politics. This bridgehead influences the manner in which modern-day pandemics are constructed, and it provides a crucial frame for understanding the trajectories of the plagues of our times, such as COVID-19.

One way of approaching the common cultural history of plagues and politics is to consider for a moment the plague-ridden affective climate of the early modern mind. Even for the likes of Thomas Hobbes (1588–1679), keeping plague from affecting the more intellectual work would have required quite a strenuous effort. Yet Hobbes was a living and sensing person embedded in his temporal context where plague was a frequent visitor for his community and family. More than that, plague was not only part of his psycho-historical path; it was a key object of his conceptual thought that was made to do work in order to persuade his readers. This is clear already from the very first page of his work. Besides the imposing figure of the sovereign, the famous frontispiece of Hobbes' *Leviathan* (1651) contains an engraving of an orderly community beneath the king. The walled community has a few people in it, mainly soldiers and guards. However, there are also two figures inside the encircling city walls who are plague doctors with their characteristic beak masks (Falk 2011: 247). The Hobbesian state thus seems to be on guard for different types of storms, plague being one of them.

The plague certainly caused uncertainty and horror when it swept in one great wave after another over all of Europe. The disease, together with other epidemics such as cholera, syphilis, and yellow fever, filled the imagination of those living at the time, no matter how disembodied they were as thinkers. As stated, this same imagination was the birthplace of territorial states. In descriptions of the state of affairs outside of the state, plague and its horrible manifestations offered plenty of persuasive and understandable analogies. In several ways, the emergence of the territorial state can be thought of as a solution to emergencies caused by pestilences such as plague. This brings to mind Scarry's argument reviewed in Chapter 1 that political architectures are ultimately legitimized as pain relievers. The territorial state may be seen as both a response and a solution to the uncertainty created by an unknown killer. This is supported by the historical correlation. The emergence of a full-fledged state system also spelt the end of large-scale plague epidemics in Europe. If the state developed and 'ripened' in the disease-ridden context of uncertainty, the final triumph of the state was the prelude for the vanishing of the plague from Western Europe. This parallelism must have reinforced the acceptance and legitimacy of states as somehow natural—or even supernatural or divine—entities. A part of this legitimacy is straightforward yet often missed. States could be associated with the timely implementation of the increasingly effective quarantine regulations. The earlier mentioned parallelism between diseases and the state provides an example of how political borders and borders in politics have been present in the history of disease control. This interaction between borders and disease has had a profound, if little explored, role in the history of the respective interlinked worlds.

Besides these broad sketches of parallel histories, it is possible to delineate a more coherent intellectual link between plague and anarchy imageries. Modern notions of international anarchy may be contrasted with a fundamental notion of St Augustine's (354–430 CE) influential political thought. In his *Confessions* (7:10:16), in a dialogue with God, Augustine remarks: '*Et inueni longe me esse a te in regione dissimilitudinis, tamquam audirem uocem tuam de excelso* [I realized that I was away from you in the land of unlikeness]'. This *regione dissimilitudinis*, or land of unlikeness, refers to the basic separation between the City of God and the City of Man. The juxtaposition of the realm of heavenly order with the City of Man brought forth the realm of unlikeness as a separate realm. Inherent in the realm of unlikeness is a dystopian vision of a realm at a tangible distance from the privileged level of clarity. According to Augustine's authoritative view, the events in the region of unlikeness bear, at best, likeness to entities at the superior level of the City of God—this might have been the intended meaning of the frontispiece of Hobbes' *Leviathan*, a likeness to heavenly order. However, the element of likeness in the realm of earthly politics is deeply confused because of the presence of considerable dissimilitude. By themselves, events in the region of dissimilitude are fragmentary, without identity and, therefore, meaningless. They are inherently discontinuous and unlike in the absence of the firm reference points offered by the City of God, the realm of continuity, and likeness. This leads to a twofold distinction between the two realms: on the one hand, between the realm of perfect order and the realm of unlikeness, and, on the other hand, between that aspect of the realm of unlikeness that bears likeness to the heavenly order and that aspect that lacks identity, is fragmentary, and obscures the heavenly vision in earthly matters. For Augustine, the only way to alleviate that grave and melancholic condition, the manifestations of which included war, passion, plague, revolt, fear, violence, and indeterminateness, was through a direct connection with the realm of similitude: '*Non enim locorum interuallis sed similitudine acceditur ad deum* [Not through intervals in space, but through likeness]' (*De Trinitate* 7:6:12).[10] Judging from the relative positions of the two realms, it is not surprising that the production of similitude becomes a higher morally valued goal in many subsequent intellectual endeavours. The making of likeness and removing the conditions prevailing in the *regione dissimilitudinis* were acts of pulling together disparate and scattered elements. This could be considered as an almost divine mission for a person. For Augustine, the realm of similitude—the City of God—consists of sublime proportions and hierarchical order (*De Ordine*, ii. 8.25). It is held together by the unity of the *res*-principle, producing an intelligible purity that could be understood and consolidated through faith and reason. In Augustine, the *res* is produced through a contained whole coming into existence that was more than the sum of its parts. The *res* turns otherwise disparate entities into conditions of likeness, thereby identifying each with the other.[11] In Augustine's writings, and later in the writings of Thomas Aquinas, this quality becomes a valued presence in an otherwise indeterminate earthly existence.

Augustine can be seen as operating with pre-existing conceptual configurations in setting his influential distinctions and juxtapositions. Plato (*c.* 428–348 BCE), in his *Statesman* (*Politikos*), uses a concept related to Augustinian unlikeness in the form of the 'sea of diversity'.[12] This was a place of unlimited chaos, where the voice of reason—*logismo*—is very faint and difficult to discern. This Platonic notion can be seen as influencing Augustine's later conceptualization of the 'region of dissimilitude'. This effect may have worked through the direct weight that Plotinus (*c.*204–270 CE) had on Augustine's reading of Plato (Dahlberg 1988: 28). The importance of dissimilitude as an early template for the later idea of the 'state of nature', which was the template for 'international anarchy', becomes clearer when Augustine describes the region of dissimilitude as characterized by a lust for domination, erratic passion, profound discontinuity, indeterminateness, and haphazard communication (Brown 1965: 3). Augustine's idea seems to be that *res*—an orderly collection of things—should be brought about in any self-containing political community.[13] When a political community loses its order, or its *res publica*, its composite parts get scattered. The familiarity and alikeness slip away when remoteness, dissimilarity, and chaos in the form of violence and disease stream in to engulf what was once a polity.

This Augustinian imagery also seems to be present in Hobbes' work. Going deeper into the visuality of the underlying template, it is possible to see that beyond the walled city and its surrounding countryside is a sea from which a storm is threatening:

> The scene is bright and sunny—conditions on land are offset by the threatening storm clouds out to sea, beyond the state's territorial waters—and it is near the middle of the day, to judge by the shadows cast by the buildings and trees.
>
> *(Poole 2020)*

The approaching storm might be enemies or plague. The mythic sea imagery is important in this connection as the template for the coming into being of modern political thought's notion of anarchy. The sea of dissimilitude as an antithesis of a polis or polity can been seen widely present in the underpinnings of classical political thought. Two influential examples suffice for the purpose of illustration. First, in Plato's pedagogic myth concerning the submergence of Atlantis, an imperial community suddenly caught in a violent deluge, Plato's emphatic warning seems to be that common sense is easily submerged by expressions of the darker side of human nature, by belligerence and avarice. Second, the foundational myth of Athens links the polis to sea vortexes. The notion of a sea of diversity is seen as being present at the birth of Athena. As the Homeric hymns express it, Athena emerges from a sea that swirls in confusion. Thus, fluidity and flux and other Poseidonic qualities are abundant in Athenian iconography. Fittingly, the 'great movement'— the Peloponnesian War—unleashed by Pericles' Athens is interpreted figuratively by Thucydides as a 'chaos, terrible flux, a destructive kind of motion' (Monoson and Loriaux 1998: 291). In Chapter 3, I will discuss the importance of sea imageries for Thucydides, who was perhaps the most influential early proponent of the plagues and politics template, the foundational root of the present-day pandemic scenario.

Mythic ideas concerning the sea of diversity found their way to modern times mainly through Hobbes' sea, water, and vortex conceptualizations. The most influential of these was the state of nature. In his *Leviathan*, published in 1651, which was aptly named after a biblical sea monster, Hobbes remarks famously that the life of man in a state of nature is 'solitary, poor, nasty, brutish, and short'. This endlessly echoed phrase should be seen in its larger context in the text. Its immediate textual context details important aspects of Plato's and Augustine's ideas concerning the 'sea of diversity'. Confusion is pointed out by lack of navigation and other instruments of moving, measuring time, and mapping:

> There is no place for industry; because the fruit thereof is uncertain: and consequently no culture of the earth; no navigation, nor use of the commodities

that may be imported by sea; no commodious building; no instruments of moving, and removing, such things as require much force; no knowledge of the face of the earth; no account of time; no arts; no letters; no society; and which is worst of all, continual fear, and danger of violent death; and the life of man, solitary, poor, nasty, brutish, and short.

(Hobbes 1982: 3:11)

Furthermore, Hobbes' ideas on the state of nature as a state of confusion and violence are indebted to Thucydides' portrayal of stasis in Corcyra and the Plague of Athens (Manicas 1982: 676). For Hobbes, the idea was to provide persuasive political pedagogy to facilitate the creation of order from chaos. For Thucydides, the advice for future generations was on how to discern when the grand scale of things proceeded from order to chaos. It is not a coincidence that Hobbes felt heavily indebted to Thucydides' description of the regressive grand vortex.

In a way, Hobbes, who translated Thucydides' main work into English in 1629, passed the classical conceptual configurations concerning the bleak and brute state of nature into early modern times and beyond.[14] In this mission of rescuing Thucydides' achievement, the plague imagery and the narrative of the Plague of Athens played an influential role (Brown 1987: 33). The two most influential accounts by Thucydides on how societies can decompose and dissolve are the Stasis of Corcyra and the Plague of Athens.[15] The two sub-narratives of the overall vortex of the hegemonic struggle have influenced not only Hobbes, but also, via his translation, many of the modern-day realist thinkers worrying over threats from within and outside human communities (e.g. Monten 2006: 3). At least from this tradition, the lineage leading to the present-day image of 'international anarchy' is related to that which takes place inside a single political community under conditions of extreme random violence and epidemic contagions. It is clear that the themes of civil strife and pestilence found their parallels in the political imagery of Hobbes' contemporaries. It can be argued that these themes became integrated into the way people felt about life outside of the state. Life as nasty, brutish, and short could easily find its most concrete examples in the religious wars of the time and in its plague-ridden, collapsed communities.

The staying power of Hobbes' *Leviathan* message is indicative of its embodied quality. It can be suggested that its persuasiveness was not just due to its conceptual clarity; rather, it was supported by the larger mythology of political thought in the Barthesian sense, and because it was felt and sensed in the vivid, real-life human dramas of its day. Among the most tangible of such embodied elements were the rampant plague epidemics of the time. The state of nature became understandable and representable because it could be understood through the decomposing somatic effect of plague on the human body, life, and communality. The loss of judgement in both the sense of political authority and individual incontinence is the end result of the deadly epidemic and violence. Hobbes sought to highlight this in his progressive support for an orderly state. It is in this history of imageries concerning politics and anarchy that the politosomatic nexus between somatic and political bodies is anchored.

The region of similitude, as opposed to the dis-eased region of dissimilitude, is gradually given an increasingly earthly content through the concepts of city, empire, state, sovereignty, and even wider governance structures. The term 'state of nature' initially referred to a paradise-like and harmonious state of being, in that people were independent and free of domination, rather than wanderers living in destitution and uncertainty. However, it can be claimed that this belief became increasingly hard to defend in the face of plague and religious wars, with the result that the sombre Augustinian view of the nature of man as one of confusion and hardship was introduced. Consequently, the optimistic analysis of human rationality and morality was modified considerably (Skinner 1988). In this way, the notions of a political community and those of a state came to be contrasted with terms descriptive of confusion in a way that brought Thucydides' and Augustine's bleakness back into the foreground in the writings of Hobbes and his followers.

Moving on to the more modern-day concept of international anarchy, the inheritance of the state of nature and the persistence of Augustinian themes are easy to discern. For example, Caporaso's (1997: 564) views echo what can be called the modern version of Augustine's tale of two cities. He argues that it is common to think of the '[d]omestic society and the international system as demonstrably different'. Whereas the 'international system relies on self-help and power bargaining to resolve conflicts', the domestic 'society (not system) is, by contrast, rule-based'. Bartelson (1998: 295) notes this same tendency:

> [I]f the identity of the international domain has conventionally been defined in terms of its composite states, and the discipline of International Relations in terms of the relationship between these states, then questioning the identity of the state is tantamount to questioning the identity of the international domain itself as well as that of International Relations.

It is equally characteristic of the tradition that the way to deal with the distinction between the domestic and international—the two 'cities'—is to link them. Just like Augustine and most others, modern thinkers also often succumb to the attraction of drawing an analogy between the two realms. The happenings in the region of dissimilitude can at best resemble those of the 'intelligible' realm and thereby become understandable through this correspondence. Donelan (1978: 78–79) critically summarizes this ancient line of thought, which renders international relations 'a wasteland' of war and of 'disease, famine and beasts', in the following sentence: 'The separate states of the world are islands in a sea of evil'. Donelly reiterates (1986: 602) this phrase in the form of 'islands of order in the sea of anarchy' to refer to 'structured regularity' in international relations based on regimes. Deudney (2008: 245) echoes the often-used metaphoric expression in the form of a 'world order composed of islands of hierarchy in a sea of anarchy'. Statements like these become meaningful against the background of the earlier discussion. The mythology contained in it is identifiable in the long tradition of political thought. And the references of plague and other pestilences reinforce the sense that the conceptual frame of the state of nature and anarchy are embodied through human experiences with them. The abstract is turned into memorable by connecting it with bodily experiences of pain and suffering and the need to contain and ward off 'external' anarchies ranging from enemies to disease agents.

The Emergence of Pandemic Security

With the aforementioned scenario wherein plagues, bodies, and politics display overlapping characteristics, I will next turn to a short overview of the historical effort on the governance of international public health. I will review the main themes of this history from the perspective of the plague—politics nexus. The historical efforts to build an international regime of public health can be viewed in two ways. They are usually narrated as a progressive history detailing the milestones in the eradication of a disease and in the emergence of the public health perspective that replaced older, more political, conceptualizations. This narrative is one of success wherein the failures of today's pandemic containment are difficult to place. On the other hand, they are also seen as reflections of age-old imageries whereby various political authorities have tried to frame the world as a hierarchical locus of borders and contained political entities. This alternative history is based on the creation of international hierarchies and domains of power by influencing popular perceptions concerning the global patterns of disease spread, susceptibility, and communicability. This alternative history is one in which global order as a secure and resilient form of life tries to find its justification and legitimacy. In a way, the two histories—one of governance and the other of power—come together and also receive combined blows when global pandemic efforts fail.

The origins of international health cooperation are usually traced to the nineteenth-century International Sanitary Conferences, which, according to many modern commentators, 'represented the earliest examples of international health cooperation, culminating in the establishment of a permanent international health organisation' (Siddiqi 1995: 14). Having said that, it is important to note that there were formal coordination mechanisms that preceded the International Sanitary Conferences. It is possible to argue that the roots of international health cooperation are as old as, if not older than, the state system itself. For example, in September 1652, Genoa and Toscana reached an agreement to stop the spread of plague and to integrate their quarantine regulations. This agreement resolved a crisis, the antecedents of which had to do with the intense political and economic competition between the two city-states and which had escalated into a mutual imposition of quarantines that hindered trade. Although this convention is a telling sign of the tight and early connection between international relations and epidemics, it

> has passed totally unnoticed by both general historians and historians of medicine—and yet it represents a revolutionary and enlightened idea which,

in the interest of 'the common health', envisaged international control and the voluntary relinquishment of discretionary powers by fully sovereign states in the matter of public health.

(Cipolla 1981: 34)

Even before this agreement, which drew in other Italian city-states as well, there were active networks for information sharing between health officials and unofficial coordination of policies in order to smoothen the flow of commercial activities. Furthermore, the brief history of the agreement proved that it was possible to channel the actions of states away from unrestricted competition to cooperation in the best interests of all the parties involved. The diligent, persistent, and unfailing implementation of quarantine regulations in the name of common interest soon became an arena for competition between 'respectable' states, instead of giving priority to openly self-serving political and economic objectives, giving states a first taste of the societal side of international relations. Any failures in implementing the control measures against plague resulted easily in economically crippling countermeasures that could readily be used as an excuse for achieving self-serving objectives by neighbouring states.

What makes the ignorance of these early attempts deplorable is that it confuses the less significant need for chronological progress, culminating in the WHO of today, with the more significant breadth and depth of the interaction between states and epidemics that is not limited to international conferences and organizations but originates from the ways in which states engage in power-politics in the context of diseases. It could be argued that the most common and powerful influences that affected the origins of international society emerged out of the plague years. From this perspective, the power-political games within the European international society have much to do with the development of common means to control plague and coordinate policies against it. The core of international order has to do with overcoming the demoralizing, subdued and opportunistic resignation to anarchy and with learning to control the uncertain international environment in the same way as states learned to coordinate the measures against plague that were considered impossible and even sacrilegious initially. The fledgling international society contained prominently the idea of control, demonstrated particularly by its use of 'reason' and 'science' as signifiers to overcome prior conceptualizations which were characterized by unpredictable changes in fortunes and misfortunes in the context of unrestricted competition and the equally fortune-like recurrences of plague.

Thus, the beginnings of interstate coordination of health measures had already developed in the seventeenth century. There were several reasons for the internationalization of health, which stemmed from interest conflicts between states and their elite groups. For example, the interests of the rising merchant class were incompatible with the myriad quarantine regulations imposed on trade by the multiple authorities. In this extremely complex situation, it is difficult to imagine that even a maestro of statecraft could have served all the interests satisfactorily. The belief that the main objective of a government was not to arouse fear among its own population or to show weakness in the face of rival states motivated careful management of the knowledge of the existence of different epidemic diseases. Political intrigues highlighting the sinister motives and hostility of neighbouring states were often used in the face of quarantines and *cordons sanitaires* imposed by the neighbouring states. These measures often led to the cutting off of vital food supplies. In these conditions, any disease control measures imposed on the other states led easily to retaliatory measures that further escalated the situation. To complicate matters even further, the fear aroused by quarantines was often as great as the fear of plague itself. Attempts by officials of city-states to impose restrictions on movement often resulted in situations in which people in quarantine had to choose between harsh punishments for trying to escape or starving to death (Pullan 1992: 115). Therefore, the primary way in which the local communities and states responded to outbreaks of plague was to try and hide them. People who notified the health officials of a local outbreak were easily retaliated against. For example, Cipolla (1979: 13) says that during the plague epidemics that hit Northern Italy in 1630–31, 'the doctor in Busto Arsizio who was bold enough to report the presence of plague in his town in 1630 and by implication requested quarantine controls, brought arquebus fire on himself and lost his life'. This tendency to hide for the sake of self-interest and status is very much present even today, as evidenced by SARS and COVID-19.

Stemming from a very complex situation, the idea that controlling plague was in the common interest began to gradually gain ground. The development of a centralized authority and administration, first in city-states and later in states, opened up new avenues for controlling plague. The arrival of plague control at the inter-state level was made possible by new views according to which, rather than simply committing oneself to religious piety, more earthly measures could be initiated against plague. Although it was still generally agreed that plague was essentially divine punishment, the idea gained prominence that plague came about through natural channels and worked through physical causes. These new ideas provided administrators with the novel conceptual tools to at least attempt to control the physical side of the plague by implementing changes in its physical context. Moreover, as it became evident that the plague posed a common threat to all emerging states regardless of their moral status, there was growing acceptance of the idea that states should cooperate to control the effects of the disease, not only to individual health but to the economy as well. Because they strongly interfered with foreign trade, the varying quarantine regulations had become somewhat a burden for flourishing commerce with the result that the anti-contagionist arguments and disease downplayers soon found strong supporters among business and government communities. There existed no clear-cut scholarly proof that showed diseases such as yellow fever and cholera to be contagious. However, the main motive for government interest, especially of the big maritime powers, to argue for the eradication of quarantines was economic. The hegemonic needs of these great powers required coordination mechanisms. At the same time, those states that were located close to the main routes of transmission, Russia and the Eastern and Southern European countries, were generally supportive of the quarantine measures. Thus, there seems to have been very eclectic usage of medical views, depending on one's political and economic self-interest, from the very beginning of international health cooperation.

As contacts between European and non-European states increased during the eighteenth and nineteenth centuries, the protection of 'civilized' Europe from the more 'barbarous'—less hygienic—countries became a primary concern of international sanitary measures. This can also be formulated the other way around: the intimate contact across distances could be easily framed negatively in disease language due to the inherent sense of lowering boundaries and introducing foreign elements. In this way, the epidemic diseases of different eras have been used to 'border' the emerging geopolitical map: dangers were seen as stemming from the world outside of Europe, where the political systems had supposedly defeated pestilences.

From the European perspective, eastern countries such as Turkey, Egypt, and India were a cause of much worry (Zacher and Sutton 1996: 56). For instance, the cholera that swept Europe during the 1830s was generally thought to have originated in India and Turkey. Consequently, much of the attention of the first International Sanitary Conference in 1851 was focused on such issues as the Muslim pilgrimage to Mecca or to the sanitary problems in Egypt, not because the European countries were only worried about the well-being of the Muslim pilgrims but because, on the one hand, the perceived interests of European countries were at stake and, on the other hand, the detection of problems in faraway places allowed for states such as France and Britain to showcase their own sanitary skills and mastery that were thought to be signs of high status, civilization, and hegemonic privilege. Much of the writing at the time reflected the idea that the well-being and interests of the Western European countries required that they have the means to control and isolate 'barbarous' oriental countries that spread diseases (Delaporte 1986: 97). The Western powers, 'under the guise of international control, sought to lay their hands on the entire system of sanitary protection against the Ottoman Empire, which in turn was regarded by Turkey as violation of its national sovereignty' (Schepin and Yermakov 1991: 55). In this way, international health cooperation was plagued from the outset by political squabbling (Rao 1992; Schepin and Yermakov 1991; Siddiqi 1995). The emerging area of health expertise turned the epidemics into spectacles, into a contestation between the hegemonic Western health regime and the perceived premodern and misguided efforts by the non-Western states and communities. Power and status were revealed in one's ability to contain diseases at home but were also instrumental in extending 'legitimate' governance in foreign places.

The imaginary storyline that outlines the history of international health cooperation as progress from the disharmonious initial steps through multiple crises towards efficient organization can be seen as representing the desire to distil politics out of international health. The official WHO narratives detail in a progressive spirit the beginnings and expansion of international health cooperation:

> Largely provoked by the cholera pandemic of the time, threats of plague and the ineffectiveness of quarantine measures, many European leaders of the mid-19th century began to recognize that controlling the spread of infectious diseases from one nation to another required that they cooperated.
>
> *(WHO 2007a: 90)*

These conventional accounts, which highlight the role of the enlightened apolitical collective responsibility, not only are instructive about history per se but also reveal much about today's international health cooperation's inherent historical ontology and assumptions concerning the nature of politics. This progressive ideological premise is often made in the historical accounts of the international health regime. For example, Siddiqi's (1995: 15) otherwise very informative work on the history of international public health institutions makes the following point concerning the first International Sanitary Conference:

> At the first Conference, the interconnection between world health and world politics was self-evident: each state had sent one physician and one diplomat, each of whom had one vote in the proceedings. . . . All physicians were subsequently excluded from the second, third, fourth and fifth International Sanitary Conferences, at which only diplomats discussed disease and its consequences.
>
> *(Siddiqi 1995: 15)*

Against this background of what he considers to have been undue politicization, Siddiqi fails to appreciate the true extent of the power-political nature of diseases and their containment. The experts, as an epistemic community, were later left alone to deal with pandemic containment. However, at that point, the needs of the globalized system and its coordination were shared between the expert community and the hegemonic political paradigms. It is possible to claim that the situation was one of mutual co-option rather than rational and functional separation between politics and pandemic security.

Siddiqi points to the gradual rise to prominence of expert knowledge, especially under the institutional rubric of the WHO. He also makes clear how the medical expertise paradigm broadened to include other related realms of expertise: 'The inability of medical experts alone to eradicate malaria suggested a role for previously unwelcome non-medical experts, such as economists, sociologists, anthropologists and geographers' (Siddiqi 1995: 195). This progressive version of history amounts to perceiving an imagery 'emplotment', proceeding from a Machiavellian political power world towards increasingly technical and specialist regimes of functional cooperation that keep undue politicization in check. The inherent hope of this framing has been that the repeated positive experiences of cooperation in functional organizations would make possible a more 'constructive' international cooperation, not hindered by over-politicization. Furthermore, an important argument of this progressive or functional theorizing is the view that the breaking up of the globe into separate sovereign political entities is the main cause for difficulties and failures in maintaining peace and maximizing welfare.

Making a much longer history shorter, the next stage was the emergence of new diseases, most notably HIV and AIDS, in the 1980s, which challenged centuries of progress in eradicating and containing serious pandemic challenges. The setbacks continued in the 1990s as Ebola emerged and in 2003 when SARS threw up new variants of viruses that were hard to tackle as they used the global mobility system itself as their main vector. COVID-19 saw the failure of the surveillance and preparedness systems but also revealed that the underlying tendencies for secrecy and enmity were still present in the global health system, not much unlike how they were present in the first Sanitary Conferences.

Pandemic Security's Containment Dramas

As an ideological construct, public health can be said to share an element of compassion with humanitarian discourse and tradition. To a large extent, public health is compassionate participation in the perceived betterment of humanity where the object of compassion is globality and its dis-ease. However, it may be suggested that the emphasis placed on the sense of containment makes global public health practices a historically and ideologically distinct mixture of compassion and containment. Diseases have been and still are conceptually tightly interwoven with borders, bounded entities, contained wholes and clear hierarchies. Their outbreaks and immunity from them are seen as indicators of the health and legitimacy of the political system itself as well as its underlying civil region and civilization. To illustrate this, during the early 1830s, a sense of national self-confidence and belief in its high level of civilization was tangibly present in the attitudes of the French towards the advancing cholera epidemic. Apparently inspired by a sense of national or civilizational pride, one French citizen proclaimed that cholera could not conquer France because 'in no other country of (the) globe have civilization, industry, and commerce achieved a higher degree of perfection and in no country but England are the rules of hygiene more faithfully observed' (Larrey 1831: 28). In the end, the high degree of 'civilization' that the French and the English attributed to themselves did not spare them from the cholera epidemic, which reached London and Paris in 1832. However, it did, for a moment, allow the French to regard themselves as a first-class immune nation at least in comparison to such 'corrupted' and 'disorderly' countries as India and Turkey (Delaporte 1986: 16). The status of being disease-free and immune was attached to a high state of culture; however, the presence of disease was seen as a telltale sign of low status and a lack of healthy culture. In several important ways, the perceived patterns of the disease spread are translated into a supposed hierarchy of political order and to reflect one's higher location and status in the perceived hierarchy of nationhood and civilization. As the religious explanations of pestilence were gradually complemented and then supplemented by more secular beliefs and attitudes that had to do with administrative and scientific effectiveness, the underlying coupling between perceptions of decay and decline and outbreaks of epidemics remained in place. The legitimacy and viability of a state became dependent on its ability to avoid serious and widespread outbreaks with the result that the asymmetrical distribution of diseases—that is, the ability to keep in check a disease that was rampant elsewhere—was considered to be a powerful legitimating factor. In a sense, the uneven spread of an epidemic disease translated into what can be called 'containment dramas'. The dramatized disease maps representing levels of immunity and contagion seemed to reveal at a single glance something very powerful about the underlying politically pertinent 'truths' and the sustainability of the prevailing political order.

Political compassions entail closely interwoven practices and associated modalities, for example, in the form of humanitarian and human rights discourses. These can be seen as separate from power-politics. However, a historically aware overview of them is bound to conclude that the various phases of the humanitarian movement correlate with the periodization of world orders. It seems that compassionate practices and world order go hand in hand with the result that they can be seen as mutually expressive (Aaltola 2009: 1–10). There are many historical examples of the compassion—power nexus. For example, the so-called white man's burden got much of its substance from racial and evolutionary 'scientific' doctrines. This enabled the discourse during the colonial period that the West was not in Africa to conquer but to help (Brantlinger 1985: 167–8). Imperial power gained a compassionate modality. and the betterment of people's health in the colonies became a sign of legitimate imperialism: 'Ostensibly removed from the realm of land and politics, colonization viewed through the lens of salutary medical aid was made to seem essentially humanitarian' (Kelm 1998: 101). World order shapes what is regarded as legitimate forms of compassion, and the practices of compassion enable particular kinds of legitimate political hierarchies and hegemonies. This intimate relationship can also be formulated as follows: the generalized object of compassion may be regarded to be the world and its order. One can, for example, feel compassion towards the general state of the world.

However, the definitions of humanity vary and can be equated with a particular epoch's hegemonic hierarchy. This also defines whose suffering is seen as meaningful, as worthy of compassion. As COVID-19 hit China first, aid was sent in, but mostly the world watched how China coped with the disease, and it was anxious about the initial failures and secrecy. Unlike in the case of usual humanitarian crises, the next in line for the first wave of COVID-19 were developed countries in Europe and North America. Compassion was no longer outwardly directed but took a turn inwards. Compassion took on national characteristics, and attempts to deliver aid were seen through the lens of 'corona diplomacy'. Pandemic diseases can lead into worries and compassions for the world order that is seen as legitimate but under stress and pain. However, as COVID-19 demonstrated, compassion had relatively limited scope. If there was any wider compassion, it had a distinctive political characteristic. The pandemic worries ranged from worry about other alternative rising orders and competing hegemonies to concern over the sustainability of global life as a whole.

What constitutes a global mobilization of empathy? What are the various ingredients in its construction? It is evident that bursts of compassion, for example, in the form of humanitarianism, may have widespread consequences in world politics. Cases such as Bosnia, Somalia, Kosovo, Darfur, and Syria demonstrate that compassions can be used as bases for international interventionist actions that are framed as helping and pain-relieving. Besides being the grounds for state-level action, the politicization of visible mass suffering may lead to compassionate mobilization at the societal grass-roots level. In many cases, these mobilizations are routed through the transnational community, and their impetus may provide a strong sense of legitimacy to the various humanitarian non-governmental organizations (NGOs). Acts such as urgent appeals for donations, publishing of dramatic eyewitness accounts and views from the ground, and testimonies of inhumanity are constituent elements of such mobilizations of compassion. On the other hand, under certain conditions, these mobilizations may include a more or less prominent state or international aspect. Governments and their organs are propelled into action in international mobilizations of solidarity for people who are perceived to be suffering. In some cases, the solidarity is not limited to international emergency aid, coordination of donations, or intergovernmental meetings but proceeds along the path of humanitarian intervention and crisis management. Thus, the construction of humanitarian compassions involves factors that influence how human suffering becomes an issue in world politics and how the precise nature of the prevailing world order influences the form and directionality of compassionate activity.

Although political compassion often portrays itself as a genuine, instinctive, human emotion, the more culture-specific synthetic aspects of 'compassion at a distance' should not go unrecognized: political compassions are not general and equally directed. Rather, they are constituted by nuanced iconographies, sophisticated 'figuralities', and intricate patterns of who is in charge. Moreover, the resulting politically synthetized forms of political compassion tend to have a strong relationship with the different configurations of world order and with the epochal sentiments therein. As humanitarian actions often target those at the more peripheral and marginal positions, they also involve the reconstruction of geopolitical imageries, such as who is at what level and position in the prevailing hierarchy of order. These spatial and hierarchical imageries identify who is who and by what means the different levels of the power hierarchy legitimately interact, communicate, and alleviate suffering. From this perspective, the suffering bodies are also diverse, ranging from destitute and persecuted people and minorities to nations, ethnicities, and religions. The direction of compassion can be towards individual sufferers as supposedly ahistorical and apolitical entities. However, it is often the case that compassion is directed towards bodies that are deemed to be suffering because of their religious, ethnic, gendered, racial, and sexual markers that are recognized as injustice in accordance with the prevailing moral frameworks, which are themselves associated with power. The ways in which some pain and suffering are 'seen', 'acknowledged', and 'recognized' start to take on dimensions that implicate not just the basic humanness of the sufferers but also the more political modalities of the suffering. The suffering becomes recognizable through place- and time-specific political lenses. Moreover, the political dimensions of suffering may highlight the historically conditioned sensitivities of the 'caring spectator' and the spectators' identity and status expressions. These sensitivities and expressions, in turn, are often given shape by the national contexts of the spectators and their respective positions in the world-order hierarchies.

The way in which the sufferers of 'compassionable' and 'comprehensible' pain and fear are constructed at distant places is closely connected with the earlier mentioned political power sensitivities. The relative individualization of the sufferer in modern secular public health, humanitarian, and human rights discourses marks an important watershed in the history of the construction of the sufferer. The modern sufferer of compassionable pain is often framed as a relatively contextless apolitical figure, who exists in the heavily temporalized situation of an emergency. If they fit the markings of compassionable suffering, such figures are made to represent all of humanity. They are given identity by being humans at the mercy of prototypical inhumanity stemming from antagonistic rogues or from mutating agents of destruction. The spectating gaze 'zooms in' to the emergency zone and sees individuals who, at the same time, allow for the construction of the epicentre of suffering as a frame, where the voiceless sufferer communicates only through the externally visible language of human pain. The complexity—for example, the historicity of various groups of suffering people, their self-understanding, and their socially shared meanings placed on the collective suffering—recedes to the background, and the definition of the sufferer 'as a singular category of humanity within [the] international order of things' crops up (Malkki 1996: 379). The distant sufferer, with distinct and shared memories, beliefs, and myths about what has happened, why and for what end, and how to rectify the situation, is cleansed when the figure is refined into a Westernized form to which the spectators can relate (Malkki 1996: 380). It would appear that for a distant sufferer to become a member of the general human polity with specific characteristics, they have to show the markings of the right kind of suffering, the kind that is deemed worthy of assistance. Paradoxically, the sufferer is reconstructed as an apolitical and ahistorical figure in this zooming in, and they have to be denied membership of other narrower political communities with collective historical narratives concerning particular political ideologies, beliefs, injustices, and enmities. When they are thus apoliticized, they are simultaneously politicized as members of specifically understood humanity that has its roots in our contemporary sense of world order.

The 'zooming in' movement of the humanitarian compassions contrasts starkly with the tendency to 'zoom out' in the pandemic security tradition. Pandemic suffering is not humanized. Instead, it is seen as an omen of bad things coming closer and closer. The focus is not on individual sufferers' compassionable pain. The focus is on the macro level, on the containability of the contagion that the 'carrier' is manifesting. Pain is recognized, but it is acknowledged as something that must be contained and walled off. The outbreak zone does not lead to a rush to help but to a cordoning off. People escaping the zone or being allowed out are viewed with suspicion and treated with distancing. Compassion is shown towards those who are vigilant in containment efforts and effective in sealing off the danger. Instead of being framed as an apolitical and ahistorical sufferer, the figure of the disease carrier is politicized and historicized as members of a community of reckless spreaders and objects of fear known from past encounters with plagues. They easily come to embody all the things that led to the infection and are made to stand as a symbol of the misgovernance of their community, locality, or nation.

Besides being opposite, there are similarities between the containment of and compassion for the distant sufferer/carrier. The conditions inherent in both emergency imaginaries are comparable to those produced by the 'anti-politics machine' referred to by Ferguson (1990: 17). The term 'anti-politics machine' refers to the 'industries' that apply presumably 'technical solutions' to such political problems as conflict, poverty, suffering, and hunger (Ferguson 1990: 19; Ferguson and Lohmann 2016: 185). The machine—the interlocking repertoire of established 'solutions' and the infrastructures or networks of actors involved—renders politics whose subjects are further off into a series of rational or technical problem-solving exercises. Although this production of subjects is itself a political act, it is political in a specific sense of the word: it is politically privileged and shielded by its appearance of being apolitical. Further light can be shed on this mindset through Ronald Barthes' (1980: 45) concept of 'depoliticized speech'. The practice of depoliticized speech is based on rooting the political out of one's actions and turning them into something that is self-evident and natural. For example, in the rush of the vaccination campaign during the spring of 2021 against COVID-19 in the US and the EU, the acceptance, procedures, and vaccination order of people were set by expert authorities. However, it is clear that much politics was involved. There were discussions concerning European solidarity, vaccination nationalism, export bans, and other status- and power-related acrimonies. At the same time, the process was 'authorized' by apolitical expert bodies. The machinery was seemingly apolitical—also for good reasons—and speech about the issue was tight-lipped and depoliticized. The sufferer/carrier/vulnerable person was produced as a subject in the apolitical governance language of the national, regional, and global agencies administering them and the emergency situation.[16] However, such speech only hides the deep power-political significance of this way of constructing the bodies in pain.[17] The rendering of an emergency into a realm where perceived expertise and ethics, not politics, matter enables specific types of action and also their co-option by actors in whose interest it is to turn the situation into a relatively apolitical emergency and object of technical intervention.

Paralleling the construction of the sufferer or carrier, two other framings tend to take place. First, the staging of the emergency drama involves the building of two images—a self-image as the do-gooder and helper and an other-image as the 'spreader' or 'rogue'. These enmity constructions feed back to the understanding of the sufferer/carrier and to the workings of the anti-politics machine. The dis-embodied sufferer/carrier's existence is implicated in the 'high-expertise', 'high-vigilance', 'self-sacrificing', and 'good Samaritan' actions of the intervening or containing actor. The communal-level dynamics start to prevail over the sufferer/carrier's real characteristics so that their real dis-ease is of secondary importance to the communal stock narratives of status and of one's civilizing goodness. Those inflicted bodies that are related to the categories of 'spreader', 'super-spreader', and 'carrier who participated in [the] super-spreading event' are not empathized with; they are regarded in relatively uncompassionate terms that highlight the need to quarantine and to close them out. This process of uncompassionate othering is both global and domestic. Disease is seen as spreading from somewhere and by 'some' people. In the domestic context, it is associated with some groups and with their unhealthy habits.

Plagues have had a tendency to cause bursts of civil religious righteousness focusing on re-establishing supposedly broken borders. In pandemic emergencies, the focus is on the sufferer/carrier as a spreader. The infected or possibly infected individual is seen as being bounded by and as a part of a communal body. They become members of a sufferer community, or citizens of a polity of the infected, able to travel and spread the contagion. They are seen through the lens of a bounded in-group, a political body, that is imagined as healthy and immune if the other community could somehow be cordoned off and distanced. More often than not, this group of infected people is equated with national boundaries (Reicher *et al.* 2006). The persons infected in China during the first months of the COVID-19 pandemic were referred to as Chinese, and as the disease spread to Italy, the patients were termed 'Italians'. They represented infected people but also dis-ease and the failures of their respective national communities. The iconography of such individual and national bodies in pain has a long and rich history. Extending the pain to a political body provides an important embedding for a national type of suffering:

> Narratives of pain materialize an abstract entity like the nation-state to its citizenry, transforming it into a body that is symbolically connected to that of the individual . . . the frequency and intensity of the pain-filled language and the historical persistence of conflicts over sovereignty indicate that the wounds are spread throughout the body politic.
>
> *(Burns* et al. *1999: 122)*

In this culturally significant genre of political pain, the whole polity may be in pain and dis-ease. This suffering is a signifier of wider human suffering, and, as a result, it often takes precedence over the individual's body in pain, in which the pain language is turned into a symptom of something bigger and more meaningful taking place at the level of the more encompassing political body. Visuals of individual pain become contextualized in terms of the wider national group's pain and the danger emanating from it.

Let us consider for a moment how the contemporary imageries of an emergency provide a context for the construction of dis-eased political bodies. There are different types of emergencies: natural (hurricanes, earthquakes, tsunamis, and pandemics), technological (industrial accidents), and political (genocides, wars, and conflicts). However, the general format of the emergency drama is to an extent shared by them. Whereas in traditional international wars, crises, and conflicts, a spatial feature is essential, the contemporary emergency situations often involve a heightened sense of scarcity of time when the window for effective intervention seems to be closing. Thus, emergency situations are first and foremost temporal rather than spatial dramas. Pandemic scares provide good examples of such temporalization, when all attention becomes concentrated on one critical moment in time. Time becomes increasingly salient when the rush to find solutions—cures, vaccinations, or cordoning—is accompanied by an accelerated tempo of events. In its stereotypical ideal form, the emergency plotline suggests temporalized imageries of a sequence of events: the initial triggering event, intervening curing activity by the legitimate 'authorities', and eventual restoration of normalcy. That said, the sudden disappearance of the regularity inherent in emergencies has also a spatial dimension, which leads to a collapse of vastness and into a sudden and alarming combining of the 'here' and 'near' with the 'far'. Whereas spatial distance is a buffer from the effects of international crises, the distance related to emergency dramas turns into something to be crossed by outsiders rushing in to heal the situation while it is still containable in the emergency area, while also minimizing the contagion vectors to the outbreak zone. In this sense, the geography of the onset phase becomes concentrated in one tight epicentre or ground zero. The rushing in dynamics constructs a situational agency: those able to do so become important protagonist embodiments, while those hindering this activity get marked as antagonist elements.

Humanitarian emergencies, unlike pandemic emergencies, seem to compel involvement, breaking the usual 'nearest is dearest' boundaries and allowing emotional bonds at a distance. There has been a considerable amount of research on localism and the emotional dynamics of 'nearest is dearest' (Smith 1998; Bryant 2021). Compassion, identification, and a sense of attachment seem to be at best mid-range emotions. They are contained and conditioned by the familiar and the recognizable. Glover (2000: 28) points out the inherent contained nature of political sympathies: 'Claims to be treated with respect are often linked to standing within a group. The claim of an outsider may be minimal. Sympathy has similar limitations. The sympathies which really engage us are often stubbornly limited and local'. Similarly, Ginzburg (1990: 49) refers to a tradition of pity extending as far back as Aristotle, which equates geographical and cultural distance with strength of feeling. Ginsburg states that extreme distance in space or time leads to indifference. What is implied in this statement is a horizon, the end of identification at the intermediate spatial or temporal distance. Thus, there are two contradictory tendencies. The temporal closing of the window when something can be done clashes with lack of motivation to rush in to save the situation. For example, the US faced this dilemma when there was a significant Ebola outbreak in Western Africa in 2014. President Barack Obama was accused of not closing connections to the outbreak regions and putting US troops in danger by sending them there to provide security and to build field hospitals. Donald Trump, then a prospective presidential candidate, in particular was critical of the US response and demanded a more restricted approach.

However, a temporalized emergency can momentarily change the distance limitations of compassion. At the moment of an emergency, the 'we-communities' theorized by Richard Rorty (1989) may be able to extend their self-identity and political solidarities beyond their conventional national and cultural bounds. Even in cases of pandemic emergencies, compassion can extend to outside communities, as in the case of US agencies rushing in to stop the spread of the 2014 Ebola or 2003 SARS before it reached the US.[18] The global scene of emergencies often animates and empowers wider political embodiments, especially in we-communities that regard themselves as having a global role or being leading nations. As the emergency extends we-communal boundaries vis-à-vis distant sufferers/carriers, it also extends the we-communities into global embodiments. In this sense, the global can turn into the hegemonic or the Western as the agencies of Western governance are seen to be able to act and eliminate the danger. While the world zooms in to the epicentre of an emergency, it zooms out to embody itself in a highly power-political way. Examples of such dynamics are numerous in recent pandemic discourse:

> Once again, nature has presented us with a daunting challenge: the possibility of an influenza pandemic [avian flu]. . . . Together we will confront this emerging threat and together, as Americans, we will be prepared to protect our families, our communities, this great nation, and our world.
>
> *(Whitehouse 1 November 2005)*

President George W. Bush focused on the emergency caused by the avian flu scare by embodying it in an encompassing template of 'America's world'. A pandemic emergency can be said to contain both these movements as the rushing to zero in is accompanied by zooming out to imagine the encompassing political body implicated in an emergency. The emergency situations can also compel actions because they allow opportunities for demonstrating global status instead of being merely compassionate activity.

While keeping in mind the movements in and out that embody those involved, I will refocus on the nuanced theme of compassionate engagement. It may be argued that besides the political mobilizations for engagement, the politics of global indifference comprises a culturally established tradition. The compassion-eliciting 'images of the heart' are based on skilled mobilization of codes and signifiers that can be used to manage the different outcomes along the action–inaction continuum. When powerful sentiments manage to create alarm and an overarching sense that something must be done immediately, they do so because they are strongly reminiscent of the culturally shared gallery of images, signifiers, and sentiments associated with past emergencies. It is suggested that the practice of emergency engagement consists of combining the right past imagery with current images—for example, the famous image of starving Bosnian Muslim men behind barbed wire in 1992, which reminded people of the images of the Holocaust. The same discursive power is involved in the creation of sanitized or messily confused images of distant mass suffering that will not connect or combine with the older gallery of emergency imagery in ways that would mobilize people and resources for action. In the hybrid idea of 'humanitarian war', both these aspects of political skills come into play simultaneously.

The patterns of being indifferent also implicate a third option: the practice of containment, one of distancing, avoiding, and removing. This discursive dynamic manages, restrains, and keeps in check the patterns of engagement in ways that, in general, lead to distancing and to the erection of physical and/or imaginary boundaries that maintain and signify the distance. Although different from compassion and much more limited, containment can be seen as another form of engagement and involvement. The practices of containment involve highly controlled regulation of contact aimed to stop the communicability of a perceived dangerous element such as a pandemic disease out of the epicentre of an emergency. Or, if deemed uncontainable at the source, the containment barrier is created around the domestic community.

One way to approach the difference between movements of compassion and containment is to briefly consider the objects of worry and care in both. The history of political compassion poses an important question concerning the ultimate nature of compassion: is it altruistic behaviour or is it masked selfishness? The logic for compassionate actions might arise from one's own interest: 'What is happening to the other person might happen to me one day; therefore, I have to help'. This type of compassionate interventionism is based on recognition of mutual self-interest and a reciprocal type of solidarity (Slim 2001: 325). On the other hand, the imaginative act of placing oneself in the position of the sufferer may allow one to better appreciate the other person's suffering so that one gains better appreciation of the situation that requires helping action, irrespective of any selfish considerations. Thus, the basis of compassion may be the better understanding of the other's situation instead of 'what if this were to happen to me' type of thinking. The imaginative communicative channel that opens between the spectator and the sufferer has often been thought of in terms of the signs of suffering that allow for a strong sense of identification and blurring of the boundary between us and them. Compassion can be seen as an altruistic and natural moral reflex. This doctrine centres on the notion of compassion being an irresistible human attitude (Fiering 1976: 196). The doctrine of irresistible compassion has competed with more sceptical and cynical perspectives concerning the fundamental nature of compassion. These critical views have been wide-ranging. Some have pointed out the less than altruistic nature of basic instincts, while others have stressed the calculative human capacity to co-opt suffering. The scepticism is more pronounced in the cases of pandemic emergencies where the helping and assisting actions are easily seen as ways of preventing the contagion from spreading closer to home.

These two scenarios of compassion blend partially in a third important way of understanding compassionate engagement with sites of distant suffering. The tendency to equate compassion with a relatively naturally occurring emotion or with a selfishly motivated calculative sentiment contrasts with the view that compassion is a synthetic sentiment that is embedded as one modality in larger political scenarios with multiple overlapping characteristics. For example, acts of commiseration can be given communal status whereby they stand for a modern enlightened and sophisticated identity. Helping can also be a sign of the high status of a responsible actor. This compassionate identity is often an empowering embodiment in today's Western culture. Formulated in more normative terms, the more synthetic compassion may be viewed as an enlightened stage in human social evolution. These naturalistic and cultural modalities are part of the multidimensional and polysemous discourses of political compassion where containment also finds its place.

Containment as a form of controlled engagement is not that different from compassionate interventionism. Containment can also be formulated in terms of it being a selfish, self-regarding activity. For example, the severing of flight connections with Mexico during the spring of 2009 or with China in 2020 because of pandemics can be seen as motivated by the desire to stop the spread of disease from a particular country or place. On the other hand, it is possible to see a pandemic emergency as an instigator of compassion for the more encompassing political identities. I have already discussed the ways in which compassion is often directed primarily towards various types of in-groups or we-communities—ethnicities, nations, empires, civilizations, and hegemonies. It is important to see how a particular hegemonic world order can become an object of compassion. It is also clear that human polity or humanity may be regarded as an object of the containment type of worry and care. These wider, more encompassing political embodiments are the emergent properties of a pandemic emergency. The practices of compassionate containment can be seen as stemming from such compassion, instead of being only self-interested we-communal activity. However, one should note that the practices of containment also contain worries over narrower and more specific definitions of we-communities. It is often the case that the narrow and more encompassing sentiments are nested within each other as was indicated in the earlier mentioned remark by President Bush about avian flu: 'Together, as Americans, we will be prepared to protect our families, our communities, this great nation, and our world'. Such sentiments can form an interlocking concentric whole when hegemonic we-communities extend themselves into the wider definition—for example, the West can easily turn into a definition of humanity where the US has a special privileged role that requires leadership actions in the case of a major pandemic outbreak. However, in the case of COVID-19, the hegemonic competition between China and the US reframed the self-identity of both the US, which was largely missing in action, and China, which, instead of appearing to be a supporter of a harmonious world, found itself struggling in a controversial role and status.

To shed more light on pandemic-related compassion as a form of containment, it is important to further examine the general nuances of compassion. Donini (2010) refers to the three Cs of compassion: compassion as 'other'-regarding work, compassion as a movement for social reform, and compassion as a world order conserving and retaining activity. The third option may entail, for example, making sure that excesses of power are mitigated so that the world order does not spin dangerously out of control. A more conscious form of compassion as containment refers to 'the deliberate incorporation of humanitarian action in the world-ordering and security strategies of the north' (Donini 2010). The possibility of compassion fulfilling a containment function has been noted influentially by Duffield (1998: 156), who said that humanitarian action can become integrated into the world order 'to manage symptoms of global polarization and exclusion'. To reiterate, the containment tendency of compassionate action can surface in at least three interrelated ways: containment of the alarming trigger perceptions and imageries, mitigation of some of the most painful characteristics of a world order (such as the birth of the International Red Cross movement or the possible reform of the WHO after COVID-19), and the more ethical and high-minded strategies that give a good name to the underlying power-politics.

In international public health discourse, the importance of the move to contain is explicitly articulated. The containment tendency finds its expression in the various overlapping scenarios of 'containment zone', 'quarantine', 'outbreak zone', 'distancing', and '*cordon sanitaire*'. These practices can be seen as forms of compassionate, humanity-oriented containment. That said, one should not forget the element of indifference—the fact is that even though pandemic diseases are framed as emerging or re-emerging diseases, many of them have been continuously present in many areas of the world. They are easily seen as contained if they do not climb up the global hierarchy towards the key regions and their hubs as they did in the case of SARS and COVID-19. However, I will concentrate on the various momentary resolutions of the double moves to contain and to show compassion while also keeping in mind that pandemic emergency situations are highly differential and selective. The imageries of containment, compassion, and indifference provide tangible substance to the present-day world order, especially now when there are tensions and worries about the transformation and disruption of the present global order. The power-political territories of fear, anxiety, and worry animate and make tangible the politosomatic substance of international public health.

The Hegemonic Containment Dramas

The starting point is that containment experiences are vital for the embodied extension of political life: the socially shared and often personally lived containment experiences—for example, at international borders—greatly influence the way in which people understand their belonging and non-belonging to a global hierarchy and to diverse nested national, local, and global we-communities. Containment as lived life dramas contain an important political pedagogy based on selective processing and filtering. These dramas of selection that take place, for example, at airports or hospitals are not just physical. The main relevance of these dramas is not in that they may be of decisive importance to an individual. The individual dramas are part of a larger cultural schematic, the inherent logic of which is acknowledged in the way people leave it relatively unquestioned. The prioritization of vaccines to certain groups under a pandemic scare is not so much about the content of that particular drama; rather, the main element is the seldom questioned premise on which such containment, selection, and bordering are undertaken. Besides acknowledging the basic legitimacy of the schematic, people also implicitly acknowledge and recognize the authority of certain political bodies, which carry on with the containment as natural and necessary. When people were quarantined in their hotels during the 2003 SARS scare in Hong Kong or in the apartment complexes of Wuhan in January 2020, they knew and feared their possible fate. The worldwide audience which saw them surely felt some pity, but the act itself was mostly recognized and acknowledged as 'what naturally happens under pandemic situations'. Moreover, such a salient case of isolation could have also been conducive to a certain sense of security in that some authorities were seen as acting and doing what should be done in order to prevent the spread of the disease closer to the audience. The emergency drama sets the imaginary templates for acknowledging the logic and authority therein of separating people into various entities and of crafting hierarchies from them.

It can be argued that the state has always benefitted from the silent acknowledgements and recognition inherent in the dramaturgy of inclusion and exclusion. They have been at the heart of what state sovereignty means. Because a sovereign state's power can be said to be at its most definitive and explicit at the places and situations of containment or bordering, the recent change towards an increasingly well-structured, hierarchical, and globalized world order has had wide ramifications. The change in 'what is learnt from the containment dramas' is indicative of the deep qualitative transformation of the global system. The most distinct places for the containment used to be the political borders that separated states. In the global world, such borders have lost some of their importance. A seamless sky and free movement prevailed until the COVID-19 outbreak. However, the scope of containment dramas has expanded to cover new global issues such as pandemic diseases or climate change. These dramas of containment scares spell out who is who and at what level they stand in the global hierarchy of power. I will briefly examine the central stock figures and the underlying dramaturgy of the containment spectacles and trace the landscape of the contemporary world-order imagination where pandemic scares have found unique expression.

During the twentieth century, the spread of the universalistic ideal of citizenship partly replaced the older stock form of containment dramas, which were based on more particularistic and elitist notions. For example, international border practices started to be, at least nominally, based on a system of random checks, whereby most, if not all, people were inspected for travel documents and for security. Similarly, international health was, at its face value, based on universalistic humanistic ideals. In this spirit, various large disease eradication programmes were undertaken to defeat major pandemics in the developing world. But the fledgling international hierarchy after the bipolarity of the Cold War arguably brought about a marked change in this trend. Since the early 1990s, international containment has been defined by a perceived imperative to classify, differentiate, and separate the various flows of people. This takes place, for example, at international border-crossings, at hospitals, and in works of popular culture such as movies and books. Individuals are classified and profiled, their movements differentiated, and the flows of groups of people slowed down or stopped. They are categorized in particular types and classes according to the risks that they pose. The risk groups are in a realm of governance wherein the central rights associated with being a human and citizen can be considerably restricted.

Pronounced and consequential spirals of suspicion and distrust saturate this atmosphere. This personally experienced vortex of danger, fear, anxiety, disease, and anger provides an effective setting for politically relevant conditioning and for the contemporary spectacles of power. The border imagery has spread from that of territorial political borders to other realms of bordering between the various levels of the global hierarchy. However, much of the discursive dynamics can be interpreted to have remained the same. The fact that most people have personally experienced the crossing of borders gives containment-related memory images and stories a high degree of relevance. This heightened importance makes it understandable that the prevailing hierarchical world order is saturated by the 'semiosphere' of the multidimensional physical as well as imaginary border-crossings.

At these places of bordering and border-crossings, people experience, learn, and memorize the effectiveness and status of the order. Are the borders 'leaking'? Are they secured? Who are the suspicious and risky types? Who is authorized to move smoothly across borders and by whom? Who are the figures whose life is made difficult by the containment? Who are the privileged and preferred ones? How thoroughly are people being checked at the security checks? Are pandemic security concerns being addressed by the border officials? Who were checked more closely than the others? How was I treated? Who looked like illegal immigrants, illegals, drug smugglers, traffickers, or terrorists? Did anyone sneeze on the plane? Who can fly, and who has to swim, run, or dig? Who has to hide and conceal their identity? These questions and doubts are reinforced by popular culture— for example, movies and news—which provides the visual rhetoric needed for memory and storytelling. Profiling defines a practice whereby people are reduced to figures in a hierarchy of types based, for example, on their skin colour, clothing, background, religion, ethnicity, region and state of origin, socio-economic status, and spending habits. My argument is that the micro-level containment sentiments are inherently linked to the macro-level world order and security-related demands. An individual at the multilevel border-crossing becomes a personified abstraction, which derives its meaning partly from the security concerns of the hegemonic world order and partly from the specificities of the more regional and individual dynamics.

The contemporary political environment in which people's reduction to types intertwines with the worldwide production of security is often anxious, tense, charged, and dramatic. At their most dramatic, the occasions of containment are highly publicized spectacles. The terror-related frames containing no-fly lists, red flags, diverted or stopped flights, and intercepting fighter planes accentuate these captivating stories. CNN carried the following news on 12 May 2005:

> US authorities have released a passenger and his family detained after their transatlantic Air France flight was diverted to Maine Thursday afternoon when the man's name matched one on the US 'no-fly' list, federal officials said. . . . A federal official told CNN that the man's date of birth matched that of a person on the watch list, and the names were a 'nearly exact match'. But he was allowed to continue on his way Thursday evening after being questioned, a US Customs and Border Protection official told CNN.

Pandemic scare imagery can become very much like the terror-filled drama of May 2007, when the world followed the tale of a tuberculosis-infected man who took multiple flights despite having been ordered not to do so:

> Federal health authorities said Tuesday that they are looking for people who may have been exposed to a rare and potentially fatal form of tuberculosis from an infected passenger during two trans-Atlantic flights this month. The man, infected with the extensively drug-resistant form of TB known as XDR TB, departed Atlanta, Georgia, on May 12 aboard Air France Flight 385 and arrived in Paris, France, the next day, said Dr Julie Gerberding, director of the Centers for Disease Control and Prevention. The man, who has not been identified publicly, returned last Thursday to North America aboard Czech Air Flight 0104 from Prague, Czech Republic, to Montreal, Canada, then drove into the United States. 'During these two long flights, the patient may have been a source of infection to the passengers,' Gerberding told reporters.
>
> *(CNN, 29 May 2007)*

During the early days of the COVID-19 outbreak, there were stories of infected people travelling from Wuhan. There was a heightened need to identify those spreading the pandemic. Such presumed 'close encounters' or 'super-spreaders' stimulate and excite the security sensitive imagination. Such dramatic situations are easily turned into morality plays: containment dramas as morality plays involve fights by the protagonist—often presuming the guise of all humanity—against the bad minority of rogues and socially 'unintegrable' people such as terrorists or disease carriers.

The figure of the 'rogue' is one of the foremost descriptors of the sources of worry in the contemporary world order. In the 1990s, the term 'rogue state' came to signify illegitimate existence outside the international community and its accepted behavioural norms. Interlinked with the idea of the roguishness of a state are the terms, 'failed' or 'failing states'. Whereas rogue state carries the charge of intentional evil, failed or failing states have a more passive connotation, yet one that highlights similar dangers. The US National Security Strategy, for example, poses that outlier—'rogue'—states such as Iran or North Korea can unleash unconventional attacks in the form of bioterror. Failing or failed states or regions may pose a more passive threat by creating situations conducive to an outbreak of pandemic diseases.

Etymologically, the term 'rogue' derives from various sources; however, it can be partly traced back to the medieval term 'ragamuffin', which refers to a demon or devil and later to a ragged and disreputable person. In the same spirit, Darwin (1859: 32) used the term 'rogue' in reference to a plant that deviates from the 'proper standards' in horticulture. The important role played by the rogue figure in the cultural imagination was noted by Jung (1973: 10), who generalized that a rogue in the figure of a trickster 'haunts the mythology of all ages'. In this light, present-day rogues may be detected in the world political discourse as 'evildoers', 'enemies of freedom', and 'agents of terror'. Moreover, the root of the term highlights both 'devilishness' and 'ruthlessness' (Spitzer 1947: 90). The trickster imagery allows for the embodiment of pandemic diseases as well. During the plague years, the attention was on witches, well poisoners, and various other forms of evil disease carriers. The advent of modern medicine placed disease carriers inside human bodies. Various microbes were considered to be invisible enemies trying to defeat the body's defences and modern medicine by mutating. Such shape-shifting disease agents are also present in the contemporary imaginaries of (re)emerging disease and mutating new variants, which can penetrate boundaries of immunity. These connotations of the term evoke the figures of an 'infidel' and a 'heathen'. These meanings capture well the contemporary politico-religious definition of illegitimacy in international relations. Whether in the form of a state, terrorist organization, or mutating disease, the rogue figure seems to share some common features.

Thus, the rogue element is not static. 'Monstrous', uncontained rogues are seen to be able to change their shape. This 'mutability' was also one of the most important ingredients of the Western enemy images during the Middle Ages (Harle 2000: 55). In keeping with this imaginary, both the conceptual and temporal characteristics of hybridity have also been present in the figure of a 'foreigner': the foreigner is a figure that is partly recognizable but natively always a stranger, an unrooted figure that has shifted its identity and can continue to do so. It is telling that foreign minorities were often accused of spreading diseases. Minorities, as the cases of Jews, Muslims, and, later, gypsies indicate, were repeatedly massacred in public rites of pestilence 'control' during the European plague years (*c.* 1346–1721). Closer to our times, states and communities do not like to announce their epidemic diseases for fear of commercial impact and loss of prestige and image. If a disease crosses into wider publicity, the most common reaction is a pattern of blame avoidance and blaming others (Farmer 2006). Ultimately, violent epidemics are foreigners' diseases. They embody 'we' versus 'others' distinctions in making sense of what has happened. The knowledge inherent in them opens up in the imagined geographies of suffering. The hybrid and mutable figures find their associative connections in the supposedly contaminating and polluting groups of people who are easily connected with poisonous, thick, and cloudy air. Miasma, or 'mal' air, was thought to form in places where the air did not circulate or where no sunlight penetrated. The qualities of a plague 'atmosphere' were ripe with associative connections to poisoned political and religious power relations. Patterns of blame were predictable only to a degree. Much was left to combinatorial plays of the popular imagination, which innovated with contemporaneous issues to form an embodiment of a disease. However, pre-existing patterns of animosity and hostility provided the main fuel for this creative blame game.

In modern popular culture, rogue defines a continuum along which there exists a whole variety of types—for example, disease carriers, risk-taking travellers, conspiracy theorists, and anti-vaccine groups. The protagonists of these dramas include such stock figures as watchful authorities, alert border guards, efficient surveillance or security agencies, and politicians 'who did their job'. Rogues stand in opposition to these protagonist figures. From a general perspective, morality plays involve a communal verdict, a passing of a judgement about the moral status of the participants. Morality plays can be said to put the limelight on the actors' moral characteristics and their ability to make the right choices. In many ways, morality plays stage events in a manner that highlights the sense of being at a crossroads. The main question becomes how well the actors choose: Do their choices reflect progressive or regressive moral characteristics?

Questions of this type are answered at tense, critical moments. From that moment onwards, there is a strong sense that events can continue either negatively or positively. Another way of looking at morality plays derives from the iconic Western notion of the Protestant ethic. It can be argued that one major way of doing morally virtuous labour in contemporary times is by sweating over security concerns. The perspiration connected with the feverish agitations of the globalizing world provides the setting for the staging of containment-related morality plays. These morality plays contain a stern moral lesson about the disastrous consequences of laxness and lack of vigilance. In this respect, morality plays are not so much focused on punishing the wrongdoers as on teaching correct behaviour and the virtues and values of 'proper' figures.

Although good and evil are each illustrated by different and distinct figures, there exists a tense atmosphere of surprise. This is particularly true of the pandemic dramas that seem to demand constant vigilance against the unknown. The drama turns into a telling gauge of polity's underlying conditions, which is read through a mythic lens. The tension puts the emphasis on the moral worth and judgement of the respective actors. The set of figures becomes Manichean: those trying to do their utmost to stop the looming doom and those who contribute to the decay of the world community's moral character. In an important way, the unforgettable dramaturgy and visual rhetoric of 9/11 has set the stock plot for subsequent plays, especially in the US. Although striking, the elements of this drama are as familiar as they are ancient. Deviant figures managed to hijack and pervert the sacred icons of modernity—airplanes and skyscrapers. The visual rhetoric of the images was one of distortion and collapse. The inversion of icons portrayed the image of a disintegrating world. The theme of sacred symbols turning into their opposites is an old practice in morality plays—for example, sheep and wolves—which points to the disintegration of reality. The anxiety deriving from transgressed and violated boundaries provides another related ingredient for the plays. They become the setting for attempts to maintain and restore wholeness. At the level of the polity, the dramatic tension is one of a fight against the decline and collapse of the presumed sacred essence of the community.

As a theatre of proof, a pandemic offers in essence a revelatory way of demonstrating the existence of unquestionable power, which can conquer the hostile, rogue element of a pandemic. The bystanders gain confidence that there is a particular method inherent in global governance which can secure them. One should note that the suspense built into the original theatre of proof was largely artificial. Its conductors knew beforehand what was going to happen. Drawing from this intentional building of drama, one could say it comprises the fourth element of the pandemic theatre of proof. The setting is such that the outcome is known beforehand. It might be because of this that it is not surprising that pandemic scares have thus far turned out to be just scares. I am not trying to imply that there is a conspiratorial tendency inherent in the machinery of global health. Rather, the staging of the field drama is construed in a way that naturally flows from the cultural premises of plague and people. The reason why, for example, the spread of HIV and AIDS is not framed as a hyperbolic drama similar to that for SARS or COVID-19 might have to do with the instinctive desire to produce theatres of proof that demonstrate legitimate authority.

Pandemic emergencies, as containment spectacles and theatres of underlying global 'proofs', are intense and engrossing events in which the power of modern states and their international health regimes are being tested and are supposed to be managed by diligent—highly visible and dramatic—applications of modern health expertise. When the management is effective, as in the case of SARS in 2003, power is being revealed and felt at a personal level. When failure becomes apparent, as in the case of COVID-19 escaping containment, worries, fears, and bitterness ensue and feed a sense of a world in dis-ease. Moreover, the performer of 'health' is a figure, an embodiment, who is supposed to objectively and securely meet the external hostile reality. By proxy, the effectiveness of this performance reveals the 'true' and 'authentic' foundation of the Western political bodies. In this historically well-rehearsed way, any successful act of the health theatre turns into an empowering foundation for the Western political power and its global extension. It is the high political stakes involved that give the pandemic emergencies their central feature. From this perspective, the staging of the theatre of proof is meant to produce an acknowledgement that there is a technology of life which has a precise nature, definitions, and protocols and is embodied by states or by the hegemonic order of the global polity. The field of a pandemic contains the highly culturally salient and visible signs of this life-sustaining technology: medical personnel in white protective suits, masked doctors and concerned citizens, hovering helicopters, field hospitals, and military presence have been constant features of post–Cold War epidemic imageries and their more fictitious portrayals in popular culture. Another fairly constant feature of the pandemic spectacles has been the culling and burning of animal carcasses—for example, cows (BSE) and birds (avian flu). From the perspective entertained here, these visible demonstrations are needed because the pandemic scare is turned into a moment that challenges the underlying truths concerning who possesses life-sustaining technologies. For example, the images of SARS in 2003 provided a drama that demonstrated the goodness of organizations such as WHO, while China was held suspect when it came to its trustworthiness in an increasingly interconnected world. COVID-19 revealed WHO as an under-resourced and ineffective agency and China, again, as a dangerously secretive nation. The demonstrative pattern revealed at a single glance to the average Western spectator the presence of the threat and what was being done about it. The frame of the pandemic theatre of proof conveys power and ideology in these seemingly non-political acknowledgements of who is who on a particular type of disease map. This pedagogic aspect makes it evident that what is done in the name of disease control and eradication is inherently beyond doubt. It recreates a particular way of defining humanity in terms of an inherent power hierarchy. Pandemics are refined into governance exercises that are thought to be beyond politics (Siddiqi 1995: 196; Symonds and Carder 1973: 157). However, a closer examination reveals the close co-optive relationship between the demonstrations of health technologies and hegemonic political powers.

Notes

1 Compassion may be viewed as the general sentiment motivating actions at a distance and across global space—of effectively influencing far-off events without being in close contact. These practices have gained influence as legitimate practices in the global context, where political borders have lost their place in the foremost practices of containment.
2 The epidemic is named after Emperor Justinia I who was infected by the disease but survived.
3 For a more detailed debate on why plague disappeared, see Cliff et al. (2009).
4 WHO Interim Protocol (2007b).
5 NSS 2015.
6 NSS 2017.
7 Appeasement, as a reciprocal gesture, aims at bringing about valued and advantageous tranquillity and calm, which guarantees the overall status quo, albeit at the expense of some other principles, goals, values, or needs. Soothing or pacifying an imperialistic state entails conciliatory efforts and gestures to overcome hostility and the need to change the status quo. These conciliatory gestures are considered minor compared to the probable disadvantage caused by major changes in the prevailing order. The main risk of appeasement is that it reciprocates demands for changing a status quo with actions more

befitting to demands for minor adjustment within prevailing power relations (Morgenthau 1955: 60).

8 K. Kiple (2001) examines the issue of unequal distribution. Immunity against yellow fever is acquired. So, if you have the disease once, you will develop immunity. However, the 'black' population seemed to have an extra immunity, which Kiple calls 'special'. S. Watts (2001) attacks this view of inherited immunity, calling it racist, because Kiple's view suggests that yellow fever originated in Africa and that 'blacks' are natural workers, better able to adapt to harsher conditions than 'whites'.

9 The association between yellow fever and the slave trade was strengthened by the fact that the final horrible stages of the disease brought along vomiting of a strange blackness, which was believed to be a clear sign of guilt.

10 The dangerous, difficult, and antagonistic nature of travel along the main commercial sea routes further reinforced the sense of unnatural connection (Curtin 1964).

11 See Dahlberg (1988) and Barr (1962).

12 In Augustine's work, the lack of res at the spiritual level refers to the existence of demonic forces. The earthly counterparts of the demons are, for example, law breakers and criminals or people who break the earthly order.

13 Benjamin Jowett translates this term as 'infinite chaos'. However, Harold N. Fowler uses 'boundless sea of diversity' in the Harvard edition. See also Dahlberg (1988: 27–8).

14 For example, Book x of Confessions.

15 See, for example, Sowerby (1998) and Slomp (1990).

16 See, for example, Brown (1987).

17 See Malkki (1996: 378).

18 For example, in a magazine interview, Clarence Peters, the head of the Special Pathogens Branch of the Centers for Disease Control and Prevention, made the following statement: 'When [Mr. Peters] learns of an outbreak, he asks a series of questions: Is the problem here [in the United States]? How easily can it get here? If it gets here, how easily can it spread?' (*Business Week*, 21 August 1995: 72–3).

3

UNDERSTANDING GRAND VORTEXES

The Classical Model for Politics and Plagues

In the search for an encompassing politosomatic schema, I will turn to Thucydides because he presents a classical account of large-scale hegemonic enmity, which emphasizes its all-encompassing nature extending from collapsing communities and plagues to grand convulsions at the level of hegemonic competition. Thucydides regarded large-scale enmity as a great motion in human history. He describes, with deep worry and compassion, how the vortex of war engulfed all of Greece, causing strong convulsions in both big and small poleis. The intensifying, regressive flow led to strong passions, which, in turn, helped to intensify the flow. Sudden emergencies such as the Stasis of Corcyra and the Plague of Athens, Thucydides claims, were emotion-laden sub-motions of the overall regression. In a neoclassical reading of this model, I intend to build a comprehensive model based on the idea that political enmities provide the foremost vector for intensification of the motion that holds different political bodies in the thrall of unstable power-political flows. Caught in the pains of the global structures, people sense their anxieties and project them onto various pandemic scares. The scares fit their global contexts and eras tightly and should not be understood only from an epidemiological perspective but as politosomatic processes as well.

William McNeill's (1976) seminal work, *Plagues and Peoples*, rediscovered vital insights concerning the nexus between diseases and politics. These re-emerging neoclassical conceptualizations have been largely overshadowed by McNeill's masterful account of how diseases enabled the Spanish conquest of the Americas by devastating the native populations faster by spreading diseases among them than the Conquistadors' firepower.[1] Contagion was rushing ahead of the invaders' horses, spreading like wildfire from city to city, village to village. Yet McNeill's main contribution is his skilful combined narrative, which pulls together seemingly incompatible sub-histories of conquest and disease into one grand narrative of moving contagion, germs, horses, soldiers, and horses. Standing on the shoulders of great

DOI: 10.4324/9781003169147-3

historians such as Thucydides and Herodotus, who were the subject of McNeill's doctoral thesis at the University of Chicago, he turns the language of politics into epidemiology and the language of contagion into a description of colonial relationships. Through this combinatorial analysis, contagious diseases acquire another layer of significance, that of power, politics, and conquest, which feeds back and recontextualizes the biological causative mechanisms and disease vectors. It seems that the biological nature of disease and the dynamics of contagion and infection appear only rarely in a political and societal vacuum. McNeill's argument goes even further: there are no single self-contained histories, all strands of history intertwine and entangle with outside factors such as 'plagues'. The opposite is equally likely too: lethal epidemic diseases do not appear in a vacuum, insulated from the layer of politics. 'Plagues' reflect the power-political patterns of hierarchy present in the global realm. The pattern of disease spread abides by specific global power contours. Diseases turn into registers, or characteristics, of an intricate fabric of power, which also enables conquest.

In the neoclassical strand running from Thucydides to McNeill and beyond, disease agents are given a role in the human drama:

> In any effort to understand what lies ahead, as much as what lies behind, the role of infectious disease cannot properly be left out of consideration. Ingenuity, knowledge, and organization alter but cannot cancel humanity's vulnerability to invasion by parasitic forms of life. Infectious disease which antedated the emergence of humankind will last as long as humanity itself, and will surely remain, as it has been hitherto, one of the fundamental parameters and determinants of human history.
>
> *(McNeill 1976: 296)*

Encounters with 'plagues' should not be isolated into exceptional episodes and demarcated into analytically precise categories within different fields of study. They should be seen as parts of world history and international politics. The very essence of a 'germ' is to combine, spread, and mutate—as a disease agent, its main aim is to just survive. It germinates, comes into existence, spreads, and develops. It readily combines with the valences—openings allowing for combinations—inherent in co-occurring political processes. In a non-linear way resistant to analytical reduction, different types of plagues combine with varying political processes and feed, in some cases, a vortex-like emergency scenario, which contains even more valence. On the one hand, plague has a combining power with politics, as seen repeatedly in world history. On the other hand, there is a logic to it, a combinatorics, provided by the sedimented histories of plague and people. One such combinatorial logic is that plague catalyses existing patterns of political enmities. Another characteristic of how plague and people combine is that the unevenly distributed markers of contagion and immunity register the pattern of power disparities. In McNeill's account, the power of the European invaders was deeper inside their veins than previously studied. It was also through the diseases that the Europeans were carrying—to which they themselves were largely immune—that they had the power to coerce.

Much before scientific knowledge about invisible disease agents was brought forth by the Pasteurian revolution in the late nineteenth century, people were fully cognizant of the power-related features of diseases. The particular patterns of disease spread were read as signs of authority and legitimacy. Before the age-old discourse acknowledged states as the containers of authority and legitimacy, politico-religious practices attributed the pattern of disease spread to communal, religious, and earthly authorities. The religious interpretation of diseases construed them as divine punishments and trials. These punishments depended on communal piety and impiety. This interpretation was able to 'explain' the spread of deadly diseases in a way that gave meaning to individual fear, physical suffering, and death. Diseases and wars bring fear and death. The underlying traditions, practices, and policies influence how individual-level fear is communally expressed and manifested—what is held to be valuable fear or fearlessness (e.g. Desmond 2006: 359). As diseases were seen as communal punishments for a community's misdeeds and irreligios-ity, there was a pious way of dying because of 'plagues'—religious pilgrimages. As already mentioned in the previous chapter, pilgrimages have long caused epi-demic concerns. McNeill also points to this when he says, 'More generally, reli-gious pilgrimages rivaled warfare in provoking epidemic infection' (1976: 202). He goes on to point out a connecting valence between religious pilgrimages and wars:

> Part of the meaning of pilgrimage was the taking of risks in pursuit of holi-ness. To die en route was, for the pious, an act of God whereby He delib-erately translated the pilgrim from the hardships of life on earth into His presence. Disease and pilgrimage were thus psychologically as well as epi-demiologically complementary. The same may be said of war, where risk of sudden death—one's own or the enemy's—was at the very core of the enterprise.

The way in which a person can suffer or die well connects wars and pilgrimages, thereby offering one additional avenue to see the combinatorial possibilities of linking 'plagues' and suffering in a culturally comprehensible way.

The markers of the right kind of piety associated with disease and politics came to be read from the suffering bodies of people and from the suffering of wider communal bodies. As said, McNeill's account highlighted the relevance of the old accounts that connected disease with power. The combinatorial accounts, like Thucydides' work, of disease encounters had been largely forgotten in the twen-tieth century after the Pasteurian public health discourse turned the way in which disease was understood into matters of apolitical scientific episteme. McNeill's fas-cinating rediscovery was that the history of human–disease interaction could be divided into two categories: besides the micro-parasitic relationship of infection, there were the co-occurring macro-parasitic relationships of conquest and domi-nance from one polity to another in which diseases have played their role, with the conqueror being deadly, not only through advanced weaponry but also by being a disease carrier.[2] This insight was a fresh new articulation of the fundamental relevance of politics in disease spread and vice versa. Perhaps McNeill had in mind the parasitic relationship that resulted in what Thucydides termed *pleonexia*, referring to overreach and overextension driven by greed and avarice at the individual and communal level. What is parasitic about this is that one is ruthlessly motivated to take what does not belong to one (e.g. Schlosser 2012: 169). A war on distant places can be driven by this, and, in the context of such wars, the likelihood of keeping political governance organized enough, in the face of a rush, against diseases and disasters is lowered both at home and abroad. Maladies of the political type create openings, or valences, for political incontinence that lead to escalations and wars and, at the same time, open up opportunities for a weakened body politic and individual-level disease vulnerabilities.

To reiterate, the restored neoclassical framework brings the political modality of lethal epidemic diseases into a form that is also vitally relevant for the global era in which germs germinate through the vector of global mobility systems and air travel which are key elements of the global order. Global connectedness and interdependence are realms where concurrent processes of political contestation and epidemiological phenomena partially overlap and produce consonancies— politically meaningful and historically recurring agreement, resonance, and intensification among the two that have an impact on politics and 'plagues'. The significance and complexity of this nexus between global order and germ circulations are often bypassed and ignored even today, in the time of the COVID-19 pandemic, although its history and proto-theory are ancient, as reviewed in Chapter 2.

In this chapter, I will provide an overview of the historical and theoretical narratives that connect politics and disease. These often-ignored, yet extremely rich and at times consequential, narratives also stimulate the contemporary political imagination when a pandemic emergency scenario suddenly erupts. It may be argued that the central trigger narrative is that of large-scale world-order competition, intensification of rivalry, and rise in the potential of hostility—a spreading sentiment that things are moving on the grand level of events. What this means is that war as a cultural configuration leads to an expectation of enmity in the shape of disease, and any serious contagion catalyses underlying patterns of enmity.[3] This observation serves as a bridgehead into the combinatorial logic—that is, combinatorics—between political regression and pestilences. I will also chart other valences—such as relative capacity to unite, react, or interact—between the two as they are critically relevant for the world during and after COVID-19. It is possible to understand, for example, the earlier pandemic scares as being influenced by the general context of the War on Terror initiated by the US after the 9/11 World Trade Centre bombings in New York City, in particular how the SARS epidemic in 2003 interacted with the build-up to the Iraq War. Today, we can see how COVID-19 combined with the great power tensions between the US and China and put pressure on the overall global order as well as its rule-based governance institutions. It is hypothesized that the rediscovery of the narrative roots involved can enlighten our awareness of the overall phenomenon with which we are deal-ing. The purpose of this rediscovery is to continue in McNeill's footsteps and to define the narrative dynamics/drivers that influence the contemporary events in which these concepts come to play.

The Thucydidean Grand History Framework

Before beginning the review of the first formulation of the nexus in which politics and disease interact, a further distinction is in order. The most acute context for individual suffering and politosomatic effect is the immediate political community where a person feels (in)securely embedded. In order to understand the relevance of the local political community in a disease scenario, it is important to proceed beyond the spatially fixed, static understanding of political communities. Being part of a political community can be understood as a process in which members' lives intertwine in complex dynamics. The status quo keeps moving and develop-ing, often towards a common goal, and sometimes events become looser, more in flux, and change regressively. Regressive dynamics have always been especially rel-evant from the perspective of diseases as social constructs. The perceived communal regression and decline are often embodied through disease language—phenomena ranging from corruption, political violence, unrest, and terrorism to governance collapse are often understood through disease metaphors and metonyms. Under-stood in this way, lethal epidemic diseases become markers of communal dynamics and, more broadly, signifiers of negative intercommunal processes, change, and transformation.

The frame of politosomatics developed herein is as ancient as politics itself. Much of the current research on political processes focuses on progression—for example, sustainability, integration, and state/society building—in line with the overall progressive modernization paradigm. It should be noted that epidemics have played a marked role even in this progressive process. The successful eradica-tion campaigns against major killer diseases during the twentieth century have lent much credence to the modernization paradigm itself. The absence of disease emer-gencies has become a marker of good governance at the state and international level. It can be argued that peoples' sense of general health provides a bodily way of experiencing what is meant by good governance in their local embeddings, as they feel se-cure and less dis-eased. The success in fighting major diseases started to suffer major setbacks from the 1970s, for example, when the campaign aimed at the eradication of malaria failed to deliver. The growing alarm over the future of global health was further reinforced by the emergence of HIV and AIDS in the 1980s. Progressive interpretations have given ground to more declinist modalities in the face of recent pandemic emergencies. Despite this, however, regressive linkages and processes have been left mainly unattended. This is true of general political theory, which lacks ways of understanding political decline (e.g. Aaltola 2020). Therefore, Huntington's (1965: 415) suggestion that when it comes to the regression of politi-cal communities, 'perhaps the most relevant ideas are the most ancient ones' is still persuasive when looking for culturally significant models. This rediscovery from the perspective of the plagues and politics paradigm is the key aspect of this chapter.

For the modern mind, immersion in classical political thought may be useful for the purposes of understanding the different ways in which violent epidemic diseases have been a part of the political frame. It is likely that the paradigm still impacts us, so the mission is to make tacit knowledge explicit. The key discursive frame that ties together epidemics, political violence, and hegemonic struggle in one overall dynamic finds its most distinct and influential formulation in Thucydides' epic, *History of the Peloponnesian War*. The co-occurrence of the pestilences of war, death, famine, and plague provides a stock script that may even today be activable in situations where the occurrence of one leads to culturally laden expectations of the other three broad signifiers of political calamity.[4] Thucydides views regression at the individual level, such as somatic and moral diseases, in the dynamic context of the large-scale political movement unleashed by the hegemonic struggle between Athens and Sparta. Diseases become a way to tell a much larger story. For example, the Athenians launched a rushed and miscalculated military operation against Syracuse during the war. Thucydides narrates how badly the Syracusans treated the prisoners they took, keeping them in crowded holes exposed to the rain, sun, and cold. The prisoners became 'ill by the violence of the change (μεταβολῇ)' (7.87).[5] Such an abrupt change under conditions of war led to diseases whereby the military expedition came to a horrible end.

In his history of this hegemonic struggle, Thucydides suggests that a sense of compassion is natural in a participant observer witnessing a macro-scale war or the vanishing of order that exposes states as well as people to the varying but intertwined manifestations of regressions (e.g. Stahl 1966; Brunt 1967: 278; Monoson and Loriaux 1998: 285). Setting aside his own compassion at seeing the world around him crumble, Thucydides seems to be suggesting that passions such as anger, haste, and hatred were also among the important driving forces of the violent regressive flows that comprised the hegemonic struggle between Athens and Sparta.

Thucydides regards the decades of the Peloponnesian war (431–405 BCE) as 'the vastest movement in human history', as one violent grand movement (Greek: *kinesis megiste*).[6] Appian, in his work, *Wars of the Romans in Iberia*, uses (2000: 8, 39) the same term '*kinesis megiste*' to describe the expansion of the confrontation, revolution, and disturbances in Spain during the Second Punic War—a big grand movement including smaller side crises. In Plutarch's *Agesilaus*, the meaning of the term is in reference to a great disturbance or stir (e.g. Plutarch 2010: 3, 8). Dionysius of Halicarnassus also uses the term in *Antiquitates Romanae* (1940) when referring to a feared and very serious turmoil. Thucydides seems to refer to a grand disturbance with widening and deepening consequences at both the macro and micro levels—what may today be referred to as a world war, cold war, or hegemonic struggle. His detailed account describes how this vortex of war engulfed all of Greece, causing strong convulsions and disturbances in both big and small poleis. The pulsating, yet always intensifying, regressive flow led to strong passions, which, in turn, fed the intensification of the grand flow. Sudden emergencies such as the Stasis of Corcyra and the Plague of Athens, Thucydides can be read to claim, were violently erupting sub-motions of the overall violent regression of the primary hegemonic struggle.[7] Yet it was not a widening and deepening grand movement in only the military sense. It is crucial to understand that, for Thucydides, the deterioration as a consequence of the grand movement led to other vulnerabilities: extreme deterioration led to likely vulnerabilities to disruptions of different types such as earthquakes, droughts, famines, and plagues (1.23). The escalating hostilities blended with natural calamities such as earthquakes, great droughts, famines, and plague. The violent, rushed actions, and intensifying tempos of violence combined with disasters and diseases in a way that was unparalleled in history as the lack of stability that had prevailed during peace time made it harder to cope with the widening scope of the different inflictions. Disequilibrium that produces political disorder (stasis), so Thucydides suggests, combines with the Hippocratic understanding of disease causation, as disequilibrium of bodily humours and unbalanced passions (akrasia) feed the flux opening up at the political level. Thucydides' idea suggests a politosomatic relationship: disarray at the political level is a disease of the body, mind, and political entities.

It is important to note from the beginning that Thucydides' political ideas were greatly conditioned by the Hippocratic medicine of his time.[8] This overall model found one expression in the Hippocratic hypothesis which conceptualized bodily flux as the source of disease (Craik 2001: 102). There was a close link across the soma–psyche boundary: it is important to realize that physical movements and the imbalances caused by them were thought to be the key to human emotions as well as to physical maladies. Both human disease and human emotions were seen as co-instantaneous with changes in bodily humours. However, it should be noted that this was a two-way street—the language of politics also permeated the medical thought of the time. To highlight this pertinent connection, some have suggested that Thucydides was moving well beyond the medical thought of his time by suggesting the dynamics of contagion in his analysis of the widening and deepening effects of political malady. However, as Craik (2001: 102) points out, the 'contagion' reading is an anachronistic interpretation of Thucydides. Rather than referring to contagion, Thucydides was using a related, but different, idea of spread, flux, vortex, or flow, which he also projected to his interpretation of the Plague of Athens. On the one hand, the Plague becomes a sub-narrative that supports the main narrative of vortex-engulfed political bodies by pointing to how the plague dissolved human bodies in a similar manner. On the other hand, it is a more ambitious argument in which the dissolution of political and somatic bodies is simply what happens in times of a grand movement. Moreover, in Thucydides' time, 'flux' and 'change' were used to understand various political processes as well as in attempts to construe the realm of bodily physiological kinetics.[9]

Thucydides' idea of politics links to the body. He said that both man-made political processes and natural phenomena 'characterize both actors and events and are also devoted to supporting political, scientific, and historical arguments' (Foster

2009: 368). As the plague travels deeper and downwards in the human body, hope is gradually lost and fear becomes the key motion leading to incontinence and even madness. This is parallel to the spread of the grand movement. It spreads wider, and the knowledge of it getting closer and more serious reinforces its horror and brings in passions and motions feeding the horrors of stasis. The medical knowledge of Thucydides' time is present in his narrative about the plague, but the driver, it is suggested, is the grand movement of things where regression inside a human body and its passions were embedded. Without the context of the grand movement, the diseases would not have been as severe and devastating. The neglect of the plague-sufferers, lack of compassion, and collapsed governance also point to the added burden constituted by the co-occurring war. The grand movement added to the dehumanizing horror, catalysed it, and became a highly calamitous event.

It is significant that Thucydides considered war to be one 'grand movement', which provided the context for many other movements. Passions got unleashed in a war. These war passions caused strong impulses for smaller communal and human side-movements, which, in turn, further fed the broadening and deepening multi-level regression and unravelling:

> In peace and prosperity states and individuals have better sentiments, because they do not find themselves suddenly confronted with imperious necessities; but war takes away the easy supply for daily wants, and so process a rough master, that brings most men's characters to a level with their fortunes.
>
> *(Thucydides 3.82)*

To understand the effects of the grand movement on a political community, one needs to keep in mind the value that Thucydides placed on that most fragile of spaces—the human space. In Thucydides' political thought, the political realm is often defined as a human space. Within the confines of this space, humans can govern and manage their destinies and work towards a good life. This space is maintained in between randomness and necessity. There are, on the one hand, happenings which are totally accidental, in which there is no sensible pattern, such as natural disasters. Human communities and political deliberations do not have much power over such accidental calamities. However, a well-governed community, as a human space, can alleviate the situation and be more prepared for accidental occurrences. On the other hand, there are things that are highly patterned and human made. For example, violence, feuds, conflicts, and wars will happen. The law of the jungle can prevail. There are situations in which anything goes and everybody looks out only for themselves, where survival belongs to the strongest or the fittest and where the strong do what they can and the weak suffer what they must. In Thucydides' work, much emphasis is placed on the constant need to keep the human space prepared and guarded against these two boundaries. Moreover, the idea is to push against the two boundaries to expand the human space where and when possible—that is, to make more patterned processes dependent on human will and to mitigate the chances that accidental events would negatively impact the human possibilities of a good life. What is needed for the prudent and effective guarding of the political space is to seek to preserve time, provident/prudent delay, which grants the time needed for sound political deliberation. It is the human space that gets constricted in political regression, the end point of which is political convulsions. The motions and emotions unleashed by grand dynamics gradually erode the possibilities of having enough time for sound political deliberation (e.g. Desmond 2006: 359).

The overall direction of the political regression is clear. Different forms of lethal violence move from one community to another in the same way as plague. This is the point of the contagion present in the sub-narrative of the Plague of Athens. It is not so much a factual description of the contagion of plague as a description of how regressive political processes spread from one community to another. Thucydides read plague as a process of bodily decomposition that progressed deeper into the somatic body—starting from the head and progressing to a fatal intestinal condition—and vertically across human bodies. Keeping this reading in mind, let us proceed further along the politosomatic approach suggested by Thucydides: What happens to the somatic and mental state of a person who is inflicted with plague? The whole body becomes engulfed by the plague, as the grand movement affecting the whole of the Hellenic world. Violent heat in the head and redness and inflammation of the eyes come first, followed by pain in the throat and tongue and sneezing and hoarseness. It then affects sight and voice, as in losing the vision and voice of politics. Next the plague strikes at the heart, where, according to the then prevalent worldview, emotions were embedded. Emotions towards compatriots and even towards immediate family become erratic. Then it proceeds deeper into stomach, to the key constituents of the body, similar to the grand movement affecting the status quo of the Hellenic world and, most violently, individual poleis. The fire that spread at the macro level causing animosity among poleis found its parallel in the plague decomposing the somatic body. The ultimate effect of the plague was the loss of memory, similar to the rushed actions unfettered by conventional constraints affecting the relations within and between political communities. Virtues changed into vices, especially in the deep intestines—in Athens and Sparta—as well as in the extremities— the smaller city-states—which suffered the most violent episodes of the grand convolution.

The political conflict started from the hegemonic macro level and spread downwards, influencing bigger and smaller poleis. One notable characteristic of Thucydides' flux was the ability of regression to become more intensive as the broadening and deepening grinding intensified. It was as if the condition mutated into a more serious form until it simply burnt out of fuel, in this case human bodies. This dynamic mutability was one of increasing intensity in terms of war, but also of spreading intensity in which the underlying condition took on new forms, as in the case of stasis and plague. Importantly, Thucydides links this intensity effect partly to the fear aroused in people during the later stages, when they are more aware of and horrified by the devastating effects of the violence in other places and at earlier stages:

> The suffering which revolution entailed upon the cities were many and terrible, such as have occurred and always will occur, as long as the nature of mankind remains the same; though in a severe or milder form, and varying in their symptoms, according to the variety of the particular cases. (3.82.2)

There is an added horror in the acknowledgement of impending doom, in knowing the horrible fate that awaits them. This increasing fatalism further undermines the maintenance of the human space and affects all aspects of life, turning them into potent symptoms of impending horror. In this context, the Plague of Athens during the war turned into a politosomatic narrative of a horrid fate to come, and this sense of impending doom enhanced the plague's terrorizing effect.[10]

Thucydides uses the concept of kinesis (*ekinethe, kineo*) to refer to the overall vortex and its various side whorls (e.g. Clark *et al.* 2015). Kinesis and *ekinethe* suggest destructive types of 'movement and instability' (Monoson and Loriaux 1998: 291). Kinesis highlights the general flow-like qualities of the context. However, Thucydides seems to be referring to a more specific type of movement, a flow-vortex or spiral (e.g. Ellis 1991: 344). The kinaesthetic metaphor of a spiral-like vortex is appropriate in this context when the associated mythological connotations are considered—that is, the grand movement was set in motion by the sea power, Athens. According to mythology, the coming into being of Athens—a sea power—was linked to sea vortexes.[11] Moreover, it is highly suggestive that Plato, in his *Statesman*, uses (273d) the concept of 'sea of diversity' when referring to existence outside or in the absence of a political community. As discussed in the previous chapter, the inter-poleis space—its ether—was imagined as a boundless sea in constant flux, against which the community's governance should be on constant guard. Fittingly, the 'great movement' unleashed by Pericles' Athens was imagined by Thucydides as a 'chaos, terrible flux, a destructive kind of motion' (Monoson and Loriaux 1998: 291). For Thucydides, the vortex of conflict induces uncontained pulses, co-currents, and ripples.

Thucydides paints a scenario of grand movement: new sub-currents were likely to occur in the vicinity of the conflict's rhythmic expression of energy. The increasingly violent circular motions meant that intervals in extreme pain production became progressively shorter: violence kept coming back, cutting across and within bodies in more intense spirals, circling round and back, again and again, grinding bodies, both somatic and political, to pieces.[12] It is within this frame that the Plague of Athens became politosomatically meaningful and widely influential, for Thucydides' account and framework were later adopted by many commentators as a narrative model for a description of a lethal epidemic disease and its contemporaneous processes (e.g. Longrigg 1992: 27; Snowden 2019: 20–31). Enmity and plague became interlinked in a way that still evokes age-old political imageries and increases the probability of the one in the presence of the other.

A strong characteristic of the overall spiralling enmity scenario consisted of contagious diseases. It is highly significant that the macro-level movement did not spread only horizontally between polities. It also turned into increasingly deep vertical vortexes or, as Thucydides descriptively frames it, into deep 'intestinal disorders'. The more confusing the currents became, the more destructive were their effects at multiple, increasingly overlapping, levels. Despite the overall clarity of the violent vortexes, it was anything but clear for those involved. Among the first victims of the regressive kinesis was the collective memory of various people. For Thucydides, shared memory was fundamental for a healthy political community. Thucydides' stated mission was to help people to remember so that they might be better equipped when such violent grand movements struck again in the future, as they would inevitably. The regressing mind may lose memory altogether by reducing it to inevitable necessities—for example, the 'might is right' type of memory—or may accommodate the recollection to the immediate violent events and passions of the moment (1.22, 2.54). Thus, proper collective memory keeps safe past horrors and mistakes. The primary reason for memory is to enable a political community to function as a whole. In Thucydides' account, the same way of remembering and communal methods of recollection make for the coherence of a political community (Cogan 1980: 168). The emergence of splits in communal together-mindedness raises the likelihood of whimsical courses of future communal action. The degenerating shared memory makes it increasingly hard to rediscover the common persuasive element needed for rhetoric virtues. Aristotle intertwines alikeness at the level of common opinions to what is likely and collectively realizable (e.g. *Nicomachean Ethics* I, 1, 1355, b18). Communally controlled collective memory is key to steady governance. Communal together-mindedness is a method for alikeness and an anchor for situational decision-making in a way that leads to likeness and predictability in the steering of the community.

When a grand movement is allowed to proceed unchecked, it starts to affect people by diminishing their ability to remember and think in the same way and, at the end, to communicate without resorting to violent action. The deep 'intestinal' nature of enmity and plague may be taken to refer to deep societal movements resulting from and constituting the war, whereby poleis and individuals lost their 'reserve, the power to check their motion' (Monoson and Loriaux 1998: 292). According to Thucydides, these abnormalities referred to local-level factionalism and atomization (Monoson and Loriaux 1998: 287). The ability to plan and maintain a chosen course of action was overwhelmed by the increasing complexity of the currents. Categories—such as personal, polis, and inter-poleis—became confounded (Connor 1984: 7). This complex entanglement further fed the vortex.

The deepening vertical vortexes led to the annulment of the constitutive elements defining individual communities. It also affected individual bodies by causing different types of political violence and suffering. However, this intestinal disorder was more radical than simple annihilation of people and their communities. It coupled with its context—the hegemonic war—and further fed it. Thucydides' description of the Stasis of Corcyra describes an extremely malignant form of political disease. On the one hand, the political community does not only disappear and dissolve, it turns into what can be called an anti-community when its community's constitutive element transforms into what can be called a de-constitutive element. This means that communal collapse does not stop at the violent dissolution of a community but leads further to the community's inversion—turning inside out—into an anti-community or, to use today's vocabulary, into a failed or collapsed state or society. Rotberg (2002: 90) can be read to offer a modern-day interpretation of Thucydidean sentiments in using the appropriate metaphor of 'black hole' when describing a failed state: 'A collapsed state is a mere geographical expression, a black hole into which a failed polity has fallen'. As it turns into an anti-community, a stasis-ridden polity still interacts violently with its surroundings through its attractive gravitational pull. The disease does not simply die out; there are still further stages after the loss of the common constitutive element. The constitutive element leads to mutually felt animosity among what were previously members of a community sharing a degree of political friendship. The shared mutual hatred provides the constitutive form for the Thucydidean anti-community. The inherent extremism

> in a strict sense, defines the mentality of stasis. The excess of disposition comes to be admired in place of its mean, and the mean to be despised as the deficiency of this excess. Having supplemented the mean as the standard, however, the extreme continuously feeds upon itself: It enjoys a striving for ever fresher extremes, a frenzied struggle to exceed one's rivals at excess itself.
> *(Orwin 1988: 835)*

Furthermore, the disorder is destructive not just for the community it strikes; it is also contagious beyond it. Thucydides puts forth the idea that the implosion of a political community is inherently tied into intercommunal warfare. A stasis-ridden anti-community directs its previously internal bonds outwards, thereby actively attracting foreign elements into the anti-community's hatred-driven internal struggle—in today's context, perhaps Syria post-2012 could be seen as an example of this. Back in Thucydides' time, Athens and Sparta were willing collaborators in the internal violence of individual poleis since they could not see the difference between the macro-level enmity and the struggles of factions in various small communities. The two were one and the same thing.

On the other hand, this violent regression spreads simultaneously to the individual level—in both the moral/psychological and physiological senses—as the striking sub-narrative of the Plague of Athens demonstrates. While the convulsions of the stasis atomized Corcyran society into factions and finally into violent, but extremely vulnerable, individuals, the Plague of Athens entailed a parallel story of somatic bodily disintegration. This sub-narrative highlights the influence of the overall 'movements' on human bodies as the loci of the soma and the psyche. The suggested direction of the dynamics is clear. The grand movement of hegemonic war gathers intensity and spreads downwards towards smaller communities, which are thus set into disintegrative motion, and to the individual level, where somatic suffering—such as disease, mass murder, or mental incontinence (rash actions, selfishness, and failure to obey sacred norms)—takes place. The extreme perversion of politics was the breeding ground for the plague as well as the ground whereby its political meanings were construed. Plague continued the intestinal degeneration by decomposing somatic bodies and further inducing an overall sense of horror and unavoidable doom. The plague continued by other means the processes unleashed by the hegemonic struggle. For Thucydides, the plague was an essential constituent as well as a consequence of the war. In the absence of the overall kinesis, the plague could not have been what it became under the grand movement.

The concept of stasis is a process that cannot be adequately understood without taking into account its intimate relationship with lethal diseases, in particular with plague. Thucydides' account of how stasis gathered more steam when it spread closely parallels what took place during the Plague of Athens: 'It first began . . . in the parts of Ethiopia above Egypt, and thence descended into Egypt and Libya and into most of the king's country' (2.48).[13] Even though the Peloponnesians were blamed for the plague due to enmity-related suspicion and paranoia, it is highly relevant that Thucydides mentions Ethiopia—the faraway, strange land—as a more 'factual' birthing place for the plague. Then the disease suddenly fell upon Athens, Thucydides tells us, and the deaths in Athens became much more frequent: 'For the plague broke out as soon as the Peloponnesians invaded Attica . . . committed its worst ravages at Athens, and next to Athens, at the most populous of the other towns' (2.54). The plague's intensity grew in a manner that reminds one of the stasis' ability to become more serious as people who were struck later know more about its devastating nature. In his highly influential narrative, Thucydides seems to be suggesting that plague is a fundamental part of a grand movement as are individual occurrences of stasis.

The increasing effect of the spreading disease at the individual level is matched at the communal level. Its regressive nature is evident in the way in which plague first affects the head and then spreads malignantly to the bowels:

> [P]eople in good health were all of a sudden attacked by violent heats in the head, and redness and inflammation in the eyes, the inward parts, such as the throat or tongue, becoming bloody and emitting an unnatural and fetid breath. These symptoms were followed by sneezing and hoarseness, after which the pain soon reached the chest, and produced a hard cough. When it fixed in the stomach, it upset it; and discharges of bile of every kind named by physicians ensued, accompanied by very great distress. . . . But if they passed this stage, and the disease descended further into the bowels, inducing a violent ulceration there accompanied by severe diarrhoea, this brought on a weakness which was generally fatal.
>
> *(2.49)*

This regressive process of gradual decomposition was accompanied by the rapid weakening of the manner in which people recognized previously important and even sacred communal creeds and norms:

> The bodies of dying men lay one upon another, and half-dead creatures reeled about the streets. . . . The sacred places . . . were full of corpses of persons that had died there, just as they were; for as the disaster passed all bounds, men, not knowing what was to become of them, became utterly careless of everything, whether sacred or profane.
>
> *(2.52)*

The power of norms and beliefs to bind the community together was replaced by open deviance from communal norms:

> Fear of gods or law of man there was none to restrain them. As for the first, they judged it to be just the same whether they worshipped them or not, as they saw all alike perishing; and for the last, no one expected to live to be brought to trial for his offences, but each felt that a far severer sentence had been already passed upon them all and hung ever over their heads, and before this fell, it was only reasonable to enjoy life a little.
>
> *(2.53)*

Judging from such excerpts, the plague affected the communal body as much as it caused suffering on individual lives, minds, and bodies. Plague was a political—as also civil religious—disease similar to stasis, which caused civic collapse: 'Stasis as a medical term was used for describing a disequilibrium among conjoined elements' (Kalimtzis 2000: 19).

Adherence to the common values decreased as individual desires and incontinences became the foremost concern during the plague. This led to changes and reversal in the meanings of central concepts in the same way that stasis leads to loss of meaning:

> Men now coolly ventured on what they had formerly done in a corner, and not just as they pleased, seeing the rapid transitions produced by persons in prosperity suddenly dying and those who before had nothing succeeding to their property. . . . Perseverance in what men called honor was popular with none, it was so uncertain whether they would be spared to attain the object; but it was settled that present enjoyment, and all that contributed to it, was both honorable and useful.
>
> *(2.53)*

This is very similar to the Thucydidean description of stasis as a process aversely affecting norms, memories, and language. One of the most striking details of the stasis provided by Thucydides is the way in which words lose their meaning during stasis:

> Words had to change their ordinary meaning and to take that which was now given them. Reckless audacity came to be considered the courage of a loyal ally; prudent hesitation, specious cowardice; moderation was held to be a cloak for unmanliness; ability to see all sides of a question inaptness to act on any. Frantic violence became the attribute of manliness; caution, plotting, a justifiable means of self-defence. The advocate of extreme measures was always trustworthy; his opponent, a man to be suspected.
>
> *(3.82)*

Thucydides continues his list, in the context of stasis, in a way that highlights the reversed nature of virtues and vices—the meanings had changed from those instituted though previous interactions to ones characterized by deep hatred, polarization, and extremism. Moreover, the stasis, characterized by loss and reversals of meaning, was contagious as it

> ran its course from city to city, and the places which it arrived at last, from having heard what had been done before, carried to a still greater excess the refinement of their inventions, as manifested in the cunning of their enterprises and the atrocity of their reprisals.
>
> *(3.82)*

The slips in meanings caused by plague and stasis were parallel processes that flowed towards private gain and desires, replacing deliberative processes as the ultimate arbiters of meaning. The judgements, Thucydides points out, are not the same in the case of fear and horror as they are in the normal contexts of political calm and sound governance. Rather, an inversion takes place through which that which makes sense under a disease is very different from the common sense prevailing under normal conditions, in which accidents and facts of nature leave space for political deliberation, choice, and action—for the existence of a governable human space. A disease can turn a political community from an area of showing together- and like-mindedness to a locus of split-mindedness in the form of unbound factious and individual desires.

In Thucydides' account, the violent bodily spasms caused by the plague, which are among the most severe symptoms, are also among its last symptoms. The disease has run its course much before the spasms. In the case of stasis, bodily spasms find their parallel in convulsions (kinesis) of the political body. These spasms are uncontrollable and can signal the imminent end of the community's and the person's life. The violent movements at the later stages of the concurrent political diseases of plague, stasis, and the grand movement are signs of isolation and apart-mindedness. Thucydides describes how people were left alone, unattended and uncared for. The condition of isolation brought about by the disease is enforced by the selfish and egoistic actions of the diseased, those fearing the disease, and those who have survived the disease. People did not indulge in any of the activities that would have reaffirmed the existence of a shared sense and common understanding in a political community. Instead, isolation and apart-mindedness prevailed. In stasis, friends were forgotten, and factious strife became the overpowering motivation.

To sum up, the idea here is that classical thought contains an influential social construct, a well-rehearsed frame of a multidimensional and intertwined regressive process. This process intertwines macro-level politics with other 'dis-eases': an epidemic as a regressive and spreading condition is inherently political, and hegemonic war as a violent vortex is always disease-like. Moreover, large-scale war predisposes the general moods of worry, fear, and horror towards perceptions of somatic diseases. The overall grand flow of hegemonic/imperial enmity brings along other passions, such as hatred and aggression, which predisposes the overall context towards an intensifying vortex-like flow. The resulting constriction of political spaces leads to ungovernable situations and opens up vulnerabilities to accidental processes such as plagues. The regressive flow starts from the macro-level movements, deepens into problems in larger and smaller polities, and ultimately arouses a situation ripe for self-fulfilling fears and scares of lethal epidemic diseases. The point here is that the 'dis-ease' at the level of the individual somatic body may be seen as a part of a larger grand movement in the macro-level political hierarchy. Occurrences of large-scale enmities and the resulting dis-ease make conditions ripe for somatic diseases.

Contemporary Power-Political Dis-eases

The Thucydidean understanding was that the energetic kinetic dynamics of a major power contestation provide a context in which governance weaknesses and fear and consequences of a violent lethal disease are amplified. This comprehensive framework can be used to shed light on our present-day ways of understanding pandemics. This bridge between enmities and disease can lead to a better appreciation of the complex entanglements that pandemics have with other major global dynamics. For example, it can be hypothesized that the present-day macro-level turbulences in world politics have recontextualized what pandemics look and feel like, and their causes and consequences. The emergence of global order after the end of the Cold War, followed by the War on Terror with its major wars in Iraq and Afghanistan, and the present-day escalating enmities among the great powers provide a varying source for anxiety that can heighten disease-related fears, scares, and manifestations. In some important ways, it is possible to claim that pandemic emergencies embody anxieties that stem from power-political grand movements.

One way of approaching this account is through understanding that the emotional charges involved in global public health—containment and compassion—provide for situational scenarios that overlap with the emotional content of US hegemony and its way of construing its enemies but also with felt life under the global order with its mobility-based transnational geo-economy. To use Thucydidean language, the feverish grand movements feed into and are fed by perceptions of major violent epidemics.

The grand kinesis is a context in which modern forms of political compassion have been redefined in comparison to the humanitarian practices that prevailed during the Cold War years. Furthermore, it can be argued that the rule-based global order has further recontextualized political demonstrations of compassion and, by definition, humanitarianism. Humanitarian mobilizations have usually been connected with single, isolated spectacles such as Rwanda, Kosovo, Somalia, Darfur, the Democratic Republic of Congo, Afghanistan, Yemen, and Syria, which are deemed to have mainly local root causes. My main working hypothesis is that this treatment of humanitarian emergencies in a vacuum, detaching them from wider violent processes, leaves out the central elements of wider humanitarian compassion. From the perspective entertained here, many of the largest recent humanitarian events are connected and better appreciated as parts of overall violent, regressive flows underlined by the open-ended War on Terror (2010s–2020s) and its escalating great power enmities. The localization of ground zeros into single countries leaves out a large part of political compassion that is directed not only to the suffering of distant individual bodies but also to the suffering of other political bodies; besides empathy for suffering individuals, this also denotes sentimental worry over the sustainability of the world order and compassion for declining nations and peoples going lower in the global hierarchy. 'I' and 'we' can worry and be concerned about sudden changes, unsustainabilities, and opening vulnerabilities that are functions of perceived enmities and power dynamics at the global level.

It has already been reviewed in the previous chapter that compassion includes a need to contain the compassionate suffering from spreading and becoming contagious. Such containment practices can alleviate the sense of the world becoming more dis-eased, which regulates the ways in which fears and anxieties are projected to external actors. A sudden need to contain and demarcate a clear boundary between us and them leads to a distinct but nuanced focus on various overlapping boundary conditions. The blend of modern ideas on humanity contains both compassion and containment. What this means is that modern compassion practices also take part in the containment of the objects of that compassion and the subjects that are seen as being in a state of compassionable suffering and pain. In an important manner, the practices of compassion, which are often deemed as legitimate and as sources of legitimacy, are also practices of containment, distinction, and 'othering'. It is in this emotional emergency, where the characteristics of compassion and containment interact, that compassion can and often does constitute a sentiment towards containment. Without this compassion–containment combination, it is very difficult to understand how pandemic situations are constructed. Pandemics are among the second-order entanglements that result from the ways in which the compassion–containment discourse interacts with the overall power-political flows of our time.

Compelling feelings for and against 'others' are a multifaceted and mobilizing, yet inadequately examined, political phenomenon, as, for example, exemplified by the COVID-19-related vaccine nationalism and diplomacy. In the study of humanitarian emergencies, it is common to reduce compassion for distant others to mere modernist, secular, and liberal ethical visions, which derive from enlightenment and humanism. However, political compassion may equally well be contextualized in much older historical strands, in the sentiments felt towards significant in-groups (such as nations and hegemonies or empires). In a sense, compassion implicates a contained group(s) that is not limited to or constrained by the suffering distant others as individuals. Compassion contains both its agent and object of action. Often, these are similar: when a state is the agent of compassion, then the object is likely to be a state. When a hegemonic actor such as the US is an agent of compassion, its object is usually a sufferer that signifies the vulnerabilities of its own hegemony, for example, the repression of democratic opposition and demonstrators or the victims of autocratic aggression.

Moreover, it is suggested that the more modernist version of humanitarianism does not work in a void. It interacts with other older traditions of compassion. Different compassions for in- and out-groups and individuals interact and, in some cases, constitute mutually reinforcing regressive flows. For example, the compassion felt towards the plight of the Iraqi Kurds and Shias immediately prior to the war in Iraq connected the compassionate parties to the internal decomposition of the Iraqi state. The larger context for this compassionate connection was the worry over the threat to Western security posed by the claimed Iraqi weapons of mass destruction (WMDs). These world-order worries blended with particular types of compassion and formed the context for humanitarian compassion for the suffering Iraqi population. The humanitarian compassion for the suffering Iraqis was overwhelmed by other compassions inherent in the power-political situation, despite millions of displaced people and tens of thousands of non-combatant deaths. Thus, in the case of Iraq, the compassion was containment based and directed to the possible suffering should Saddam Hussein's Iraq be left uncontained. The fear of alarming, uncontained processes motivated a particular type of hegemonic alarm and mobilization for a war of containment.

Compassion implies containment and vice versa. However, when the combination takes place in the pandemic emergency scenario, containment sets the frame for compassions that can be felt. Compassionate containment's narratives focus on global connections and closeness, but they also imply boundaries and how people are and should be confined to the contours of their geography.

At the level of hegemonic embodiment, the politics of compassion contains worries over the all-encompassing nature of Western and US power. Often, the underlying passion for containment stems from the effects of contacts and mobilities over long distances in the global order. It is clear that such anxieties and the declinist fears inherent in them provide ingredients for the pandemic emergency scenario. With the specificities of hegemonic times that might now be passing, it is relatively easy to envision pandemics connected with the feverish agitations of the hegemonic embodiment.

The infighting and in-group versus out-group tensions at the level of the hegemonic US body politic can easily translate into visions of an overall regressive flow. US domestic discussions are full of examples of declinist images and fears of deepening polarization. Sometimes, these are easy to discern, and sometimes, they recede to the background. The worries over in-group tensions found their manifestation, for example, in the so-called culture wars of 1990. The culture wars were significant because they framed particular hegemonic sensitivities and animated such lofty fear images as Huntington's vision of a clash of civilizations. The perceptions of threat and decline in the US led to particular world-order sensitivities that were put into high gear by 9/11 and, later, during the Russian invasion of Ukraine and the rise of China. The societal regression at the level of the hegemonic body was projected outwards in the form of felt compassion towards certain types of distant suffering and suffering bodies.

Political compassion is also a notable tradition because it frames anxieties about world politics in a way that focuses on identification with sufferers and self-perceptions of being actors with high moral worth. In many cases, the positive framings are used by the actors themselves to understand why they undertake violent means, as in the case of humanitarian intervention. The Western attempts to accentuate the Afghan operations as a way to build a state where human rights would be restored to their proper place is a case in point of the tendency to find a positive framing for acts mainly driven by power-political instincts. A way to read Thucydides is that the double act of appearing to doing good as an apparent driver for interventions can turn value, compassionate politics into enmity, based on battles over reputation, prestige, and morality.

Sentiments, Emotions, and Power

The analytic typologies of various political sentiments and their relatedness are relatively meaningless in that they are not embedded into the dynamic context of political flows. Emergencies ranging from the humanitarian and terror to pandemic ones provide an important contemporary flow context in which political emotions mix and combine finding their situated, emergent meanings. Despite the apparent suddenness and ad hoc-ism, emergency scenarios are historically well-rehearsed activities. They have a history and contain a tradition wherein different characteristics combine and resonate with each other in relatively path-dependent ways. From this perspective, an emergency is a pain-laden event that suddenly surfaces for a time period and seems to compel some type of compassions and containments by the concerned actors.

It is argued that an emergency scenario that binds together characteristics from different levels—for example, macro-level political enmities, political instability, and individual-level vulnerabilities such as health anxieties—has a relatively well-rehearsed geometric trajectory. Proceeding beyond clear-cut, rational–cognitive imagery to one of political flows, movements, motions, emotions, reactive combinations, and bonding between characteristics with historical and cultural valences,

I will next expand the idea that motions between communities and in the over-all international setting are naturally unsteady, especially in an emergency frame. Unsteadiness of political flows reflects the constant possibility of vorticity, that is, the spiralling circles of expressing enmity and finally inflicting and suffering pain. In the Thucydidean tradition, the social construction of vortex-like violence is highlighted often, as, for example, in research literature where there is a strong tradition of using various signifiers of cycles to describe the patterns of political violence and war (e.g. Goldstein 1985; Minow 2002; Meisel 2016). International crises are seen through the scenario of a vortex, as unstable, downward spiral-ling flows (e.g. Hermann and Fischerkeller 1993). The presumed crisis vortex is pictured as a dynamic circular engulfing and deepening dynamic. The multiple embodied metaphors construct international crises in the dynamic context of an exchange—a movement composed of responses and counter-responses, revenge and counter-revenge. For example, Leng (1993: 74) uses the analogy of a 'school-yard fight' to characterize a pattern of symmetrically escalating enmity. There are recurring references to downward spirals that grip actors, spin them quicker and quicker, and suck new players into the vortex. This deeply ingrained mental con-struct, or cultural model, portrays the course of events defined by a downward momentum that keeps increasing and a spiral that keeps reinforcing itself and tight-ening into deeper abysses. Leng (2000: 268) calls this type of crisis dynamics a 'spiralling crisis'—a spiralling crisis escalates the situation out of control, driven and fed by what are seen as misperceptions and emotional reactions. All these modern conceptualizations can be seen as key aspects that Thucydides formulated.

Within such an unstable downwards flow, the sensing of flow currents is cru-cially important for the actors involved. In a sense, emotional sensitivity becomes a constitutive element of agency in a crisis or emergency situation. Emotional content is fed by the shifting motions of power relations and by the changing positions in a power hierarchy. The images of the emergency—such as eyewitness accounts, news stories, and photographs—turn into triggers of complex emotional judgements for both the internal actors and those beyond. It is this emotionally fed dynamics that offers a helpful, culturally embedded model to enable us to under-stand the regressive grand movement initiated as great power relations sour.

A short review of contemporary research offers evidence that the motion–emotion pairing of the classical topos continues to be relevant. The connection between power and emotions has been examined by several contemporary think-ers. Among them, Kemper's studies (e.g. 1981) are refreshing for their emphasis on power hierarchy-related emotionality. In Kemper's model, emotions consist of actu-ally or imaginatively existing social organizational or social relational conditions: 'When these conditions are met, the desired emotions will flow of themselves, authentically' (Kemper 1981: 358). More specifically, the intimate relation may be based on a close connection between power relations and the primary, instinctive, or physiological feelings of fear, anger, depression, and satisfaction (Kemper 1987: 263). Other theorists have put forth different models of emotionality flowing from social relations (Lewis 1971; Scheff 1993; Retzinger 1991; Rogalin et al. 2007).

Besides making a distinction between cognitive and more unconscious and instinctive processes, the literature often points out that some emotions, such as (loss of) respect and (mis)trust, linger on. These moods or sentiments can become chronic and recurring and differ from shorter-term flare-up of emotions such as enmity and hatred (Jasper 1998: 402).

In both power-political and emergency scenarios, two key sentiments—compassion and containment—manifest themselves in a coherent combination: the rush to contain in order to control is co-instantaneous with the compassion for one's own community or with identifying with similar actors seen as expressing some key constituent elements of one's own community. The sentiment of containment and compassion embedded in it can be regarded as a social emotion because its object is other people's emotional expressions—for example, fleeing, disease carriers, superspreaders, and keeping one's reference group immune and free of contagion—and, therefore, it occurs only as part of the dynamic patterns of social interaction (see e.g. Clark 1987: 180). However, containment/compassion is not only a constructive social emotion; it is also a potentially enmity-arousing and exclusionary political dynamic. During the vaccine nationalism phase of COVID-19 in the early spring of 2021, developing states were over-ordering vaccines to the tune of three to four times their need for their own immunization programmes, and they were also implementing export restrictions, although the most effective and rational approach would have been a globally coordinated effort to vaccinate as broadly as possible. However, peoples' compassions were directed first and foremost towards their own national/regional reference groups. The sentiment of containment prevailed, and the slogan, 'One World, One Health', was seen as meaningless in the rush to contain the pandemic. More generally, the starting point is that the motions inherent in any emergency process translate into compassionate emotionality, the objects of which range from social grounds that are near to other groups constituted by distant sufferers; these strong sentiments further contribute to the intensifying of the identification and enmity pattern flows. This definition, which is based on the neoclassical model, maintains that motions or changes in power hierarchies cause emotions. Emotions turn into motion, kinaesthetics, and they fuel movements and mobilizations (e.g. Crawford 2000: 124; Jasper 1998: 397). Emotion research has concentrated on referring to such mobilizing events as moral shocks, frame alignments, and emerging collective identities. At their minimum, political movements and flows stir the existing patterns of understanding about what are positive and negative emotions, what should be expressed and what hidden, and what constitutes adequate and inadequate responses.

The perceived sight of a pandemic suffering somewhere causes sudden jolts. These abrupt political convulsions find their embodied parallels in the expressive reaction of people recoiling in the face of an unanticipated threat. This embodied kinetics may be projected into the world of political objects. The sensibility of the recoiling kinetics pervades a pandemic emergency and constitutes situational logics for individuals and their communities. This general kinetics of containment is a scenario that is often alluded to in the relevant national, international, and supranational documents. For example, the European Union document on strengthening coordination on generic preparedness planning for public health emergencies at the EU level (COM 2005: 605) states:

> Such generic plans would involve not only medical countermeasures, such as diagnosis, isolation and treatment of cases and the administration of vaccines and prophylactic drugs to at-risk groups and the population at large, but also public order measures, such as restriction of movement and border controls, closing down premises and the cordoning off of specific areas, civil protection measures such as rescue operations.

The attention clearly is on creating geographical obstacles and distance in order to stop the spreading patterns of infection and contagion. The dynamics of contagion has a cultural history that links it with failing states and with practices of bad governance as the following quote from the US 2010 National Security Strategy illustrates: '[W]e seek to mitigate other problem areas, including . . . the threat of emergent and re-emergent disease in poorly governed states'. Such scenarios actualize in specific interventionism practices vis-à-vis failing or badly governed polities, which are deemed as risks to global health security. The fact that failure to manage health in some local communities is a common source of insecurity for the rest can be seen as leading to a specific type of containment blended with interventionism.

Political emotions in the vicinity of stirring flows empower by translating influence and status into power, that is, into the capacity to produce intended and foreseen effects (Willer *et al.* 1997: 573). The emotions produced by power structures vary, from enmities to compassions (Kemper 1991: 330). It is equally clear that emotions of animosity can be expressed through the language of more compassionate sentiments because the international affective climate favours rhetoric through solidarity and helping to induce identification. So it is much easier to express the emotion of enmity through the language of compassion. For example, vaccine nationalism was expressed at the European level as a common vaccination programme that emphasized European solidarity. This seemed, in its own temporal context, inherently positive, but it also meant that vaccination became harder in other parts of the world. The same applies to public attitudes in other vaccine-producing nations and blocs. The needs of one's own citizens had to come first; compassion for others was seen as the next stage. Emergency scenarios produce prioritization that is based on the sentiment of containment expressed through the language of hierarchical compassion. For example, one can state the compassion felt towards one's own local community, nation, or even Western democracies, in a more legitimate way than one can express open hostility towards some more distant group. This language of compassion provides another example of how the sentiment of containment is signified in the contemporary rushes inherent in emergencies. This 'emergencisation'—the process of turning a situation into something unusual and extraordinary—has a pattern that provides this work a comprehensive research method.[14]

The sudden disappearance of regularity that is inherent in emergencies has a spatial dimension as well, which leads to a collapse of vastness and to a sudden projection of intense close-at-home sentiments into a condensed 'faraway place'. Whereas spatial distance acts as a buffer from the effects of international emergencies, distance as related to humanitarian emergencies turns into something to be crossed by outsiders rushing in to ameliorate the situation. The emergency-embedded compassion annuls distance and calls for accompanying sentiments of containment. For example, the supposedly compassionate intervention implicitly makes sure that the distant sufferers are contained to the location of the emergency. In pandemic-related emergencies, the containment of people into a specific geographical location is explicit and encouraged by public reaction. Containment is stressed over compassion, while acts of separation and isolation are framed as compassionate from the viewpoint of overall global health.

Conflicts—external and internal—have often been constructed as passionate movements in methodological nationalism or internationalism. Sentiments ranging from disdain, superiority, hostility, and anger to compassion are equated with the movements and with the changing power relations signalled by them. The general idea is that changes in power hierarchies trigger emotions and stimulate participation in further flare-ups of collective feelings. The power status differences are established, challenged, and reinforced by emotions (Lutz and Abu-Lughod 1990: 14). In this way, for example, the social practices of shame and mourning may channel open anger into emotions that strengthen factional or communal solidarity (Durkheim 1965: 443). This type of channelling seems to be quite common. But emotions also have a darker side, as when they feed antagonisms and mutually exclusive in-group cohesions and divisions between oppositional out-groups and power-holding in-groups.

Emergencies contain unique temporal and spatial embeddings with associated characteristics such as containment, rush, cyclical patterns, flows, and acute vulnerability. Whereas a spatial feature is essential in conventional international crises and conflicts, the contemporary emergency practice involves a heightened sense of scarcity of time, the opposite of what Thucydides recommended for good governance, that is, provident delay. The window for effective intervention seems to be closing. This pervasive closing-in sentiment leads to a compelling expectation that something needs to be done, and done now. Politicians do not have the option of doing nothing. A sense of urgency favours a mood of rapid action and the normative preference of haste over time-consuming deliberation. All attention becomes concentrated on one critical moment in time. The scarcity or lack of time becomes increasingly salient when the rush to find solutions is accompanied by an accelerated tempo of events. The overall impression of an emergency suggests a temporalized context of a specific sequence of events—the initial triggering event, rush to contain, effective management activity, and the eventual restoration of normalcy.

Yet this expected trajectory can turn on its head in emergencies where the situation spirals seriously out of control.

The underlying necessity of containment is an integral part of compassion-laden practices. Political sympathies remain limited to conceptually containing national and cultural identities. The sight of pandemic sufferers arouses compassion, but it takes the form of severing of ties of contact. The suffering of a person with an epidemic disease is a sight that can lead to the political sentiment of indifference, failure to identify, and even fear. The immediate and first worry is for a community that is closer home. A pandemic emergency as a political spectacle brings to the fore embodied scenarios that highlight existing boundaries and necessitate the erection of new ones. The compassion for distant suffering is instinctively relegated to secondary status. Thus, a pandemic emergency blurs 'normalcy' in a way that underlines containment over compassion. The erection of various we-communities is a constitutive element of the downward flow involved in pandemic emergencies. And the emotional motion gives rise to a unique pandemic ethics, where the rush for finding a solution and erecting boundaries become an essential virtue. Pandemic emergencies produce complex considerations of connectedness, a sense of complex entanglement, and negative interdependency. In this way, contagion engrosses the popular imagination as it envisions scenarios of temporal regression and spatial entanglement.

When Contagion in Politics Combines with Contagious Diseases

It can be suggested that public health issues are easy to use as excuses for other forms of (mis)governance because public health appears to be an apolitical field of expertise.[15] There is a valence between public health and power politics in that public health can be co-opted for power-political interests and for the co-current trajectories of enmity. The flow of power-politics, especially when fixed by security concerns and when there is a perception of a power struggle, easily adapts public health concerns to fit the overall general dynamics. Furthermore, the overall dynamics' main anxieties are always regarding patterns of political animosity and the internal coherence of particular we-communities.

It is because of these likely focuses that health-based power-political co-options may be seen as a register of a larger ongoing power struggle: for example, the increasing enmity between the US and China formed a scenario in which COVID-19 could become a register and signifier of the underlying conflict. Therefore, it is useful to examine first the potentials for co-optive patterns of pandemic security. International health efforts can offer ways of diverting attention from problems closer home and co-opting them for the purposes of bringing about a sense of more coherent and legitimate governance at home and its projections more globally.

As a starting point, one can say that just as there is bad public health governance in the developing countries, there are equally acute problems closer to the hegemonic heartlands of the West. The public health systems in the developed countries are under much stress. For example, the emphasis on curative health and on individual health can come at the expense of more general public health measures. The number of uninsured people in the US can be seen as a major public health risk as also the lack of pandemic preparedness planning and capabilities. Another major health issue is the misuse and overuse of antibiotics and other drugs that can lower the ability to contain major diseases and lead to the development of drug-resistant superbugs. This poses the risk that drug-resistant forms of HIV and AIDS or tuberculosis might become rampant. It is clear from these examples that health governance is experiencing problems in the developed parts of the world too, not just in the developing regions.

However, there are deeper patterns of co-option thrown up by the contemporary pandemic threats. These reasons have to do with power trajectories in the key we-communities. The underlying group identities might be experiencing difficulties and strains that require externalization. Different diversionary uses of external interventions often stem from the dynamics of in-group solidarity, the need to create rally-round-the-flag effects.

One important in-group problem dynamic that sheds light on the political usefulness of the different forms of interventionism is offered by the practice of diversionary actions, or foreign campaigns, as a pretext. There is a long tradition of the state—both the hegemonic and the other—initiating seemingly legitimate interventions for ulterior motives (Goodman 2006: 107). The image of 'humanitarian rescue' can offer attractive opportunities for a relatively safe expression of enmity. Diversionary practices offer insights into the underlying linkages that push and pull different actors to engage with each other. In the COVID-19 context, the seemingly other-interested protective equipment and vaccine diplomacy were at least partially motivated by the need to demonstrate China's or Russia's capacity to safeguard the health of others and thereby show domestically to their citizens the more effective nature of their government and to other citizens that their governments cannot be as trusted to take care of them.

At first glance, the diversionary tactics seem far removed from the practices of global international health. Nevertheless, even when health interventions do not form the primary avenue of diversionary interventions, they are part of the gamut of different types of interventions. Furthermore, it should be noted that public health measures can be used as a pretext for exporting different sets of values in the name of public hygiene and good health governance. The US HIV- and AIDS-related President's Emergency Plan for AIDS Relief (PEPFAR) programme in Africa was accused of spreading traditional American values, for example, in the form of 'abstinence only' measures (Aaltola 2008: 69). These conservative values were part of the domestic US culture wars and were very necessary for the coherence of a particular in-group in the US during the George W. Bush administration. The associated strand of conservatism was heavily influenced by the evangelical movement and the emergence of the religious right in the US. In this sense, it often refers to the programmatic idea that Christian values should be applied in the public life of the nation. In this context, themes such as abortion, homosexuality, and abstinence education have functioned as rallying calls, and these religiously founded ideas have led to strong movements of political mobilization. From this perspective, the PEPFAR programme was co-opted by evangelical groups in their missions in Africa. The internal political dynamics came to be projected outwards in the form of various public health interventions.

Lebow's (1981: 23) general pretext model for foreign interventions includes appeals for wide domestic support as well as for signalling to other states the legitimacy of the actions taken in the various target states. In terms of rational choice, the diversionary model can be defined as follows: leaders faced with domestic troubles, who anticipate being contested, often choose to undertake foreign interventions and campaigns to create domestic social cohesion and to divert attention from their domestic problems and to embark upon aggressive foreign policies and wars (Smith 1998: 625; Levy 1988: 666). The basic rationale of an actor engaged in such externalizations of underlying domestic strains stems from the belief that in-group cohesion tends to increase with the onset of foreign interventions. According to this model, the existence of compassion or containment-related arguments lowers the pressure for other actors to resist the intervening state. Therefore, it is in the strategic interest of a diversionary state with in-group problems to argue for action based on compassion and containment, for example, on the grounds of humanitarianism or public health. However, since political emotions are involved, the action is never solely based on rational power-political calculations. Rather, the diversionary action might flow naturally and even unnoticed when an in-group is stimulated by the specificities of political problems and governance regressions in the perceived emergency area.

Most formulations of the diversionary dynamics tend to be rationalistic. Diversion refines the choices available to a political leader, different regime types are differently disposed to diversions, and different types of domestic contestations and conflicts have different diversionary outcomes. Gelpi (1997: 256) argues that when faced with internal problems, state leaders have at least three approaches from which to choose. First, they can appease the domestic opposition through dialogue and concessions. Second, they can repress and bypass the opposition by more coercive means. Third, they can try to restore a favourable status quo by cohesion-creating diversionary activity abroad. Pandemic emergencies can offer an avenue, to a degree, to carry out such missions of vaccine diplomacy. A foreign diversion and its accompanying rally-round-the-flag effect may offer a solution to the early symptoms of in-group troubles. When the in-group troubles have escalated to the point of internal violence, foreign war may not seem a viable option. For a disintegrated domestic in-group, anything 'foreign' is already conceptually problematic. These places can become the targets of other less regressed states' 'benevolence' in the form of humanitarian campaigns, health interventions, and military action.

Thus, domestic reasons can lead to various diversionary interventions. The reasons constitute the 'push factor' of diversionary practices. The directionality of the diversionary actions is often determined by the 'pull factor'—certain places and groups within these places are more identifiable in their suffering or in their enmity. The pull of these target groups can determine what direction the diversionary and co-optive tactics take within the general enmity scenario where pandemic emergency is one dominant characteristic.

Approaching the issue from the Thucydidean neoclassical viewpoint entertained here, regressive communal trajectories have a tendency to get entangled. States experiencing in-group problems are fixated with them. They become sensitive to seeing the signs of similar regressions in other places. At the same time, failing communities that are further along the regressive slope actively draw in outside interventions, diversions, and co-options. In line with the argument delineated here, diversionary practices can be approached from a less strategic or rational perspective, which is more sensitive to the different in-groups' identity dynamics. It is notable that in the rationalistic models, the direction of causality is thought to be straightforward: domestic strife encourages foreign aggression (Dassel and Reinhardt 1999: 56). Besides the push factor of the domestic in-group problems, the pull factor of the site where the projection takes place has been rarely considered. It could be equally likely that highly visible problems in some out-group communities stimulate or pull other actors into diversions in the form of highly visible interventionism. The pull factor of a failing political community caught in the vortex of spreading and deepening violence offers further insights into the patterns of co-option between different actors. This general regressive nexus provides a dynamic context for the broader understanding of pandemic spectacles. On the one hand, pandemic scares are reflections of broad anxieties in the viability of the present hegemonic in-group. On the other hand, the interventions made in the name of global health security become ingredients in the overall complex entanglements of a world in crisis. In a world where the distinction between the nearby and the distant becomes blurred, various forms of containment-based interventions are in high demand. It is in this world that pandemics become extremely scary and their powerful visual rhetoric starts to express other types of enmities. In this complex entanglement, the threat posed by a foreign actor can start to resemble a lethal epidemic disease.

The largely non-cognitive nature of the push–pull effect means that diversionary practices may become less strategic as states drift down the intervention-enabled slope.

The contagion models of political conflict shed additional light on the push-and-pull dynamics involved in diversionary intentions and co-optive tactics. The term 'contagion' refers to the idea that political agitation in one location influences the possibility of similar political contestation in another location either by increasing its likelihood or by causing increasing immunity (Li and Thompson 1975: 63). Contagion in politics and economics often refers to the rapid transmission and spreading of disturbances throughout a region in a way that eludes 'efforts to control its scope, speed and direction' (Koslowski and Kratochwil 1994: 215, 247). Contagion is a metaphor, or a metonym, in political language, especially in scenarios of growing major enmities. For example, blaming China for COVID-19 combines two elements: the actual physical contagious disease and a sense of China's growing influence as a type of contagious danger. This combination of actual and political characteristics is partially tactical. However, this combined contagion dynamic is also quasi-cognitive—it refers, in this sense, to the flows of emotional content, to the spread of a mood, sentiment, attitude, and judgements. The contagion dynamic can assume different forms. Besides the spread of technical mimicry, the transmission of symbolic– 'performative' content is central to this type of contagion under the emergency rush. The contagions can be understood as stimulating and agitating content that seems to make sense in a particular temporal context irrespective of the underlying facts. It seems that unconscious and habitual political dispositions and dynamics matter (Mayer 1969: 294).

Pandemic Dynamics and Trajectories of Enmity

The discourses on contagion and diversion illuminate crucial elements of the underlying directionality of the regressive flow. They also provide ways to understand how pandemic emergencies and enmity practices—such as diversions, pretences, and co-options—can become constitutive elements of the overall flow.

Pandemic scares provide opportune moments for channelling underlying great power enmities as well as domestic pressures. There are two general reasons for this. The first reason stems from the tendency of global health governance and security to remain relatively apolitical. Their more political content remains relatively under the radar of global attention and, therefore, the pandemic practice offers the ideal excuse for political co-option. For example, the explicitly humanitarian language of health development has been tightly connected with colonial practices. As a frame, it helped in creating the perception that the colonial powers were in the business of helping Africa, rather than conquering it (Brantlinger 1985: 167–8). Imperial expansion was turned into a necessary curative and apolitical movement: 'Ostensibly removed from the realm of land and politics, colonisation viewed through the lens of salutary medical aid was made to seem essentially humanitarian' (Kelm 1998: 101). Besides noticing the intimate connection of public health with empire or nation-building, it is important to note that this political function made the related field of expertise very powerful in the domestic context. Its job was to maintain the general perception of curability in the more constricted sense not only of epidemic control but, in a broader sense, of political progression and health. Among the important demonstrating grounds of curability was what Bruno Latour terms the 'theatre of proof' (Latour 1988). The core of this health theatre was essentially a laboratory experiment, which became an essential testing ground for modern state governance expertise, transferred into the field—for example, into the African landscape. The colonial practice offered 'fields' for the demonstrations of efficacy. The related interventionist practices gained political legitimacy when fields, such as in Africa, were made to visibly show signs of Western-induced health.

The second reason is that the language of pandemics is part of the more general rubric through which enmity is felt and made tangible in international relations. From this perspective, the ways in which lethal epidemic diseases are made understandable and significant are inherently similar to the ways in which political threats are perceived. Consequently, 'disease language' tends to acknowledge and reaffirm the existing patterns of political authority and the beliefs about 'natural' power hierarchies separating different actors (Gwyn 1999; Larson *et al.* 2005; Nerlich 2007). Moreover, political violence and its sub-categories are commonly treated in terms of a disease (Spilerman 1970). In their treatment of state failure, Zartman (1995: 9) states that '[s]tate collapse is a long-term degenerative disease'. There are numerous additional examples equating extreme political violence with a disease-like regressive process. Most and Starr (1980) refer to 'war disease' when they discuss the diffusion of war. Holden (1986: 875) connects the related phenomenon of aircraft hijacking to 'skyjack virus'. Hamilton and Hamilton (1983: 41) state that the main paradigm in terrorism studies holds that 'terrorist incidents may encourage further violence through a process of imitation or diffusion, giving rise to a dynamics of terrorism analogous to that observed in the spread of a contagious disease'.

The general disease discourse offers a useful template for making events in the international realm seem tangible. The embodied object world evoked by using the disease metaphor is everyday enough for people to tangibly understand the intended meaning of political rhetoric. There are umpteen examples of this. Former US president Jimmy Carter stated in a speech on 4 January 1980, soon after the Soviet troops rolled into Afghanistan: 'Aggression unopposed becomes a contagious disease.' In today's context, these words are meaningful through the analogous associations that they contain. They draw from the dynamics of disease in explaining the meaning of international events. They hyperbolize the importance of the otherwise distant place with individual-level danger, immediacy, and urgency due to diseases. This same frame was used by former US president Barack Obama, according to the book, *Obama's Wars*, by Bob Woodward (2010). Obama stressed that 'we need to make clear to people that the cancer is in Pakistan'. The gradual failure of Pakistan, a nuclear state, coupled with the fact that the US' prime enemy, the Al-Qaeda, had established a stronghold in Pakistan, was made concrete by the use of disease language. In his speech of 1 December 2009, Obama stated, 'We're in Afghanistan to prevent a cancer from once again spreading through that country. But this same cancer has also taken root in the border region of Pakistan. That's why we need a strategy that works'. Former US president Donald Trump's talk about COVID-19 as a 'China virus' had important political precursors, as regressive political influences are often seen in terms of contagious diseases. A further variant of this is seeing diseases as a cause of political regression. Obama's speech in New York at the Millennium Development Goals Summit on 9 September 2010 nicely illustrates such parallelism: 'When millions of fathers cannot provide for their families, it feeds the despair that can fuel instability and violent extremism. When a disease goes unchecked, it can endanger the health of millions around the world.' Because political enmity and physical diseases have historically been conflated, the arguments for the relevancy of each and/or both can be used in close proximity without betraying any sense of mixing apples with oranges. To further examine the parallelism enabled by the embodied sense of diseases and pandemics, the following text from the White House pages on the progress of Home Land Security is illustrative: 'Attacks using improvised nuclear devices or biological weapons, as well as outbreaks of a pandemic disease, pose a serious and increasing national security risk. We will focus on reducing the risk of these high-consequence, non-traditional threats'. The integrated approach to meeting the threats of rogue states and terrorism subsumes many of the defences against naturally occurring diseases. The probable result is that the occurrence of natural epidemic diseases heightens security concerns and recontextualizes the epidemics in a quasi-security language.

The contagion parallelism demonstrates the reactive combinability of somatic-level epidemic threats. The various situational scenarios of both naturally occurring pandemics and politically conceived enmities overlap in ways that result in the perception that pandemic threats contain a significant political enmity-related knowledge modality. The most significant consequence of this is that security-centred language and the language of physical disease share a vital embodied modality without which neither frame is fully meaningful. This sharing between the two overlapping frames can be used to understand present-day perceptions and incidence of pandemic scares—that is, scares in the absence of significant disease outbreaks. The heightened security environment of the last decade easily leads into imagined pandemic embodiment since the template for them is actively present in the figurative discourse of political rhetoric, strategy, and practice. Thus, pandemic scares and governance interventions against them are a natural consequence of the overall power-political flows of our time. In the context of the growing great power contestation, one can echo Susan Sontag's claim that notable diseases are always ideally comprehensible in their own time. And this political modality of the recent incidences of pandemics renders them as something other than how they appear in medical textbooks.

A Synoptic Approach to Pandemic Emergencies

The constancy and integrity between processes can be entangled in the context of major emergencies. When the situation is ablaze with unfolding actions and reactions, the increasing tempo recontextualizes processes that were earlier considered politically and analytically sedate. Apples combine with oranges, to use a saying that I often employ to teach my students how proper analysis should be done. Yet there are situations where this clarity and integrity would do no justice to the comprehensive entanglement of issues that do not usually combine. The message of Thucydides' method seems to be this. I started this book with a quote from Shakespeare referring to plague leading to extreme remedies. However, another quote from Shakespeare's *Julius Caesar*, 'That every like is not the same', offers important insights into the Thucydidean method. The words of Brutus in the play yield an explanation for his sudden change from loyal friend to assassin. Larger unfolding series of events overwhelm underlying micro-level loyalties and provide an answer to the amazement inherent in the question, '*Et tu, Brute?*'[16] The brutal dis-eased reality of things is unravelled as the component, which, though it previously had its own separate character, suddenly becomes recontextualized in the stirring roughness of the emergent kinetic impulse.

The kinesis can lead into stasis. The integrity of processes and of people suddenly changes, as they did in the aforementioned stasis of Corcyra: '[A]nd so there fell upon the cities on account of revolutions many grievous calamities, such as happen and always will happen while human nature is the same' (3.82). A similar temporal process overtook Rome when it entered into the civil war that led to the demise of the Roman republic.[17] The situational requirement of that clash overpowered normality and the categorical separations inherent in prototypical situations. To paraphrase Thucydides' idea of war as a violent teacher, a situation is a pedagogical setting, and emergency scenarios, as temporal contexts, are teachers of fear, reversal of virtues and vices, loss of memory, uncertainty between domestic and foreign, and tendency towards rushed and striking actions (3.82). This recurrence of a scenario with specific frames, flows, and situational abnormal/regressive requirements is also the key to Thucydides' description of the Plague of Athens:

> All speculation as to its origin and its causes, if causes can be found adequate to produce so great a disturbance, I leave to other writers, whether lay or professional; for myself, I shall simply set down its nature, and explain the symptoms by which perhaps it may be recognised by the student, if it should ever break out again. This I can the better do, as I had the disease myself, and watched its operation in the case of others.
>
> *(2.48)*

This echoes Thucydides' overall method in the book. Certain situational scenarios with a blend of political, social, and psychological characteristics are likely to occur again. He gives us an account of these scenarios so that we can recognize them in time, learn from them, and act in time to avoid the worst implications of the bruteness they bring in their wake.

Drawing from the Thucydidean insights, pandemic emergencies can—depending on their political context—be revelatory moments and catalyse such revealed situational requirements as the 'thing to do' now and here. They reveal and initiate temporal instants during which the normal leeway for political actions and sources of legitimacy can change. Policies are innovated and power reconfigured. During the avian flu emergency, the idea of interspecies mutability caught widespread attention. The engrossing images of dead birds and animals being culled carried with them a profound message about the meaning of the times and what should be done, but only as a function of the right circumstances. The situational characteristics offered ways of understanding the pandemic scare in a more innovative and transformative way.

In the following chapters, I will delineate case studies that emphasize particular political dynamics, situational requirements, and combinatory features of epidemic and pandemic emergencies. This work is based on historical analysis but draws from the comprehensive method that Thucydides applied in his analysis:

1   Emergency scenarios do not happen in a vacuum, and they are resistant to analytical categorization or functional separation between fields of expertise. There are multiple global scenarios—such as wars, conflicts, terror attacks, other outbreaks, natural catastrophes—occurring at the same time. The pandemic scenario can be the prevailing emergency scenario; however, it can also be nested within and entangled with other co-occurring scenarios such as great power enmity. These combined or nested characteristics between a pandemic scenario and other scenarios change the nature of what aspects of a pandemic scenario are seen as real, important, and consequential.

2   The pandemic emergency scenarios have characteristics that combine with other concurrent scenarios in a relatively path-dependent way. These key historically well-rehearsed combinatory aspects are, for example, 'hostilization' (turning the pattern of a pandemic into something that fits patterns of enmity), localization/nationalization (the disease is associated with one locality or nation), ethnicization (it is seen as related to certain practices and customs), internationalization (it is seen as having a relationship with international institutions and outside states), sexualization/moralization (it is seen as the consequence of 'bad', 'immoral', or 'civil irreligious' habits), and speciesism (it turns the interspecies boundary into something that is inherently hostile and unnatural). This means that there is a logic in the situational combinations that a pandemic gets. This combinatorics—logic of situational combinations and historical combinability—is one key to a more comprehensive analysis of pandemic emergencies.

3   A pandemic cannot be approached as a single self-contained process: an analytic approach usually follows two general patterns. First, studies can satisfy scholarly interest through initial mapping of implicit and explicit knowledge so as to better allow for a subsequent, more nuanced explanation and model building, weeding out more stable and relevant elements from a mass of observations and different data sources. However, this simple two-step analytic approach is best suited to cases in which the phenomenon is a single self-contained unit in itself—that is, it does not consist of an open-ended bundle of multifarious linkages and seemingly incompatible characteristics. Although this approach is often used in scholarly articles that seem to require such a delimiting approach, the real scenarios of global life are often much more complex and entangled to allow for such a clear-cut method here. Second, it is possible to overview different overlapping scenarios and discover a synoptic variety and to see how the combinatorial possibilities are actualized in them (Cioffi 2010: 301). This second type of synoptic overview applied in this book

answers to different types of scholarly puzzles than the first analytical alternative. What are of interest here are the synoptic potentials, valences, which need to be approached from diverse angles to build a fuller understanding of how the actual, potential, and circumstantial are interrelated (Wittgenstein 1980: 37). The overview approach utilized here suggests a discovery process that is based on an examination of historically and coincidentally established combinatorial possibilities. This discovery is done by (1) trying out how different scenarios are combinable historically and conceptually and (2) detecting how these possibilities and valencies are relevant in contemporaneous events. So the synoptic overview method applied here contains a kind of game of discovery and innovation unbound by customary ways of arranging and containing knowledge. An overview of synoptic plays is instrumental in drawing novel associations—and in gaining insights. Associated facts and co-occurring processes are collated and shuffled with the expressed intent to reveal novel combinatorial possibilities. In this sense, the first step of the synoptic method is to discern the prevailing myths of why some aspects of global life merit volumes of attention from one particular angle, while others are left relatively unstudied. This includes why pandemic emergencies are usually treated outside of their relationship with power-politics and the fears elicited in us as political animals.

Notes

1 For a more recent account in the same genre of grand history, and world history, see Diamond (1997).
2 Jared Diamond's *Guns, Germs and Steel* (1997) further reinforces this point by pointing out how virulence, rather than virtuosity, led to European dominance of the world.
3 It is noteworthy that the Greek root concept, 'nosos', describes both the condition of political chaos/confusion and the outbreak of epidemic disease.
4 See Greenwood (2020) for examples of Thucydides' growing relevance in the times of COVID-19.
5 Richard Crawley translation of Thucydides. In Hobbes translation: 'by reason of the alteration, into strange diseases'.
6 Or kinēsis autē megistē.
7 Aristotle also uses the medical terminology of his time in relation to political violence. For him, stasis refers to the coming into being of a stop in the overall motion of a polis. The emergence of multiple contradictory movements halts the overall telos. This equation of stasis with the medical disequilibrium of a body was also shared by Plato (Kalimtzis 2000: xv, 19).
8 On how Hippocrates' ideas have affected Thucydides' political thought, see Jouanna (2012: Ch. 2).
9 For example, Aristotle (Pol. IV.16 1300b35–38) uses kinesis in terms of negative, badly managed changes. See also Skultety (2009).
10 'When the god was asked whether they [the Lacedaemonians] should go to war, he answered that if they put their might into it, victory would be theirs, and that he would himself be with them. Events were supposed to tally with this oracle. For the plague broke out as soon as the Peloponnesians invaded Attica, and never entering Peloponnese

(not at least to an extent worth noticing), committed its worst ravages in Athens, and next to Athens, at the most populous of the other towns' (Thucydides: 2.47).

11 In the Homeric hymns (nr. 28), the sea swirls in confusion (*ekinethe*) at the birth of Athena. Thus, fluidity and flux and other Poseidonic qualities are abundant in Athenian iconography.

12 'A more fitting image of stasis motion would be to visualize it as movement that has strayed off the main highway . . . travel along the side roads leads to nowhere, for these are endlessly and hopelessly looped' (Kalimtzis 2000: 125).

13 During this period, Ethiopia was viewed as the furthest part of the world—as something far, far away (see Herodotus: 3.114).

14 On emergencization, see, for example, Wenham (2019: 1093).

15 On the contention between politics and apolitical governance, see, for example, Louis and Maertens (2021).

16 Shakespeare had likely studied Thucydides through the first translations into English (e.g. Franko 2009: 234). Another direct influence between Thucydides and Shakespeare is through Plutarch.

17 See, for example, Peer (2015: 71).

4

GLOBAL MOBILITY-BASED ORDER

The Disruptions of SARS and COVID-19

The bridgehead into this chapter is constrained and contradictory: diseases know no borders, and the global mobility system crosses political borders in a relatively seamless way, yet national politics is still based on an archipelago of contained political entities. This tangled order is now being challenged by a new menace. The corona family of viruses that caused the SARS in the spring of 2003, the MERS in 2012, and coronavirus disease (COVID-19) in late 2019 seems to be uniquely adaptable to the vulnerabilities of the present global order. The key contagion vector has been the global mobility system, in particular its human mobility through air travel. The signifier of the global order suffered a major setback with the recognition that COVID-19 arrived in all the countries of the world except China mainly through air travel. For good and bad, the medicalized sphere of our existence has expanded hand in hand with the increasingly interconnected global economic and political order, thereby heightening the exposure between individual bodies and the wider global order of things. In particular, the encounters with SARS and COVID-19 have brought medical and security scenarios of daily life together with an acute understanding of their global scope. A politosomatic relationship has opened up wherein individual-level anxieties feed into worries concerning the dangers of the global political order and its corresponding distance-crossing mobility structures.

It seems that 'we have entered a new era of deep microbial unease' which includes 'the growing tendency to articulate international health policy in the metaphors and vocabulary of security' (Elbe 2011). Pandemic security scenarios readily and reactively combine with other scenarios such as global order and security, the great power contestations, and other more regional and national perceived insecurities. In Chapter 3, I reviewed the historically influential Thucydidean proposition wherein conflicts and plagues can be parts of the same overall entangled scenario and that they can be combinable if they occur in the same temporal framework,

DOI: 10.4324/9781003169147-4

one increasing the likelihood of the other. Chapter 3 also gave an account of the method whereby we can study the consonantial—non-causal and non-linear—interactions between politics and pestilences. This chapter focuses on the importance of the global mobility system embodied in the worldwide hub-and-spoke system of air travel, its linkages with contagious diseases, and the overall combined effect that delegitimizes the underlying premises of the coupled and interdependent globalized world.

In the case of pandemic emergencies, while pandemics are securitized and politicized to fit the contemporaneous patterns of enmity, simultaneously, the security situation and political order interact and adapt to the medical and epidemiological realm's processes and authorities. The scenarios interact through, for example, the wave patterns the contagious diseases can take on and through medical attempts to control the severity and spread of the disease through, for example, practices of containment, physical distancing, lockdowns, and vaccination efforts. The 'blend', 'combination', or 'bonding' of the otherwise relatively incompatible elements of order, security, and health happens because of the high stakes involved in the intermeshing of the pandemic emergency scenario with the scenario of the world order in flux, or under challenge, while the sense of human vulnerability has heightened.

The SARS of 2003 can enlighten us on how contagion and security can interact in an already unstable and contentious global political climate. Let us consider for a moment the following scene from the spring of 2003, when the then US secretary of state, Colin Powell, gave a much anticipated and hyped-up speech to the United Nations Security Council on 5 February 2003. The aim of the speech was to convince and persuade: 'My colleagues, every statement I make today is backed up by sources, solid sources. These are not assertions. What we are giving you are facts and conclusions based on solid intelligence'. Powell concretized the WMDs particularly through their biological disease-related dimension, arguably to make the threat easier to understand: 'Saddam Hussein has investigated dozens of biological agents causing diseases such as gas-gangrene, plague, typhus, tetanus, cholera, camelpox, and hemorrhagic fever. And he also has the wherewithal to develop smallpox'. The point was that Saddam, as an antagonist figure, had turned plagues into weapons:

> There can be no doubt that Saddam Hussein has biological weapons and the capability to rapidly produce more, many more. And he has the ability to dispense these lethal poisons and diseases in ways that can cause massive death and destruction. . . . Less than a teaspoon of dry anthrax, a little bit—about this amount. This is just about the amount of a teaspoon. Less than a teaspoon full of dry anthrax in an envelope shut down the United States Senate in the fall of 2001. This forced several hundred people to undergo emergency medical treatment and killed two postal workers just from an amount, just about this quantity that was inside of an envelope.

Powell's use of contamination and contagion imageries was meant to legitimize the necessity of decontamination and containment through a large-scale military operation against Saddam's Iraq. The military action that ensued as a result of this combinatorial act was framed as a practicable and reasonable yet existential exercise, just like a doctor treating a cancerous growth in a patient. Historically, examples abound of using the threat of lethal contagion as a reason for military intervention and operations, thereby setting the stage for valence between contagions and political/military acts of containment. It should be noted that the 2003 SARS epidemic was concurrent with the Iraq War. It provided the backdrop that reinforced the imagery rather than providing a key part of the lead-up to the large-scale troop mobilization in the Persian Gulf around Iraq. Rather than providing a seemingly revelatory part of the argument, the fear of pandemics provided a persuasive characteristic that added value to the overall scenario's comprehension.

In this chapter, the key question has to do with the mobility-based global order rather than a more specific military scenario. How have SARS and COVID-19 changed our ways of understanding the sustainability of the globalized rule-based order or, more specifically, its underlying logistical mobility systems? Has the mode of global governance changed? Or is it viewed now as less legitimate and more vulnerable because of the two pandemic shocks?

All tense temporal contexts in world politics have synoptic potentials whereby seemingly unrelated processes can form surface-level or deeper confluences, which need to be approached from diverse angles to build a fuller understanding of how the actual, potential, and circumstantial are interrelated. The comprehensive approach utilized in this chapter suggests a discovery process that is based on an examination of not-so-obvious combinatorial possibilities. This discovery is done by (1) examining their historically entangled trajectories (see Chapters 2 and 3), (2) permuting the possible scenarios to discover the likely linkages/valences, and (3) discerning and comparing past cross-cutting confluences between distinct and separate categories of events.[1] This chapter compares and contrasts the mobility-related characteristics of the 2003 SARS and 2020 COVID-19 cases using this method to answer the key research question concerning the likely consequences of the disease scenarios for the now prevailing global order.

Separate Yet Entangled: Contagious Diseases and World-Order Mobilities

It is clear that treating global processes as separate, self-contained, and closed bundles with no interaction would be analytically satisfying. However, this would distil away many relevant and consequential entanglements that provide meaning at a particular moment in time. International events have a modality of promiscuity that involves relative contingency and association between conventionally dissimilar processes at any moment in time. More precisely, instead of conventional and conceptual clarity, the co-occurring and simultaneous sequences of events entangle with one another and other incidental characteristics. Any comprehensive scenario building has to take into account the consonantial dimension across simultaneous dynamics. The combinatorial connections are based on these consonancies whereby different bundles of events interfere and resonate with one another. Against this background, the mobility-based global order can interact with a pandemic disease. Moreover, as explained before, the interaction is not without historically well-trodden and rehearsed paths.

Global and regional orders are characterized by regular patterns and shaped flows of raw materials, goods, people, services, and data. The key pattern to many of these global and sub-global flow systems is a hub-and-spoke system with megahubs, regional hubs, national hubs, and spokes of various types. That is to say that the regularity is distinguished by infrastructural, logistical, and operational power with regard to regulated and sanctioned mobility from one place to another. National political and economic success is seen as depending on the ability to act as efficient hubs or relay nodes for such defining global flows as trade, resources, and finance. Moreover, the mobility of people is seen as a key part of this, as they negotiate, agree, and manage the mobility system and the value-add that can be gained through it. It is not only tourism but the movement of people to do business that has been vital for the functioning of the system.

Along with the people's flows, economic, technological, commercial, trade, and, related to this, international diplomacy and political power are also on the move, and these find their expressive language in the varying tempos of the mobile bodies. The humming regularity of the national, regional, and global air mobility systems is often used to constitute and signify the power of the 'movers and shakers' in the global economy and politics. The opposite is equally true: the regular disturbances and disruptions in the hub-and-spoke dynamic translate into lack of or decreasing power-related activities. For example, Northern Italy is a fashion and textile industry powerhouse. However, the goods designed there are not produced there but through complex production and value-add chains run by people. A significant amount of the production takes place in the Wuhan region of China. The smoothness and intensity of this flow of activities run by people caused the disruption—the fast spread of COVID-19 from Wuhan to Northern Italy in the first weeks of 2020 through the vector of global air mobility. For the added economic value to be produced and for people to enjoy their designer clothing at relatively cheap price points, there had to be a smooth flow of a kinaesthetic assemblage of people. However, these people—who can be called road warriors—were also somatic; they were as vulnerable as anybody else to the new SARS variant spreading in Wuhan towards the end of 2019. Instead of being road warriors sustaining a particular industry with their mobility, they turned into (super)spreaders in the onset phase of COVID-19, as it started to hit the industrially developed parts of the world.

The usual protagonist figure, the global order's road warrior, is a figure embodying the qualities of innovation, initiative, and leadership. This figure is a professional citizen of the seamless skies. Moreover, the figure is multi-mobile and does not get stuck in airports or hotels but blows ahead aided by a sense of duty and rewarded with air-mile cards and airport lounges. This nomadic protagonist of the global order embodies leadership that is deemed lacking at the more constricted and stationary local and national spoke levels. When flights were scaled down due to the pandemic's flight restrictions, the empty airspace, flights, and airports signified the opposite—the vacuum at the leadership level. The pandemic emergency also produced passive and paralysed subjectivities, a full range of stranded figures. These subjectivities were described as hopeless, enraged, tired, and in disarray at the global airports and hotels. At this stage of the lockdowns, the antagonistic figure was one of marked indifference—people who were still crossing boundaries irrespective of the disease and the health guidelines. They were bypassing the containment through side links and back channels.

Anecdotes and travelogues reported during the travel restrictions offer a window into the embodied aspects of different people as they moved across continents and inside regions in, to a degree, an improvised and experimental manner because of the historical-scope disruption. Many were trying to get back to their homes or travelling for work that could not wait. Sometimes they were suddenly ordered home because of the decisions to stop flight connections. These resulted in crowded airports, long queues, and contagion. Politics and people's bodily vulnerabilities were suddenly combined in the filled airports and in the sudden twists and turns in political decision-making. At the same time, travel was a must for some people. The world could not just stop. There was much emphasis on the security aspect of this strange multi-stop and stop-and-go journeys back to home and back to distant places to negotiate and make deals and guarantee the flow of goods. The protagonists suddenly turned into possible carriers were many, and there were many maligned figures of tourists taking risks to go on vacation and possibly bringing with them newer variants of COVID-19. People were on the move even as the contagion spread. Diplomats were taking risks to make the system run; decision makers had to meet under changed circumstances. At the same time, there were the adventurous few who were taking risks because of their lifestyle choices—continuing with their cosmopolitan lives or holidaying as per usual in faraway places. While most people were staying put, those on the move risked becoming the antagonist figures of border transgressors and disease spreaders. The moral panics were on, as was the blame game. The environment was full of rash decisions motivated by lack of preparedness and the political need to outsource blame. COVID-19's tides interacted and entangled with the established styles of living and the modes of political systems, disturbing the established value hierarchies. The open and seamless skies suddenly turned into restricted and empty skies, reversing the virtues and vices of the 'old normal'.

The near coming to a halt of the global air mobility system was a reminder of its risks, if not the mortality inherent in it. It had happened before, during 9/11. Back then, the empty airspace and diverted flights sent out a message or set a scale of harm. International airports and flights provided the sudden scene for the declinist drama, contrasting with the ideology of globalization and the modus operandi of the mobility infrastructures. In doom and gloom imagery, submergence under global influxes of 'terrorist[s]' is a signifier of not only being overwhelmed by 'corruptive' influences but also being left an acute apprehension of being unable to cope with a spreading contagion of 'carriers'. Although the imagery is largely attached to the influx of immigrants and the mixture of incompatible elements, the root metonym has to do with spread and regressive contagion as embodied in an infectious disease. For example, Huntington (2004: 30) points to uncontained borders and migration flows as a source of potential regressive decay in a political community. He was not directly talking about a dangerous spread but about a transgression by incompatible elements in terms of the regressive impact of the American creed, its civil religion. He was talking about political contagions associated with border-transgressing globalization. According to Huntington (1997: 38), contemporary linkages and mobility systems do not cut immigrants' umbilical cords in the same way as they did during previous migration waves. Links and contacts remain like a disease vector in Huntington's largely xenophobic analysis, turning people coming from different civilizations into bridgeheads of decay and erosion. It is fitting to the later anxieties related to COVID-19 and SARS that Huntington (e.g. 1998 and 2004) directly evokes medical metaphors in connection with border transgressions by equating linkages with decaying civilizations, cultures, and countries with schizophrenia; he frames the alien cultural influence as a 'virus' (e.g. Perry 2002: 40). This 'disease'—political contagion—is a symptom of allowing foreign elements into domestic environments. He paints an inherently regressive image of globalization and its ideology of diversity. For Huntington, this is a sign of submergence because it creates mixtures composed of people who are incompatible. This fits well with one strand inherent in the proto-theory of politics described here in Chapters 2 and 3—that the hybridity, border transgressions, and vectors formed between the domestic and the too foreign can supposedly lead to dangers.

In contrast to this type of civilizational ideology was the ideology of an increasingly seamless world, with the lowering of borders. After the end of the Cold War, the spirit of the times emphasized the creation of a global system of flows and mobilities that was inherently transnational and cosmopolitan. Trade liberalization and the opening of markets spread and were institutionalized in organizations such as the World Trade Organization (WTO). The wishful thinking was also that the world would democratize, and the major powers would eventually assimilate, and share similar political systems. A further idea was that the state would normalize, contain the competition to the field of the global economy, and would stop harbouring expansionistic ambitions towards its neighbours. Integration and trade liberalization were seen as leading to a peaceful world with lowered tensions. Accordingly, borders became easier to cross with some areas, such as the Schengen region, offering free movement of people and goods, which was seen as of inherent value, not in just the economic sense but also in the wider political sense. Seamless mobility systems, if efficiently governed, were seen as signs of health and progress instead of alarm and danger.

The pandemic security system after 2003 as encoded in the changed IHR of 2005 envisaged an effective system of pandemic control that did not stand in the way of the economic and political benefits seen as stemming from the seamless global system. The 2005 IHR was a response to the calls to reform one of the backbones of global life that had turned into a tangible and painful vulnerability and contagion vector—the nexus of serious contagious diseases and expanding global air travel. When the new IHR was established by the World Health Assembly in 2005, the aim was 'to prevent, protect against, control and provide a public health response to the international spread of disease in ways that are commensurate with and restricted to public health risks, and which avoid unnecessary interference with international traffic and trade' (WHO 2005, 2016). The IHR struck a balance between pandemic security and unnecessary interference with traffic and trade. As such, it tried to achieve coordinated measures that also took into consideration the need to ensure smooth flow of traffic, commerce, and trade.

The attention shifted away from containment at the state border to containing an outbreak at the local source, at the sub-state level, and flexibly throughout the air-traffic system.[2] The global pandemic security system was supposed to work based on (1) quicker local reaction on the ground based on national health, surveillance, and control measures; (2) fast alerts on serious outbreaks to WHO; and (3) a distributed system whereby the blow could be cushioned at the key global airport hubs and border-crossing places, such as harbours and land borders, by containment measures once the local outbreak containment efforts had failed (Andrus *et al.* 2010; Ferhani and Rushton 2020: 458). Important changes in the overall strategy had to do with emphasis on a tailored and flexible approach instead of the pre-SARS response pattern that was deemed to be not sensitive to the specific characteristics of the outbreak. The flexible system focused more on the spokes—local outbreak contexts—and the profiling of the disease carriers throughout the hub-centric system. At the same time, though, pandemic security had been, since the 1990s, increasingly integrated into the national security strategies that had become more comprehensive in nature. Pandemics had been nationally securitized (Ferhani and Rushton 2020: 458). This meant that the national borders did not recede to the background in a way that would have been optimal for the flexibility of the IHR if it was really going to work in a serious pandemic situation. States and the learnt history of politics and plagues still mattered. The lack of openness, the tendency towards secrecy and non-notification, and the instinct to re-establish borders were still present in the system.

Equipped with the IHR, the mobility- and circulation-based world was supposed to have a flexible framework and actors that reacted quickly and in a coordinated way to an outbreak in a manner proportional to the outbreak but still sensitive to not causing too many disruptions to the global economy and its main arteries. However, the experience of SARS left significant doubts concerning the effectiveness of the new framework. Although it had mainly naming-and-shaming-based sanctions against states failing and delaying notifications, it was not a strictly enforceable regime. Global pandemic health still depended on the cooperation of national authorities, and when the outbreak zone was located in the area of a great power with a fully developed and integrated national security culture, the cooperation could be compromised by other factors such as the need to maintain status and place the blame on others.

China's rise to a global hub position was accompanied by lingering suspicions about the 'safety' of such a rise. Would the inclusive and supposedly seamless new global health framework be efficient in the case of China's production and manufacturing linkages? In case of SARS, China was seen as hiding the true extent of the outbreak for weeks. With COVID-19, China again, initially, failed to deliver on full and quick accountability. Outside China, the system that was supposed to respond flexibly to limit the spread of the disease did not work and failed to check the contagion from becoming fully developed outbreaks in many places. The disease carriers were difficult to recognize since they could be asymptomatic; the testing was not immediately standardized; and the symptoms, such as fever and a running nose, were quite common symptoms and similar to those of, for example, seasonal flu. Clearly, the responsibility could not be delegated to the whole network if one spoke connected to key hubs became the source of infection. Whereas SARS as the first significant outbreak of the corona family of viruses came with the message to create a more secure and resilient global mobility system, COVID-19, a variant of SARS, seems to reveal the not-so-resilient nature of the fixes created after 2003.

A Seamless Sky and the Sudden Return of Borders

Just like diseases know no borders, the idea has been that the global aviopolis should be based on flows that are as smooth as possible. The cleavages and bottlenecks between state-level and global institutions were not the only failure in the management of SARS and COVID-19. The guardianship of the global air mobility system is divided between various international organizations. These organizations have not only their own roles but also the common aim to create smooth travel and trade flows. As global air flows have become a key part of globalized life, WHO, the International Air Transport Association (IATA), and the International Civil Aviation Organization (ICAO) have cooperated to play a vital role in creating an efficient, reliable, and secure critical infrastructure from setting best practices and rules to standardizing the technical and operational aspects. In response to SARS, a working group composed mainly of ICAO, WHO, and IATA developed under the auspices of ICAO a set of anti-SARS protective measures and guidelines for regular inspections.

The control and reduction of the risk of pandemic pathogens that can spread via air travel is mainly the responsibility of WHO, but ICAO and IATA also play key roles.[3] IATA is the official trade organization for the world's airlines. It has a Medical Advisory Group that specializes in aviation medicine or occupational health. Besides advising IATA on health issues related to air travel, the group liaises with WHO and ICAO on medical matters. It cooperates with WHO in order to facilitate the control of pandemic diseases. For example, IATA gave its review on the 2005 IHR in the aftermath of SARS caused by a coronavirus (IATA 2005). It is telling of its role that IATA expressed its concerns about 'inappropriate and unnecessary governmental fines and penalties'. ICAO and IATA have a long history of cooperation, for example, in training programme to promote safety, security, and sustainability standards.[4] WHO works closely with ICAO and IATA to provide accurate epidemiological data in a timely manner to further reduce the risk of diseases spreading through the air travel vector. To prevent SARS from spreading through air travel and in order to rebuild the confidence of the travelling public in the safety of air travel, ICAO set up, for example, the Anti-SARS Airport Evaluation Project. ICAO's aim has been to restore public health best practices and also increase travellers' confidence in the aftermath of SARS. The Anti-SARS Airport Evaluation Project was aimed at making airports compliant with ICAO's anti-SARS measures and to maintain preparedness against the possible resurgence of SARS and other communicable diseases that use air traffic as a vector (Finkelstein and Curdt-Christianse 2003: 1207).

The WHO regulates the global pandemic surveillance and response system. It provides technical assistance and guidance for the international community and member-states. Its leadership role is reduced by the fact that its advice, recommendations, and coordination are not binding. However, WHO's IHR is a binding agreement even though it lacks ways of enforcing them and proposes relatively weak measures against states that break them. The IHR expanded the international regulatory mechanisms to include new tools and new diseases. It also made it legally binding to provide timely and accurate information to the WHO on public health emergencies:

> Each State Party shall notify WHO, by the most efficient means of communication available, by way of the National IHR Focal Point, and within 24 hours of assessment of public health information, of all events which may constitute a public health emergency of international concern within its territory in accordance with the decision instrument, as well as any health measure implemented in response to those events.
>
> *(WHO 2005)*

Instead of enforcement powers, WHO has normative powers. It can name and shame actors although its funding is dependent on the key member-states, which makes the use of its normative tool box politically sensitive. For example, in the COVID-19 case, WHO refused to name and shame China but, instead, applauded Chinese efforts to fight it as helpful. The understandable aim was to make states collaborate in the common effort to maintain cooperation in the management of a situation that was quickly getting out of hand.

The strategy of a 'seamless sky' or a 'single sky' encompassed the reaping of 'economic benefits' by creating an efficient air traffic system with acceptable safety levels while respecting 'individual State's Sovereign territory' (ICAO 2011). The promotion of an open and seamless system was seen as valuable in itself and an interoperable system valuable in the promotion of greater economic value and growth. The idea itself is a radical departure from the patchwork on the ground where state boundaries create discontinuities. The texts concerning the strategic goal talk of the creation of 'a homogeneous continuum of upper airspace that promotes harmonized air traffic management with the same level of performance and significant benefits for users, States and service providers' (ICAO 2019). In the vast seamless airport hub system, no airport or airport authority wanted to be a weak link. Being a choke point would mean that the airport would be bypassed through alternative routes in the vast air travel network. This resulted in an incentive to harmonize regulations in line with the rest and to take what amounted to a 'liberal' attitude towards regulations and any hindrances to the smooth flow of people and cargo. WHO, ICAO, and IATA documents focus on the economic benefits with just one caveat, environmental protection. It seems that besides air safety, the security scenario included climate change and took into account the need for the industry to decrease emissions. However, pandemic emergency scenarios are not the first-order priority. In fact, the documents use 'disease' in a wider, more metaphoric, sense. For example, air mobility congestion is seen as an 'insidious Disease' (e.g. CANSO 2015). The emphasis on single, seamless, and open skies was to cut down on costs and carbon emissions. Although sovereignty was recognized, it was seen as a problem that needed to be bypassed rather than dealt with and managed. Why would Europe need some 30 air traffic control systems when the system could be handled much more efficiently? Sovereignty was an issue, a sensitive issue. COVID-19 made it clear to everybody that lack of attention to the fast spread of pandemic agents via air travel left the problem and the final bill to be handled by the states. After the fiasco of letting the coronavirus spread, it should be clear to all involved that the restoration of air travel can happen only when such bills to support airlines and economies will not be put on the shoulders of the tax-payers, especially in the developing and fragile regions of the world.

Once COVID-19 broke out, the guarding of borders became paramount. The declinist fear of submergence turned into the level of micro-parasites. Suddenly the cosmopolitan visions of open skies and seamless global connections seemed out of place and came to be viewed as sources of insecurity. Of course, there are precedents to the rapid decline of air travel, cutting off of flight connections and health checks. Apart from 9/11, the European experience in April 2010 with the Icelandic volcanic ash that stopped flights in the European airspace demonstrates the importance of air travel in many sectors of life. Since power and mobility are highly interchangeable terms in the canon of Western modernity, such episodes are easily used to signify lack of preparedness, declining status, and loss of leadership. Although Europe often experiences direct political crises and shocks, air mobility shocks are increasingly personally felt because of the centrality of air travel in modern life. Air mobility specificities are about people making sense of their regional and global surroundings. Disruptions to these surroundings have become a type of scale akin to Richter of what is happening around us and in places to which we are connected.

The anxiety and nervousness about the global order were revealed in the 9/11 context through airplanes used as weapons and through the disruption caused to air travel with more checks, stop-and-go mobilities, profiled borders, and no-fly lists. The disease carriers were not micro-parasites but harmful radicalized terror cells, an embodied image close to describing a disease of a political kind, radicalization. Back then, the interrupted flights crashing into buildings become signifiers of proto-theory, and in memory and meanings, 9/11 was embodied by airplanes, airports, and air traffic. Ellis (2002: 377), for example, in her travelogue, signifies the crux of the events taking place with striking air travel memory images. The impact of the day registered as frame-breaking in contrast with the suddenly old normal, with what she previously took for granted—her smooth flow through the international airport. Ellis continues her personal story at the airport by recounting the difficulties of placing a call, the impossibility of collecting luggage, the people gathered around TV screens, the long lines at the rental car area, and the relief of finally getting a car. The entire North American airspace was suddenly halted in an emergency. This language concerning 9/11 is now being rehearsed with talk about the new normal and the return to the new type of normal after COVID-19. The emergency scenario was made meaningful through sudden halts that represented not only bodily kinaesthetic smooth flows though the mobility system but, abruptly, with the disrupted global order. This meaning of 9/11 is also one key modality of COVID-19. The mobility systems that had been taken for granted were disrupted as well.

The eerie similarity between 9/11 and the Icelandic volcanic ash episode as precursors to COVID-19 spelt out some political meanings relating to the global order, such as the dangerously crowded airports as transatlantic flights got cancelled suddenly in the spring of 2019. The disturbed and torturous flight connections during the COVID-19 pandemic illustrate a problem of global space, yet they also send out an ominous message of movability of the global order based on fast movers and smooth flows. The order itself was seen as being shaken by COVID-19. The analysis focused on de-globalization, de-coupling, major power rivalry, and increased human health vulnerability. This is something Thucydides would have noticed as ominous symptoms of a political order being under heavy stress, and his prognosis would probably have been bleak.

The global mobility system is not a consequence of the contemporary political order. The geo-infrastructure is the crux of it. Daileda (2008: 225) makes a valuable point about the speciality of air travel vis-à-vis the new expanding notions of the 'final' frontier of modernism: 'Finally air travel made distance a completely manageable obstacle'. The expansion of the horizon, the final frontier, was not a physical barrier but a function of making power and economic growth as movable as possible and, in practice, engineering various technologies of transportation and mobility to solve the obstacles for the emergence of a truly global and distributed mobile form of what can be called imperial or hegemonic power.

This logic of global order on the move led inevitably to the establishment of a relatively de-territorial and decentralized structure based on what can be called a network empire that is seen as the global order (Hardt and Negri 2001: xi–xiii, 160). It is based on the standards and rules of mobility and on the underlying values driving the virtues of infrastructure development. It is telling in this regard that China's Belt and Road Initiative (BRI) is seen as a key signifier of its rise as a global power. Similarly, the US response to the COVID-19 outbreak included major economic support packages. The biggest of these packages was announced by US President Joe Biden in spring 2021—a large-scale plan to develop US infrastructure, domestically as well as globally:

> In fact, it's the largest American jobs investment since World War Two. It will create millions of jobs, good-paying jobs. It will grow the economy, make us more competitive around the world, promote our national security interests, and put us in a position to win the global competition with China in the upcoming years.
>
> *(Biden 2021)*

The COVID-19 response was not just health based. It was seen as a reason to mobilize resources geopolitically, as a call to investment in the mobility system.

COVID-19 as Order Disruption

The local intensity and regularity of such global flows and their security as well as resilience are increasingly a crucial indicator of a state's economic viability and its political influence. When COVID-19 hit, it undermined the system and opened up vulnerabilities. Securing steady access to such global flows poses a different set of domestic and foreign policy challenges to states in general, and especially to smaller states, than the challenges posed by the traditional Westphalian model, which has been rooted in territorial notions of international order. States are increasingly caught in a cross-current between these two co-existing realities, as the dynamic, flow-centric model emerges and the older territorial state-centric model recedes. Global circulations of activities are challenging traditional state-based security cultures and strategies, rendering older policy solutions—for example, increased national self-reliance and related national strategies—increasingly ineffective. However, at the same time, over-reliance on global mobility networks can lead to harm, as was revealed in the spread of COVID-19 and the rush to secure access to PPE and later to vaccines. The cross-current of contradictory tendencies is one of the messages that the pandemic has brought with it, and it is likely to be one of the most lasting yet puzzling lessons learnt. The key puzzle is how far actors can rely on the global mobility order in their resilience strategies and in what ways and aspects they should find national, regional, or bloc-based solutions.

The recent confluences between contradictory tendencies have led to the emergence of global health and pandemic security practices. The way in which pandemic emergencies are presented in public debate turns them into exceptional and heightened security episodes to be managed through medical means (e.g. Elbe

2006: 125). Medical expertise is turned into a containment force that is supposed to make global interconnectedness more resilient. Such a medically more secure and smart form of global order is a likely trend that is not only going to continue but will be enhanced by encounters with coronaviruses. Yet, at the same time, there has been a heavy crisis of confidence in the viability and sustainability of the medicalized security and securitized medicine. Disruption is deep because of the politosomatic ramifications. It is not only the modes of pandemic security but the combination of somatic vulnerability and doubts about the 'order' in the global order that are the drivers of the increasingly confusing and wide-ranging emergency scenario(s).

Thus, against the background of the emerging pandemic security practice looms a mission to make global society more 'resilient' to mutating and invisible microbial threats. This involves a quest to reform the existing global networks as well as the patterns of political solidarity and trust. There is likely to be a major movement arising from what are perceived to be errors, co-options, diversions, mismanagement, and distortions of the global order. In the increasingly feverish global order, an increasing number of national as well as international and global actors have to be (re)sewn into a more accountable and resilient global fabric, or the fabric's seams will come under increasingly serious pressures and begin to fray.

The demand for epidemiologically resilient globalization is encompassing and also consequential to many realms of global life. The emphasis is on a 'somatically safe' and more welfare-centric world based on new and reformed relationships between various domestic, international, and transnational actors, as their global relevance and safety levels are evaluated against the high standards of their pandemic preparedness. The preparedness and ability to adapt in an accountable way to these high standards are spread unevenly around the globe. As a result, the global order is bound to become less global and broken down into regional or bloc-based arrangements. Furthermore, reaching high levels of preparedness means taking actions proactively when there are no acute pandemic threats. In this sense, medicalization has changed the way in which security practices are understood. This scenario of reconfiguration has different key characteristics. A large bundle of insecurities is countered through politico-medical expertise and practices. Politico-medical institutions increase status in the who's who of security, while security practices adapt, on the one hand, to new technological methods, such as digitalized bio-surveillance, that have a bearing on people's freedoms and rights and, on the other hand, to practices that accentuate state-level national priorities, such as stockpiling, security of supply, and self-sufficiency (e.g. Elbe 2011: 848).

First and foremost, the expansion of the medico-security paradigm can highlight the need for state-level 'immunities' against pandemic threats from naturally occurring diseases as well as strategic use of biowarfare and terrorism. The term 'resilience', denoting an alternative modality of security, is likely to be integral to this endeavour. Resilience has one key origin in the ability of materials to bounce back and recoil after an impact. This shock-resistance may also refer to the ability to absorb sudden change(s) (Carver 1998: 247). The resilience language spread to social studies under scenarios of critical infrastructure management, mitigation of ecological change, and disaster preparedness (e.g. Lundborg and Vaughan-Williams 2011). The adaptive and shock-absorbing nature of critical infrastructures—in normal, turbulent, and emergency situations—was seen as a way of being prepared in the face of a multitude of potential risks.

This idea of enduring core functions means that a system can fulfil certain key tasks even though some of its functions might be lost. At the level of a global mobility system, in which this chapter is particularly interested, the key question has to do with the efficiency of cutting connections during an onset phase to an outbreak without affecting the economic and political sustainability of the overall connectedness in the long run.

I will now turn to a more detailed study of the chronology of events in the case of SARS and COVID-19 which are related to mobility. The overall form of a pandemic encounter is becoming globally shared and synchronized (Price-Smith 2009: 192–6). Here, the attention is on whether and how the inevitable speculation by the media and by expert analysts provided the means to build scenarios of national high preparedness and underlying communal healthiness.

Case 1: SARS' Geo-Imageries of Resilience

The analysis of concrete research cases starts with the 2003 SARS pandemic. In particular, I will review the 'comprehensive chronology of SARS related events' as set out in the WHO publication, *SARS—How a Global Epidemic Was Stopped* (2006). In doing so, I will examine how the chronology frames the vulnerability and resilience of international air travel in the context of SARS through various tropes and figures.

The WHO report notes 21 February 2003 as the day on which SARS went international:

> Index case of the Metropole Hotel outbreak arrives from Guangdong; international spread of virus begins: Professor LJL, a 64-year-old physician from Guangzhou, arrives . . . to attend a wedding. He developed flu-like symptoms on 15 February, having been infected in the hospital where he worked. . . . At least 16 other guests and one visitor are infected during his one-night stay in room 911 of the Metropole Hotel.
>
> *(WHO 2006: 8)*

This item in the chronology states the profession—a professor and physician—of the index case. The chronology does not explicitly use the term 'superspreader'. Rather, it refers to 'super-spreading events' and 'index cases'. The context is an international metropolitan hotel in Hong Kong. This is significant, and the mention of the profession of the index case is used to imply two things. First, the man was probably infected in the province of Guangdong through his work as a medical doctor. Second, it also brings the disease to a new level when, instead of an average local person, a person with access to the global arteries catches and spreads a disease. The chronology accounts for one further place where this index case infected more people before dying:

> Professor LJL is admitted to the intensive care unit of the Kwong Wah Hospital for respiratory failure. Besides the hotel guests, three members of his family . . . and one nurse at the hospital are infected. Professor LJL will die on 4 March.
>
> *(WHO 2006: 8)*

The chronology can be interpreted to construct the doctor as a superspreader and both the hotel and the hospital as possible disease hubs. The next item in the chronology that indicates further international spread to Vietnam is dated 26 February 2003:

> Hanoi index case is hospitalized: Mr JC, a 48-year-old merchandise manager from New York, is admitted to the Hanoi-French Hospital. He arrived in Viet Nam on 23 February after travelling to China and Hong Kong. . . . The WHO office in Viet Nam will be notified of the case the next morning, and its advice sought.
>
> *(WHO 2006: 8)*

The profession of the Hanoi case as an international businessman is clearly meant to be relevant for both imagining how he might have been infected and gauging the potential for further spread. An infected person is also a signifier of frequent international travel, a worrying sign as it is used in the chronology. The next item on the chronological list reports the spread of SARS to Singapore:

> Singapore index case is hospitalized: Ms EM is admitted to Tan Tock Seng Hospital with pneumonia. She has been unwell since returning from a shopping trip to Hong Kong on 25 February. The 22-year-old, who stayed in room 938 at the Metropole Hotel . . . will pass on the virus to 22 close contacts.
>
> *(WHO 2006: 9)*

This index case, infected by another index case, is identified not through her profession, but through her consumption-related activity. She is a young tourist who has been on an international shopping trip. Being a tourist is regarded as a significant status for it implies possibilities of an international and, in the case of the New York businessman, intercontinental pattern of spread.

On 3 March 2003, the chronology mentions the first signifier of the global resilience system beginning to kick in:

> Dr Urbani examines Hanoi index case: In Hanoi, WHO's communicable disease expert in Viet Nam, Dr Carlo Urbani, examines Mr JC, the

American businessman who was admitted to the Hanoi-French Hospital on 26 February with a severe form of pneumonia. Dr Urbani sends a report to WHO's Regional Office, emphasizes the need for strict infection controls, and arranges for Mr JC's serum and throat swabs to be sent to laboratories in Tokyo, Atlanta, and Hanoi.

(WHO 2006: 9)

The chronology makes an exception here in naming an eventual SARS victim, Dr Carlo Urbani. His diligent and alert actions are seen in an inherently positive light in the otherwise factual chronology. He is not identified as a potential spreader, but as a disease warrior and a germ hunter. A clear protagonist of the SARS drama, Dr Urbani is turned into the hardworking exemplary hero of the chronology. Because of this position, it may be argued that his probable role in passing on the disease is not mentioned. Dr Urbani is turned into a model of how to act in a pandemic emergency. He is also used to embody the effectiveness and vigilance of the global organization he works for, WHO, and a system of notification finally working.

However, on 5 March 2003, the chronology recounts the intercontinental jump of SARS to Canada, thereby implicating global air travel as the key vector of the spread:

Toronto index case dies: Ms KSC, 78 years old, dies in her Toronto, Ontario, home. The death certificate attributes her death to heart attack. In fact, she died from SARS acquired at the Metropole Hotel in Hong Kong. Before dying, she has passed the virus on to four members of her extended family, who will then spark the Toronto outbreak.

(WHO 2006: 10)

The chronology also reports misdiagnosis and recounts its negative consequences. These errors are the antithesis of Dr Urbani's diligent work. The chronology also implies a failure in the containment and follow-up procedures since the index case's stay at the Hotel Metropole should have been suspected by then. Contact tracing was not working. This stands in stark contrast to the next item in the timeline that emphasizes tracing and functional information-sharing:

Mr JC, the Hanoi index case who has been medically evacuated, arrives at the Princess Margaret Hospital, where he will die on 13 March. The WHO Regional Office informs Hong Kong and Singapore officials about his transfer. Singapore is informed because the medical evacuation team is from Singapore. Because of strict infection controls, no health worker in the Princess Margaret Hospital is infected by Mr JC.

(WHO 2006: 10)

Although there were further alarming cases, this chronology details how the WHO got its global machinery of containment fully working. However, one should note that all this activity took place a full month after the first accounts of the disease in Hong Kong and months after the first outbreak occurred in China.

SARS blended with the tense political processes of its day and acquired modalities that seemed to exemplify alarm over the 'health' of the hub-and-spoke skeleton of the mobility-based global order. Disease-related dramas often picture things in a way that is culturally significant: What are the prominent ways of portraying protagonists and exceptionally deviant and antagonist figures and practices? These dramatizations put the relevant actors in their respective, but interactive, positions and give them roles and backgrounds. The 'vigilant' national and international actors of the SARS play, such as the US Centers for Disease Control and Prevention (CDC) and WHO, got their share of authority and legitimacy, while those authorities—most prominently, the Chinese—that were somehow connected with the origin or further spread of the disease were portrayed as illegitimate, partly by omission of evidence of effective actions on China's part.

It can be argued that vigilance was the prominent template for understanding what was meant by normatively sanctioned vigilance. The emergency scenario offered different actors opportunities to demonstrate diligent adherence to the practices of containment and their high degree of expertise. Such rule adherence and its corresponding actions can be instrumental in conveying the health of the underlying political order and reassuring the public about the chances of the actual realization of the worst-case scenarios. At the end, when the dust settled, the SARS emergency allowed for displays of new containment-oriented practices and representations of more resilient global travel and health systems. In several important ways, however, the pattern of 'hub-and-spoke' and the figure of the 'frequent traveller' became signifiers of a possible horrible failure in the emergency drama. Border-crossing fires seemed to defy the usual notions of containment, protective barriers, and *cordons sanitaires*. The containment measures tailored to air traffic seemed inherently inadequate. For example, the screening measures, although widely used and published, proved to be insufficient. The WHO recommended that travellers should be screened at airports for symptoms and signs of SARS, such as sneezing and fever: 'In spite of intensive screening, no SARS cases were detected by the border-authorities' (St John *et al.* 2006: 6). The reason seems clear. Profiling disease carriers with symptoms very similar to the symptoms of seasonal flu out of millions of travellers is inherently difficult, if not impossible. The same problem presented in the case of COVID-19 as well. There was a sense of helplessness as the severing of connections did not seem to be an attractive option because air transport is seen as the modus operandi of the global order. However, the pandemic scare led to the cutting down of flights and, more importantly, to a decrease in individuals' desire to fly, if not trying to flee infected areas (Caballero 2005: 483). Although the checks and screening created a particular sentiment of suspicion and, perhaps, counter-intuitively, an air of security, at least something 'resilient' and 'robust', was being performed. However, it was mostly ineffective and, at worst, just performative.

A key theme in the SARS emergency scenario and the lessons learnt from it problematized China's legitimate and sustainable role in the mobility-based global order. The possibility of a wider global spread of SARS allowed for media, states, and international organizations to invest time on speculative stories but also, on the other hand, to highlight the need for better preparedness for the disease's possible movement across political boundaries. The diverse speculations on the need for elastic and shock-absorbing advanced communities at the local, national, and global levels offered insights into how contagious diseases still serve one of their historical modalities: they can be used to separate, contain, and border—whether materially, socially, or politically. Much of the media frenzy and hyperbole concentrated on the caution stemming from the perceived porous nature of geographical, political, and cultural boundaries. It is also at this juncture that the term 'resilience' finds increasing mention in global pandemic security. For example, the supposedly advanced societies were often separated from the less prepared ones and from the supposedly 'pre-modern' hotspots, like southern China, where people were perceived as eating bats in a highly unhygienic and unsafe manner. At the same time, SARS provided opportunities for the narration of the dramatic dangers stemming from by now connected global peripheries and their different cultures. One possible hypothesis is that the scare was set in motion by the historically deep-seated representational potentials inherent in the imaginaries of dangerous contact between distinct politico-cultural entities—for example, West–East, US–China, and modern–premodern. In the headlines—for example, *The New York Times* (*NYT*) headline, 'The SARS Epidemic: The Path: From China's Provinces, a Crafty Germ Breaks Out (Rosenthal 2003)—China was seen as the point of origin of the disease as it spread. It was seen as a biohazard connected to the eating of bats in southern China. The disease had been reframed as a 'biohazard', a word that echoed the recent experiences with Ebola in Zaire during the spring of 1995. The Ebola scare highlighted the vulnerability of the global community to fast-spreading contagion via the international transportation infrastructure. The word 'pandemic' had also emerged wider into global awareness by the 1990s as a result of the perceived all-encompassing nature of the threat.

By the time of the SARS encounter in 2003, the important elements of a serious contagious disease had been set in place through precursor diseases. A serious contagion crossing the species boundary to humans was defined by the BSE (or mad cow disease) and Ebola (caused by bats) scares in the 1990s. The avian flu scare in 2004 and the swine flu scare in 2009 also rehearsed the idea of nature and animals being sources of a 'killer disease'. The interspecies mutability scenario developed even earlier in connection with HIV and AIDS (believed to have spread from chimpanzees). The news stories changed dramatically in the 1990s as the 'coming plague' genre took hold in public cognition with its fundamental notions of mutability of and deep vulnerability—or lack of resilience—to the disease agents. The enmity between humanity and its global order of things was seen as clashing with nature. This antagonistic genre was reinforced by similar emerging cleavages inherent in the climate change discussions where human ways were seen as disrupting the planetary system. On the whole, the global order was seen as, at least in degree, unnatural and unsustainable.

China was turned into an emerging danger because of the perceptions of its 'teeming' cities, its different autocratic ideology and culture, and its veil of secrecy on its activities. All of this was implicated as being conducive to the emergence of pandemic threats. Moreover, it is significant that the disease jumped from animals to humans for the first time in China. The speculation assumed that China could provide the location for future interspecies jumps—rightly so, in hindsight. The combination of premodern and modern practices prevalent in rapidly growing China was seen as making it the ideal 'incubator' for pandemics. Through the act of localization, China itself was, to a degree, turned into a hostile element reinforced by the anxieties connected to its co-occurring geopolitical rise. It is possible to link this sense of enmity with the high political tensions between China and the West that were present in the late 1990s. Furthermore, this assigning of blame resonated with much older orientalist images of China, which conceived of it as a mysterious place, and gave it room for corresponding medico-security speculation. From this angle, when SARS spread to other countries, the disease became different. Canada, for example, was not turned into a possible hub for a future pandemic. In this respect, the media stories treated the disease as an 'ordinary' outbreak that was being fought diligently and contained. It can be suggested that the greater geographical, cultural, and political distance to the 'host' country enabled 'wider' interpretations and prognostications than an outbreak of the disease in a familiar and close context. As stated earlier, the localization, ethnicization, and nationalization of an infectious disease is a stock story of a pandemic emergency. However, in the case of China, there is much legitimacy to the speculations. Secrecy is also very common when a disease surfaces, as the originary country's status and legitimacy are at stake.

Besides China being placed in an antagonist frame, another key-related interpretation of the SARS emergency scenario was the aforementioned air traffic vector. In popular imagery, the SARS scare of 2003 was often linked with the global age of connectedness and the increasingly tight-knit fabric of interdependency. Health Canada (2003: 1) noted this association: 'Old diseases usually spread slowly. . . . SARS, on the other hand, moved at the speed of a jet airplane. Within days of its arrival in Hong Kong, it had circled the globe'. Crawford (2007: 29) uses the term 'super-spreader' for a figure that, in technical global health language, is referred to as an 'index case': '[T]he virus spread round the globe, aided by super-spreaders (like the doctor at the Metropole Hotel in Hong Kong) and fast international air travel'. Similarly, Noun and Chyba (2008: 208) state that 'during the early stages of the SARS pandemic, a single patient, the "super-spreader", infected every one of 50 health workers who treated him'. This antagonistic stock figure appeared in the popular accounts of SARS. *The Sunday Telegraph*, for example, reported on 23 March 2003 the following dramatized scene:

As he shuffled through the lobby of the Hotel Metropole, the elderly professor was feeling feverish and faint. At the lift, he steadied himself for a moment in the open doorway before his body convulsed in a series of wracking coughs that sprayed fine droplets of saliva onto the walls and the people waiting inside.

As a signifier of global vulnerability, 'a superspreader' is a term with a loaded cultural history that connects it with the figure of 'Patient Zero' in the HIV and AIDS narratives. During the late 1980s, there was much speculation about the original Patient Zero, Gaetan Dugas, who, through his work as an air steward, was able to fly all over the world and spread HIV to others. Varying numbers of HIV infections have been linked to him: 'Dugas was a hub in the network of sexual contacts' (Mitchell 2009: 50). Crawford (2007: 20) uses another modern air mobility trope, 'city hopping', to drive home the point about the avian flu–related dangers. Evidently, the figure of a superspreader carries with it a multidimensional understanding of the failure of pandemic containment and the acute need to trace, contain, and build resilience. The term 'superspreader' ceases to be a mere epidemiological term. It turns into a signifier that blends together into one figure multiple engrossing images and then projects them into the context of major metropolitan hotels and into the global aviopolis. As a construct, it enables the underlying invisible world of viruses to be made visible and culturally comprehensible. The mobility of these dangerous types reframes air mobility networks, which have been commonly articulated in a far more progressive light of seamless skies and smooth global flows.

The vulnerability introduced by SARS seems to be at odds with the oft-repeated view that the air mobility system is shock-absorbing and resilient. This dynamic and flexible framework is in accordance with the contours of the existing assemblages of hegemonic governance and provides a major expression of what is meant by global order and its hegemonic form of hierarchical interdependency (Hardt and Negri 2001: 13–14; Aaltola 2005: 268; Agambe 1998: 123; Dillon and Reid 2000: 117). From this bridgehead, air mobility flows have become an increasingly important register of vulnerability. It is notable that the post-9/11 air mobility scenario has started to include a marked dystopian element (e.g. Knox *et al.* 2007: 267). The Ebola scare in the mid-1990s had already given content to these dystopian framings of the modern aviopolis, as it did again in 2014–15.

Case 2: COVID-19 as a Power-Political Flashpoint

In March 2021, the WHO published the first version of its report on COVID-19, called the 'WHO-Convened Global Study of Origins of SARS-CoV-2: China Part'. The report was markedly different from its earlier report on SARS. The emphasis was on finding the likely source or origin of the disease. The report offers four possibilities for the origin of the outbreak: (1) direct zoonotic spillover was deemed possible to likely, (2) introduction through an intermediate host was considered as likely to very likely, (3) introduction through cold/food chain products was considered as possible, and (4) introduction through a laboratory incident was considered to be extremely unlikely. The report was sensitive and quickly politicized—a sign of the enmities and suspicions surrounding the disease and the resultant situation. China pushed the frozen food vector so that it could establish that the pandemic emerged from outside China; the US considered a leak from the Wuhan laboratory as much more likely than the WHO report evaluated. Thus, the report was not only politicized but also geo-politicized. The tracing of the origin in the report was indicative of the overall atmosphere of paranoia. The report itself was suspected of being produced under the influence of China and conforming to its special national interests. Even the head of the WHO, Dr Tedros Adhanom Ghebreyesus, played down the conclusions reached in the report: 'As far as WHO is concerned, all hypotheses remain on the table. This report is a very important beginning, but it is not the end'. The controversy was an understandable consequence of the inherent power-political sensitivities of the time and the sense that the WHO itself was somehow compromised.

Because of the four different theories and the inability to trace the exact origins of COVID-19, the report does not reveal a clear pattern of spread but speculates on four different patterns. However, what is clear irrespective of the report is that air travel was a clear vector. What is equally clear is that the controversies surrounding the point of origin indicate another constant of pandemic politics—the point of origin becomes a blame game which places at stake the status and prestige of state-level and international actors. Although the report does not offer detailed analyses and revealing anecdotes as the SARS report did, it leaves room for the reconstruction of the pattern of spread—also a clear feature of the pattern of blame—through other trustworthy studies.

The earliest known cases of COVID-19 were geographically clustered in Wuhan, China (e.g. Huang *et al.* 2020). This probable scenario was preceded by 'a period of unrecognized transmission in humans' (Andersen *et al.* 2020: 451). This would place the time of the initial transfer of the disease from animals to humans in Wuhan to somewhere during the fall of 2019. The 'virus probably evolved in a bat host until an unknown spillover event into humans occurred' (Rasmussen 2021). The other scenarios are unlikely and mostly result from over-politicization and direct political pressure, which are of course interesting in their own right.

As the outbreak progressed in Wuhan and became detectable, the disease's transmission domestically within China and also internationally was already on its way mainly through the air travel vector. At this point of time, between December 2019 and January 2020, travel restrictions could have had an effect on the spread of the disease. Flight and travel restrictions could have had an impact when the COVID-19 incidence levels were low or close to zero (Russell *et al.* 2021). Any later, such restrictions have increasingly little effect as the local epidemics are already well under way. The clock was ticking from the containment perspective. The situation was extremely temporalized, time-critical. The first and only line of defence had already been lost or was under serious strain.

The first significant cluster of cases in Europe emerged in densely populated Lombardy in Italy. The first diagnosed case of COVID-19 was a young man in Codogno on 20 February 2020. Milan, the local hub, is one of the most densely populated areas in Europe. Moreover, it is well linked to other hubs in Europe and the rest of the world. The characteristics of the effective spread of a fairly infectious disease agent were clearly present as the Wuhan epidemic got well on its way to becoming a global pandemic. Infection was growing exponentially, and the total number of cases was close to 90,000 by the summer of 2020, putting enormous pressure on the Italian health system. Italy reacted quickly to the situation and severed direct flights to China on 31 January. It also implemented lockdown measures— full lockdown on 8 March 2020—ahead of the other European countries, thereby becoming a key reference case and a place for learning lessons on how to approach the exponential growth of cases for the rest of Europe.

Why did Italy become the hub for COVID-19 in Europe? It was well connected. It had the required population density for exponential spread. It was quick to react in cutting direct flights to China on 31 January.

> However, SARS-CoV-2-infected people could enter Italy long before this date, as was proven by the diagnosis of SARS-CoV-2 [COVID-19] in Chinese tourists who arrived in Italy on January 23. In addition, the suspension of direct flights from China could not prevent the entrance of people though transit flights from other countries.
>
> *(Alteri et al. 2021)*

The hub-and-spoke system of international air travel is designed in such a way that indirect flights can compensate for the sudden cutting off of direct flights. This is seen in normal times as a resilience capacity built into the system. However, in the case of pandemic flows, this was far removed from the sustainable forward-looking resilience.

Milan's Malpensa airport is the second busiest airport in Italy, and the surrounding region has other active airports as well. However, Milan Malpensa did not have any direct flights to Wuhan. Air China operated direct flights from Milan to Beijing and Shanghai. But there was a direct flight between Wuhan and Rome, which is a short train ride away from Milan. Overall, the passenger numbers between Italy and China were at the level of 250,000 passengers per year before the pandemic. Yet there were critical connections between Wuhan and Northern Italy in terms of industry, especially the textile industry: 'Tens of thousands of Chinese migrants work in the Italian textile industry, producing fashion items, leather bags and shoes with the stamp "Made in Italy"' (Rudan 2020). Whether tourists or workers, it is clear that there were many connections, many possibilities for outbreaks of local transmission and virus strains. Moreover, winter is a busy season for the Northern Italian and Alpine ski resorts, which became a critical link in the spread of the disease in Europe and across the Atlantic. At the same time, Italy was only one part of the confluence of factors that led to Europe attaining worst-case scenario status during the first wave of COVID-19. One has to remember that through very effective containment measures—tracing of chains of infection, isolation, and diligent epidemic work—the outbreak in Wuhan and China was already being contained. Similarly, in many other East Asian countries, the approach adopted worked much better than in Europe despite the intense air connections to the initial outbreak zones and these countries having high population densities as well.

Pandemics are not unknown unknowns. They have long histories although there are always uncertainties concerning them. What are often not known are (1) their specific characteristics—what they are like when they emerge, (2) exact timing—when they emerge, and (3) the politics and geopolitics surrounding them as the controversy about the WHO report clearly indicates. Conventionally and conceptually, therefore, they are known occurrences. In recent history, since the end of the Cold War, the human polity has had several close calls with diseases that have spread rapidly across large areas. The element of surprise in COVID-19 had to do with timing and scale: it was a temporal surprise and it eluded the initial containment efforts. However, despite the obvious epistemic challenges with regard to pandemics, we do know something about their typical temporal qualities, such as how they tend to emerge and develop over time. The shape of their temporal flow is as follows: rapid onset and politically irresistible and even compelling policy impact, followed by decreasing attention and lessening restrictive policies. The onset phase includes the sentiment that drastic action needs to be taken and should have been taken earlier on, while the later phase contains a sentiment that enough has been done or even that the actions taken were a bit too drastic and overblown.[5] The initial efforts in Europe wavered between these two attitudes. It was seen as having started in China, and it was also seen as being effectively contained there. Alarmism was present, yet the memory of SARS and MERS as well as avian flu and swine flu focused on a restrained approach that was later seen to be reactive rather than proactive.

Pandemic emergency scenarios have an onset phase with corresponding political anticipations. It is within this temporal frame that the COVID-19 scenario defined the actors and actions, and the disease became engrossing and politically embellished by mid-March 2020. Within the onset of the first wave, COVID-19 was made out to be a carrier of profound messages and of what should be done to ameliorate the (what appears to be increasingly complex) situation. Research suggests that societies overreact to and hyperbolize sudden epidemic outbreaks and that their causal consequences are overemphasized later on (e.g. Mordechai et al. 2019). However, although the disease agent itself seldom functions as a direct cause for a major transformation, it can act as a trigger for complex and non-linear cascading effects, its combinatorial rather than causal paths being well historically established.

This can take many forms. For example, serious diseases change the context and accentuate already pronounced social and political trends. They function as triggers for contemporaneous interpretations in ways that are unrelated to their biology in the human body. However, COVID-19 indicates that pandemics do have one clear causal effect. They fit the prevailing vulnerabilities inherent in the social, economic, and political fabric: 'Epidemic diseases are not random events that afflict societies capriciously and without warning. On the contrary, every society produces its own specific vulnerabilities. To study them is to understand that society's structure, its standard of living, and its political priorities'.[6] The more serious the pandemic, the better is the fit between it and the inherent vulnerabilities. The global order based on interdependency, mobility, and circulation was the key vector for the spread of COVID-19, and, as such, it could catalyse and trigger underlying challenges and pressures to this order. Partly, these underlying anxieties were connected to the rise of China, the decline of the world order's main stakeholder, the US, the rising power-political competition among the major powers, and the sustainability of present-day global institutions that rest on the world order. The EU was largely a bystander. The perception was that just like in the case of SARS and MERS, the first line of defence was elsewhere—in particular in China. The China factor might have led to even more isolated sentiments concerning the outbreak. It could be suggested that the EU's and its member-states' self-perception of being isolated from the outbreak was fed by their location higher up in the production and value chains of the global order. For several reasons, the first reaction to the outbreak was not vigilant and proactive, but passive and waiting.

Another reason for the relative passivity might have been the lessons learnt from previous encounters with pandemics. Whereas the first line of defence in the case of SARS had been in Asia and the countries there had fresh memories of the severity of the blow, Europe had had different experiences and learnt different lessons. For many in Europe, a pandemic encounter had a customary trajectory, setting the expectations also for COVID-19. A pandemic emergency scenario is typically initiated by a sudden striking event accompanied by maximum attention that is then followed by a gradually lessening focus, a fading away of attention. In fact, the attention seems to decline and fade into political obscurity in a matter of months. This pattern was seen with Ebola in 1994, BSE in 1997, SARS in 2003, avian flu in 2004, swine flu in 2009, MERS in 2012, and Ebola again in 2014–15. The outbreaks received attention and resource mobilization for several months, although, epidemiologically, the disease itself lingered on much longer or still continues to linger in all these cases. The flows of emergency events are characterized by the rhythmic ebbing and waning of public attention and international resource mobilization.

The onset pulse, at its zenith, is extremely compelling and attention-catching. During this phase, the relevant actors—ranging from local and national health authorities and governments to international organizations (such as WHO) and individual states that take on an international leadership role—are recognized and receive their relative positions as protagonists and/or antagonists of the episode. Political action is required, and accountability is demanded. Trust is being built or broken down. The situational characteristics of an outbreak are used as a momentary criterion, or a standard, against which the legitimacy and accountability of the actors and their actions are evaluated. In a pandemic situation, citizens judge their political leaders and expect measures, preferably strong measures. The onset phase in Europe was characterized by keen interest in what was happening in China. However, politics both domestically and at the EU level was proceeding mostly as usual. The escalating migration crisis between Turkey and the EU was a key focus of politics as were the election year events in the US. Until mid-March 2020, COVID-19 was followed but not yet the main worry or source of political anxiety. The usual pandemic emergency trajectory was relatively unusual in the beginning. The onset phase was delayed until things started to unravel in conjunction with the epidemic hitting Italy.

Any failure to tap into the tempo of an event can translate into a perceived deficiency in fulfilling the necessary 'obligations' of the given situation. The criticism of common European action was sharp when the level of harm was being revealed in the steady rise of COVID-19 deaths.[7] In the onset phase, there were moments that demonstrated the emergence of such situational demands and requirements and a sense of lagging behind.

Many of the failures were at the international level, which catalysed the European failures. The first was the failure to enact rapidly enough flight restrictions to the outbreak zone when such measures could have had some effect. First, on 10 January 2020, the WHO issued a notice that travel should not be restricted in response to the alarm over COVID-19: 'WHO advises against the application of any travel or trade restrictions on China based on the information currently available on this event' (WHO 2020a). This statement said that the evidence indicated that 'there is no significant human-to-human transmission, and no infections among health care workers have occurred'. The text also stated that 'Wuhan city is a major domestic and international transport hub', which means that there should have been alarm over the spread of the contagion. However, this reference also points out the high economic stakes in any restrictive measures. The IHR was drafted not only to stop the spread of a contagion but also to balance the containment measures with the high stakes involved in international travel and trade. The situation appears to have been tricky for the WHO as there was no evidence of human-to-human spread although the disease agent itself had been identified as a variant of the coronavirus that had previously produced the contagious and deadly SARS and MERS outbreaks. This link should perhaps have warranted more decisive and proactive action from the beginning, instead of a balancing of interests and adopting a wait-and-see approach as the containment measures in China were being jump-started. However, at the very least, a critical question can be asked: if the scientific evidence did not yet justify any restrictive measures, should historical experience and caution have compelled the placing of restrictions as a precaution? The struggle to control and contain outbreaks is usually balanced with the need to not cause too deep an economic and social disruption. Perhaps the economic and trade-related stakes ultimately tipped the scales to allowing air travel to continue unhampered at that stage.

On 24 January, WHO updated its travel guidance. It pointed out that human-to-human transmission in Wuhan, elsewhere in China, and outside of it too had been confirmed. However, according to the WHO, many aspects of the outbreak remained uncertain: 'Not enough is known about the epidemiology of 2019-nCoV to draw definitive conclusions about the full clinical features of [the] disease, the intensity of the human-to-human transmission, and the original source of the outbreak' (WHO 2020b). The conclusion was the same as it had been two precious weeks before: 'WHO advises that measures to limit the risk of exportation or importation of the disease should be implemented, without unnecessary restrictions of international traffic'. The extra profiling measures included screenings for symptoms at airports and other traffic hubs.

The next travel advice was released on 27 January 2020. The text included more caution and measures to pinpoint disease carriers. However, the recommendation remained unchanged: 'WHO advises that measures to limit the risk of exportation or importation of the disease should be implemented, without unnecessary restrictions of international traffic' (WHO 2020c). Finally, on 28 February 2020, WHO issued an update recommending some measured restrictions: 'Travel measures that significantly interfere with international traffic may only be justified at the beginning of an outbreak, as they may allow countries to gain time, even if only a few days, to rapidly implement effective preparedness measures' (WHO 2020d). It seemed that the WHO was stating that because the containment efforts had failed by February, the restrictions that would have been effective if implemented earlier should not be implemented any more. Moreover, the updated recommendation was notable for giving further reasons for why the WHO was against travel restrictions: '[R]estrictions may interrupt needed aid and technical support, may disrupt businesses, and may have negative social and economic effects on the affected countries'. The failure to issue a timely travel restriction is notable if judged against the standards for proper caution and vigilance.

However, other actors were restricting travel. From about mid-January 2020, the uncontained spread of the disease became clear. Several states and airlines were anxiously pondering over when to restrict air travel to the outbreak region in Wuhan and to China. The travel restrictions issued by various countries cut down the number of direct flights to and from China during the last days of January 2020 but, from a public health point of view, only weeks after the start of the Chinese New Year holiday. As China is a hub of air travel because it is a key centre of global production, these restrictions also posed a dilemma for companies and governments, even though it was known that the virus could spread rapidly through air travel. Many countries cautioned against travel not only to Wuhan but to all of China. For example, on 28 January 2020, the CDC published a warning against non-essential travel to China (CDC 2020). Two days later, the US tightened its restrictions.[8]

While the WHO remained hesitant, China reacted strongly against the travel restrictions imposed on it. The spokesperson for China's foreign ministry stated on 3 February 2020:

> Most countries appreciate and support China's efforts to fight against the novel coronavirus, and we understand and respect them when they adopt or enhance quarantine measures at border entry. But in the meantime, some

countries, the US in particular, have inappropriately overreacted, which certainly runs counter to WHO advice.

(Ministry of Foreign Affairs of the PRC 2020)

The US is singled out as the first country to impose travel restrictions on China:

> Even American media and experts doubted the government's decision, saying that the US government's restrictions on China are precisely what the WHO rejects, that the US is turning from overconfidence to fear and overreaction, and that banning the entry of visitors who traveled to China in the past 14 days is suspected to be violating civil rights instead of reducing risks of virus spreading. In fact, according to a recent CDC report, the US flu from 2019 to 2020 has caused 19 million infection cases and at least 10,000 deaths'.

However, the list of countries restricting flights and travel to China expanded to include most of China's neighbouring countries as well as Australia and Iran. Clearly, the emerging sentiment and standards for proper behaviour at the time were becoming compelling enough for countries and airlines to go against China's criticism, possible harm to future trade relations, and the value placed on open and unrestricted travel and trade.

Thus, during the initial stage, when all attention becomes focused on the outbreak, 'going with the flow' can be a compelling approach. The moment gives prominence to actions that are in step with one another simply because going against the current translates into a sense of unwise insensitivity and inflexibility in the face of decisive events. This pull of the context-dependent standard can be more compelling than economic self-interest or established institutional norms. The institutional normative structure is based on IHR. As such, the regulations tried to achieve coordinated measures that also took into consideration the need to enable smooth flow of traffic, commerce, and trade. The attention shifted away from containment at the border to containing an outbreak at the source, motivated partially due to deep concerns after the 2003 SARS pandemic over responsibility, transparency, and accountability at the national level (WHO 2005, 2016). Another important change in the overall strategy had to do with an emphasis on a tailored and flexible approach instead of the present response that was not sensitive to the specific nature of the outbreak.

The increasingly interdependent world based on mobility and circulation was supposed to react quickly, but in a proportional and flexible manner, to an outbreak. However, the actual response has highlighted three important and strong trends: (1) China's rise to a prominent global hub position in the present global order was matched by lowered trust felt regarding the 'safety' of such a rise; (2) the order that was created to safeguard against a repeat of China's secrecy during the 2003 SARS outbreak was resisted through the reintroduction of national travel bans and restrictions based on state borders; (3) the trend towards global decoupling—that is, the geographical separation of markets from industrial production—found its recent, and very potent, driver in COVID-19, as states saw the ramifications of cutting down connections to China and its position in the global value chains in a new light. On the whole, the outbreak stage of COVID-19 can be found to chime with certain pre-existing trends, such as the return of the nation-state, major power competition, and calls to decouple the global order. This is not surprising. Whereas SARS, as the first significant outbreak of the corona family of viruses, came with a message to create a more secure and resilient global mobility system, COVID-19 seems to reveal the not-so-resilient nature of the fixes and solutions created since 2003.

Conclusion

Although thoroughly interconnected, the global space is not evenly spread out. It thickens near and gravitates towards the global hubs, the key metropolitan regions usually located at the centre of other logistic access points. When this space turns into a liability in times of pandemic encounters, the tension contains the seeds for the overall re-imagination of political solidarity, accountability, and trust. The value of freedom of movement turns into demands for smarter and more secure globalization.

Pandemic diseases—diseases overarching the *pandemos*—can be co-opted for the purposes of advocating a more decoupled system that would be safer for progressive processes. While the global hub-and-spoke system is a signifier of globalization, pandemics register long-standing fears and worries that the rapid long-distance connections are dangerously dis-easing. To a large extent, especially SARS and, much more dramatically, COVID-19 came to be constructed as diseases of global networks. At the macro level, the corona family of viruses is seen as having the capacity to force the closure of modern life's support systems and turn upside down the polities that have become reliant on them. In a way, they are interpreted to have come with an ominous message for necessary political reform. It is in this context that resilience becomes the scenario of pandemic security knowledge. It is related to the main arteries of the global order. It is different from the nation-state-centred practices of 'defence'. However, it plays the same overall function of securing a political entity—in this case the system of asymmetric interdependencies and global flows.

The resilient global order highlighted in the SARS and avian flu spectacles seemed to demand the re-imagining of social organization, political authority, and expert governance and to hammer home the importance of resilience and preparedness as the key signifiers of future security. The official documents on pandemic diseases often highlighted the close connection between naturally occurring and intentionally caused outbreaks of disease. Pandemic emergencies become signifiers for more resilience against enemies with hybrid or shapeshifting faces.

Moreover, it is perceived that the measures aimed against naturally occurring outbreaks offered a way to combat possible intentional outbreaks. The preparedness over naturally occurring diseases was seen as a testing ground for developing security in the case of biological warfare or other threats posed to the global networks such as disinformation, hacking, and meddling. Resilience and hybrid threats have become to represent curious combination of vague terms describing the seemingly mutable and ambiguous environment. This combined dynamics provided a powerful undercurrent to the term 'global health security'. The discourses of pandemics are likely to be used to create a sense of security utterly unrelated to what pandemics as epidemiological phenomena are supposed to be. The stock pandemic scenario is not value neutral. It inevitably contains a particular vision of human solidarity, namely of the particular utopian vision of prepared and resilient polities that could meet the challenge of the shape-shifting mutable enemy. This often-used speculative vision promotes corresponding national and global governance structures as well as containment-oriented and resilient national communities.

Notes

1 See, for example, Wardrip (1996: 366).
2 Andrus *et al.* (2010).
3 The criticism of ICAO has focused on its non-transparent decision-making, on the limited role of its assembly, and on its technical rather than policy focus. Concerns have also been raised that the organization is part of China's rising power in the UN system (Cheng-Chia and Yang 2020).
4 IATA partners with ICAO in the management of pandemic situations. For example, the prevention and management, or Public Health Events in Civil Aviation (CAPSCA), project was supposed to bring together actors at different levels—public health and aviation authorities, airports, and airlines—to develop a coordinated approach.
5 Aaltola, Mika (2012a) 48 Snowden, Frank (2020).
6 Snowden, Frank (2020).
7 See, for example, Fiott and Zeiss (2021).
8 On 22 January 2020, North Korea became the first country to close its borders to Chinese visitors.

5

THE GEOPOLITICS OF SARS AND COVID-19

Neglect of the cross-cutting confluences between different co-occurring emergency scenarios is a notable feature in the study of pandemics and their political relevance. In this chapter, I will examine further the confluences inherent in a particular period of time and how pandemics can catalyse directly and indirectly other emergency scenarios such as great power tensions and conflicts by adding to the intensities and fever of the emotionally charged situations. In particular, I will look at the cases of SARS (2003) and coronavirus disease (COVID-19) (2020–21) to see how they fed and catalysed contagions of political regressions in the global arena as well as locally. SARS occurred in the same time frame as the Iraq War, and COVID-19's origin and waves are concurrent with both great power tensions and domestic political tensions. The claim is often made that in order to be a reasonable research interest, there should be a causal linkage and analytical model explaining the underlying mechanisms; however, regressive processes such as wars and diseases can not only accompany each other but also catalyse and fuel each other. The effective co-occurrence—instead of causality or linear effect—is not considered here to be merely a random occurrence but, instead, historically relatively well established and a path that can be traversed again. Conflicts can be seen as frames for diseases and diseases can offer frames for contemporaneous regressive political processes.

The spread of the Roman 'world order', Pax Romana, under the Roman Republic and then the Roman Empire was based on the advanced mobility networks of its time. The Roman legions, most of the time, were not guarding the limits of the empire. Rather, they were based along the roads of Rome and at sea to enforce peace, secure trade routes, and facilitate taxation. The security of the key flows from the periphery and beyond secured the sustainability of the core regions of the empire and enabled it to send its legions to foreign operations to expand the limits of Rome. However, there were unintended consequences. The spread of

DOI: 10.4324/9781003169147-5

the Roman Empire and its modus operandi opened up a route for faster spread of disease agents as well. In a way, in the very effective way that the governance was organized, there were unknown dangers that eventually began to hit the empire in wave after wave. The Antonine Plague (166–180 CE) was rumoured to have been brought in by Roman legions returning from their Western Asian campaign. The origin seems to have been the siege of Seleucia, in modern-day Iraq. Whatever the 'plague' was (probably either smallpox or measles), it was new since the Romans did not have immunity to it. The consequences in terms of human casualties were catastrophic. The epidemic happened during the reign of Emperor Marcus Aurelius, and it is worth noting that his period, and in particular its aftermath, is a key turning point in the ebbing and waning of the eventual decline of the Roman Empire.

The next major plague wave, of one of the aforementioned diseases, was the Plague of Cyprian (249–262 CE). It also caused a long-lasting breakdown in the essential security of supply systems causing, for example, food shortages. Similar to the Antonine Plague, it also influenced the Roman Empire's war-making capabilities. In his operations against the expansion of the Germanic tribes, Marcus Antonius would have needed men and resources. The Antonine Plague hampered the building up of much-needed military capabilities. The Plague of Cyprian, during its peak, killed thousands of people in Rome daily and was a turbulent period in the politics of the time. As historian Harper (2017) puts it, 'the history of Rome is a confusing tangle of violent failures. The structural integrity of the imperial machine burst apart. The frontier system crumbled. The collapse of legitimacy invited one usurper after another to try for the throne'. The plague coincided with the so-called Crisis of the Third Century, which saw political violence, failures in power transition, migration waves, scarcity, and financial troubles. As said before, pestilences often do not appear alone in a vacuum, with no spillover to other realms of life, and political regressions often lead into expanded vulnerability and open up windows of opportunity for plagues and enemies.

Unbeknownst to Rome's contemporaries, something other than smallpox, measles, and the resulting power vacuums, scarcities and migration of new populations was looming on the horizon. The migration of a rat species from South Asia to Europe was taking place along the longer trade routes. This migration was going to have a disruptive yet also transformational impact on the Late Roman and, later, European politics and power. The mix of conquest, trade, and rodent migration was the key factor in the introduction of plague epidemics to Europe (see McCormick 2003).

Plague was thus a symptom of the rise and spread of the Roman order and the mobilities on which that order was dependent. However, it was also a contributing factor in the decline and fall of the Western Roman Empire. The Late Roman period and the Western Roman Empire came to a final end with more than two centuries of waves of the Plague of Justinian (541–750 CE). This plague was the first widespread plague epidemic, as it later came to be known in European history. Although the people of the time interpreted the origin of the disease as Africa, it is most likely that the plague epidemics had their origins in Central Asia and spread west via trade routes. During the Plague of Justinian, the key Mediterranean port cities in particular were decimated by the waves of plague that killed about half the population there. It was one of the most devastating and politically consequential epidemics in recorded history.

Although the disease agent itself does not come with a message or function as a direct cause, it can act as a trigger for cascading political and governance effects. This trigger effect is hard to trace or analytically reduce back to an outbreak. Yet it is clear that many of the most devastating diseases from the Roman plagues to epidemics in the conquest of the Americas to, for example, Spanish Flu have anteceded or coincided with historical turning points. As Thucydides would probably have argued, the political space gets placed under duress and stress for many reasons, but when vulnerabilities open up, they are likely to be abused by many regressive phenomena. In many cases, the expected 'consequential' outcomes of a serious pandemic are political collapse, instability, and other regressions such as tensions, scarcities, and conflicts. Thus, an epidemic, to be consequential, has to cause a regression in the political and social order and be accompanied by and happen in tandem with war, domestic upheavals, and major power transitions.

Focusing on a single presumably self-contained bundle of security issues or processes can lead to insular notions of global security as well as to lost opportunities for security-sensitive contributions to the adjoining issue areas. Against this background, the chapter overviews the patterns of interactions during the security scenarios of early 2003: wars, for example, the War against Terror and the Iraq War, and pandemics such as SARS. The same is done in the case of COVID-19, which opened up new avenues for the use of pandemic security in the overall building of the security scenario in the context of heightened major power tensions. The overall global order scenario where the different seemingly self-contained security scenarios fit is the declining unipolarity and the rise of China:

> The shifting balance of economic power is also beginning to be seen globally, where China's economic presence in Africa, Latin America, and Europe challenges the longstanding economic primacy of the United States. China's growing global economic and political role is also likely to begin to re-shape international norms, rules, and institutions. It will, over time, reverberate across geopolitics, global trade, investment, capital flows, reserve currency status, climate change and other environmental challenges, as well as global flows of people.
>
> *(Rudd 2015: 33—34)*

From the demonstration of US power in the Iraq War to suspicions about the secrecy of China regarding the onset of diseases from SARS to COVID-19, the key is this wide overall scenario of tensions and great power enmities in the fundaments of the global order. Pandemics can easily become (geo)political and security related in such tense situations. One measure of the degree of politicization of pandemics has been the mobilization of necessary resources. Pandemic security and politics tend to rise on the agenda, and, consequently, politics becomes the driver of events instead of expertise and expert organizations (e.g. Rushton 2019: 4).

As stated in Introduction, by overviewing different and at least partially overlapping emergency and security scenarios, it is possible to draw attention to the synoptic interplay between the different scenarios and thus go beyond mere statements of non-linear relationships or one scenario catalysing the other. This approach also crosses the usual disciplinary and conceptual boundaries separating security studies, global health studies, and world-order studies. How does the context of war amplify other security concerns? What were the synoptic interactions within temporally situated 'bundles' of security-related concerns? How did the global modus operandi—mobility systems—and pandemic politics construct their combined security problematiques in the context of geopolitics and power politics? Next, I will shed light on the difficulties of managing pandemic diseases as purely epidemiological processes, on the complexities of global mobility, and on how tense situations are prone to lead to speculative projections as people's fears find different somatic, material, and political manifestations.

SARS' Confluences with the Iraq War

The spring of 2003 was tense. Time seemed to be of the essence as the affective climate was filled with much political speculation and building of worst-case scenarios. As usual, in hindsight, much of this was based more on imagination than facts, as in the case of the alleged Iraqi chemical and biological WMDs. However, some were more factual as in the case of SARS, a deadly variant of the quite common coronavirus family, although, in hindsight, even that was more of a scare than an actual killer disease. That said, it was also a direct precursor to a much larger disruption, COVID-19. As time goes on, the meaning and significance of diseases and their perceived impact evolve and are continuously re-evaluated. It is notable that the Spanish Flu has also been known as the forgotten pandemic because its memory was overshadowed by a global war (e.g. Patterson and Pyle 1991: 4). During the year 2020, it was re-evaluated because COVID-19 brought back the spectre of the Spanish Flu and made the forgotten strikingly memorable once again.

In the event-intensive drama of 2003, different scenarios overlapped. The Iraq War scenario had a pandemic characteristic. At the same time, the pandemic emergency had the war as one of its characteristics besides bringing in the global order's mobility system and the importance of flow security, both of which had implications when it came to the US-led large-scale military campaign in the Persian Gulf. Although not directly, these two scenarios—war and pandemic—were partly interlinked in the overall confluence of circumstances.

In the charged atmosphere of the overall geopolitical flux, SARS arguably reflected the prevailing anxieties over the underlying stability of the world order and its key mobility-based modus operandi. The US anthrax attacks that followed the 9/11 attacks in New York City were still fresh in people's minds:

> The emergence of SARS is the second major event of the 21st century to change the perception of the infectious disease threat in the eyes of politicians and the general public. The deliberate use of anthrax to incite terror, which quickly followed the events of 11 September 2001 in the U.S., was the first event.
>
> *(Heyman and Rodier 2004: 185)*

The talk about bioterror and pandemics was further reinforced against the background of the era of the 1990s which saw Ebola's ability to escape out of its local context and become intercontinental through the vector of rapidly increasing international air connections, the key modality of the global order, where the focus is on its modus operandi, mobilities, and standards (e.g. Child 2014: 198). Overall, there was much talk about bioterror, which recycled the pandemic 'coming plague' scenarios that had been so popular in the 1990s (e.g. Garrett 1994).

The hyperbole of pandemic imagery was notably built into the case made against Iraq when it was accused of developing military uses of epidemic diseases. In addition, the overall fears, worries, and suspicions gave specific nuances to and strengthened the alternative articulations of air mobility: the global hub-and-spoke aviopolis was increasingly seen not only as a signifier of global connectedness but also as a register of immense vulnerability. The three security scenarios—global order, war, and SARS—became entangled in a way that defied the seemingly conceptual distance between them and highlighted how any temporal context produces nexuses and bundles of security. It is vital to overview these cross-cutting patterns and the more lasting cross-cutting bridges between the scenarios. The claim that global mobility architecture or pandemic disease's directionality are connected with those of global power and security has received relatively scant research attention in international relations (Salter 2008: 245). The relative absence of thorough accounting for the interaction between different security scenarios may easily lead, on the one hand, to insular notions of global security and, on the other hand, to lost opportunities for politically sensitive contributions to adjoining issue areas. Synoptic overviews can alleviate the tendency to regard military security in an insular way. Going beyond insularity, the aim here is to discern how other concurrent phenomena are amplified by the overall global instability.

Major conflicts, indirect clashes, and wars have a clear geographical scope, yet they also have much reach in terms of cognitive associations and many metaphors of enmity talk of the resource mobilization needed for competition and conflict, especially wars. It seems evident that the sequence, tempo, and intensity of military actions might bundle distinct events into momentary consequential wholes that react with many co-occurring processes. For example, the Afghan War, which started in October 2001, happened in close sequence after 9/11. The resulting intense tempo of events leading to the Iraq War in the spring of 2003 packaged that war in the overall context of the War against Terror, regardless of the factual connections. The relative disconnect between 9/11 and the Iraq War demonstrates the confluences of wider flux within which wars happen. The lessons learnt from Iraq fed back to the War against Terror and to Afghanistan. This power to recontextualize and draw together bundles of otherwise disparate events is a noteworthy characteristic of major wars. Apples and oranges mix, and these mixes should be recognized. It is in this context also that bioterror, anthrax, and SARS provided combinatory possibilities and valences opened up with other momentary security bundles.

On the one hand, the wide reach of war has been examined from various angles. Conflicts have a reach, as Thucydides reminds us, they tend to deepen and widen. Issues become integrated into their scope. Anything co-occurring is politicized and sucked into the vortex of a major conflict. In this mixing, there is no analytical clarity, only, at the end, a flux. It does not happen in a vacuum, as pointed out by Johnson (2000), who referred to the dynamic of 'blowback' in seeing how the US' external actions can lead to violence directed back towards it that then escalates and widens the scope of enmities. Some researchers have gone beyond the usual 'violence begets violence' models to show how military actions can amplify seemingly unrelated types of violence. Hamamoto's (2002) study of the link between foreign wars and mass murders and serial killings in the US reveals the wider complexities of the 'reach of war' argument. The enmity patterns are internalized in outward acts of mass violence and how they are justified (e.g. Henson and Olson 2010: 341). On the other hand, it is not only war that has reach and that reaches out, according to the politosomatic hypothesis. Pandemics have reach too, and they are reactive with other processes. For example, one marked consequence of the COVID-19 pandemic has been the rise in domestic unrest and violence (e.g. Kishi *et al.* 2021). Diseases, just like wars, feed underlying enemy images and patterns of enmity and cause unrest and violence on the streets. Thus, in many ways, conflicts and contagious diseases reach out to each other. It must be noted that these discernible connections do not need to be causal or analytically clear for them to exert a general impact. The historical and speculative sensitivities related to the war context can affect the specific fields of expectations. This may concretise these expectations—leading to self-fulfilling processes—and hyperbolize even the smallest expectations, according significance to noteworthy events that are made to fit into underlying trends.

One further bridgehead into this study is the belief that wars are disease amplifiers. This oft-repeated reach of war has deep historical roots and has acquired additional strength in the context of pandemic scares, biological weapons, and bioterror threats (Longrigg 1992; Rollet 2014). It may be suggested that the SARS outbreak encouraged the construction of the much-feared pandemic disease expected in the context of political turbulence. The following exchange from a White House press briefing (19 May 2003) illustrates the multiple use of disease metaphors in the War against Terror:

> **Question:** She [President Arroyo of Philippines] said, terrorism is like SARS, it's almost like SARS. Is it spreading because we still have yet to find the core, Osama bin Laden?

Answer: That's the nature of terrorism. It's the nature of hatred. Hatred doesn't exist only because of one person; hatred exists. In this case, it's the most virulent hatred because it's carried out in the form of murder—murder against Americans; murder against Westerners.

The build-up to the Iraq War arguably contained all these cross-cutting tendencies. The combinatorial possibilities between conflicts and diseases were exploited: the situation was partly conceived of in terms of spiralling hostility, there was much fear of the contagion potential of the situation, and the metaphors of contagion and disease were used to construct threats. For example, former US Secretary of State Colin Powell gave a speech to the United Nations Security Council on 5 February 2003 in which he tried to convince the council that the grounds for the military operations against Saddam Hussein's Iraq were justified. The aim of the speech was to convince and persuade, and it drew from the well-established historical pattern that connects diseases with perceived enemies: 'My colleagues, every statement I make today is backed up by sources, solid sources. These are not assertions. What we are giving you are facts and conclusions based on solid intelligence'. Powell states that Saddam's 'inhumanity' is as limitless as it is cruel and also uses diseases as weapons. As a case in point, he mentions cruel experiments with prisoners. Powell concretizes the threat of the WMDs, especially through their biological disease-related dimension. Contagious diseases can be used to make related arguments tangible, more embodied. The politosomatic persuasion concretizes the points and brings it closer to the listeners' bodies; arguably, this act of combinatorics made the Iraqi threat easier not only to imagine but to feel:

> Saddam Hussein has investigated dozens of biological agents causing diseases such as gas-gangrene, plague, typhus, tetanus, cholera, camelpox, and hemorrhagic fever. And he also has the wherewithal to develop smallpox.[1]

The clear point was that Saddam, as an agent of evil, had turned the worst historically known epidemic diseases, plagues, into weapons that he was ready to use. Powell even concretizes this by actually using a teaspoon in the presentation to maximize the impact of anthrax and reminding his audience of the horror produced by the so-called anthrax letter in the aftermath of 9/11.

Biological weapons have been developed by great powers. However, the 1975 Convention on the Prohibition of the Development, Production and Stockpiling of Bacteriological (Biological) and Toxin Weapons and on their destruction prohibits the use and stockpiling of such weapons. But they are still being researched for the supposed purpose of finding defences against them. It is important to note that this argument was further amplified by the first news emerging on the spread of SARS. The epidemic was also emphasized by the White House. The vigilance of American President George W. Bush in disease control was prominently highlighted in US official press releases:

> President Bush is very aware, acutely aware, of the situation of SARS around the world. He pays very close attention to this, has frequent briefings on

it, and has particularly been interested in making sure, as you've just heard, that the finest resources of this country—our research establishment, the CDC, NIH and other of our universities and the resources that we have in this country—are effectively and immediately and appropriately mobilized to fight this epidemic.

(White House 2003a)

The contextual bridge here is politosomatic. The abstractness of power politics and geostrategy is made as concrete as possible by introducing the element of disease. This framing allowed for projection of individual fears of bodily harm to Iraq and its leadership. The framing also made the US' later use of force in the form of surgical strikes and precision weapons seem almost like medical activities undertaken to fight a serious illness, as a doctor does when treating a patient with a malign tumour.

Furthermore, the US documents on SARS often highlighted the close connection between naturally occurring and intentionally caused outbreaks of disease. It was perceived that the measures aimed against naturally occurring outbreaks offered a way to combat possible intentional outbreaks. They were seen as rehearsals for biological warfare. The preparedness over naturally occurring diseases was seen as a testing ground for developing preparedness over possible biological attacks. The combined dynamics is captured in the terms 'health security' or 'pandemic security' (e.g. Castelli 2008: 3). The documents conceive of new health threats stemming from (re)emerging diseases and biological warfare agents:

> Given American leadership in the biomedical field and Singapore's advanced research facilities, President Bush and Prime Minister Goh agreed that the two countries should explore prospects for collaborative efforts . . . [and] to begin consultations on possible joint projects.
>
> *(White House 2003b)*

From the US perspective, the SARS-related outlook was part of a larger vision to the world as narrated in the presidential directive, 'Biodefense for the 21st Century' on 28 April 2004, which

> provides a comprehensive framework for our nation's biodefense. [It] builds on past accomplishments, specifies roles and responsibilities, and integrates the programs and efforts of various communities—national security, medical, public health, intelligence, diplomatic, agricultural and law enforcement—into a sustained and focused national effort against biological weapons threats.
>
> *(White House 2004)*

The integrated approach to meet the threats of terrorism subsumed many of the defences against naturally occurring diseases. The probable consequence was that the occurrence of a natural epidemic disease, SARS, heightened the security-related framing of it. At the same time, SARS also amplified the believability of the under-lying cause for the Iraq War—Iraq's alleged WMDs. The overall amplification accentuated the need to reform Western polities to be more resilient and prepared for all kinds of risks that could be posed to the current world order.

SARS and COVID-19's Power to Disrupt the Global Order

The tensions in the spring of 2003 clearly pointed out how a mobility-based world can suddenly change into one of containment. One factor was the Iraq War. Already in October 2002, the US Congress had granted war powers to President Bush with regard to Iraq. The war itself started on 20 March 2003 with a shock and awe cam-paign to disrupt Iraq's critical defence systems and to demonstrate overwhelming force in order to demoralize the Iraqi troops. The invasion phase came to a formal end on 1 May 2003, although the situation worsened steadily for years to include internal war and the occupation. The US-led coalition sent some 180,000 troops to Iraq. This required large-scale build-up and logistics. The Rumsfeld Doctrine placed heavy emphasis on force readiness and decreased numbers of troops in the theatre of operation. The mobility system of this modern large-scale operation depended on precision combat systems, air supremacy, and nimble ground forces. An agile force supported by logistics is also key to the great powers' global ability to project force. The US military force mobilization is based on pre-positioning sea lifts but also on airlifts to deploy and sustain operations such as the Iraq War (Hazdra 2001). The global order's mobility expertise was put to use with the movability of high-tech systems and air power.

As the US use of mobility systems in war demonstrates, the global order does not seem as borderless as the cosmopolitical visions had envisaged (e.g. Guittet 2017: 209). Although thoroughly interconnected, the global fabric's mobility capa-bilities are not evenly spread, they are more at the disposal of some key actors than others. It thickens near and gravitates towards the global hubs and super-regions where you have many mobility hubs, hubs of hubs like the US. Without this posi-tion, the US would logistically not have been able to stage large-scale military operations like two wars in the Persian Gulf. The global air traffic embodies this uneven or lumpy pattern. At the same time, pandemic diseases—diseases affecting the whole of the '*pandemos*'—can embody and be used to narrate the different fears that this system might become conducive to regressive spiralling processes. The key strength of the global order, and its prime mover, is also its main vulnerability. While the global hub-and-spoke system is a signifier of globalization, pandemics register long-existing fears and worries that the rapid intercontinental connections are dangerously dis-easing. To a large extent, SARS and COVID-19 in particular came to be constructed as a disease of global networks. However, in the case of Haiti's cholera outbreak, this connection was downplayed for political and legiti-macy reasons, as we will see in Chapter 7. At the macro level, SARS was seen as having the capacity to force the closure of modern life's support systems and upset the polities that had become reliant on them. In a way, it was interpreted to have come with an ominous message for political reform. This message was often read as one of creating a more resilient and better prepared global society. COVID-19 indicated that this lesson had not been learnt adequately enough. Vulnerability remained or, perhaps, had even become more serious.

SARS and the Iraq War blended, but in a nuanced and somewhat indirect way. COVID-19 had a much more clear-cut connection with power politics and flows of power in an apparent transition towards the relative rise of China, the origin of the virus flows. COVID-19 reached all countries other than China from outside through air connections. It highlighted the dystopian images of the mobility system as a vector of harm, yet it also pointed out how connected China had become to the Western heartlands. It is clear that there is a tight connection between air travel and the spread of COVID-19 (e.g. Shen 2021). The infrastructure of built environment contributed to the initial spread of COVID-19. For example, China's BRI plans are ambitious and global. Mobility systems under fast development like the BRI are a wonder for many and a source of anxiety in the West. China is planning to further develop its air mobility networks by building more than 160 airports, and it is also looking to expand its railway networks. Since the 1990s, the US has opened only one major airport, Denver International. The rusting infrastructure of the US indicates decline, while China's plans indicate its rise in the global mobility order's hierarchy. Yet, at the same time, both SARS and COVID-19 have shown the potential of this developing global mobility as a vector for diseases. The sentiments of pandemic and terror-related declinism in the 1990s and 2000s match the realities of the 2020s.

Mobility is unequally distributed and hierarchical—it is based on power and status. The global order itself has been based on connections and interdependence and on secure arteries between the key global hubs. The aerial vision is also geopolitical as it shows the map from a different vantage point. The expansion of US power was concurrent with the expansion of air travel and the development of the hub-and-spoke system of airports. Knowledge of a geostrategic type developed while diplomats and decision makers travelled through the mobility system. This aerial vision impacted the resulting knowledge. The hub-and-spoke model of this embodied vision translated into geostrategic relationships vis-à-vis, for example, the cartwheel model of the American alliance system in the Asia-Pacific, and today, China's BRI is a version of the same vision.

Perhaps the most famous expression of this type of geostrategic vision was Robert Kaplan's influential essay, 'Coming Anarchy', in 1994. For Kaplan, the spread of diseases was just one more worrying symptom of the global governance breakdown that was emanating from the Global South through the contagion of corruptive and regressive practices as evidenced in decaying infrastructure such as railways and airports. Kaplan's cartographic imagery represents containment-type thinking where international intersections and lines of communication signify dangerous channels of contagion that should be checked and contained. These germs of decline are spreading in the physical, cultural, moral, and political sense. Kaplan's argument uses disease as a metaphor—its inherent sense of alarm, hostility, and the dynamics of contagion and mutation—in making his case for a spreading regressive political process, in making impending anarchy more real and tangible. He begins his article with the following account of a meeting with an African minister whose eyes, ridden with malaria, became the foreground for the story of a diseased land-scape and the future to come: 'The coming upheaval, in which foreign embas-sies are shut down, states collapse, and contact with the outside world takes place through dangerous, disease-ridden coastal trading posts, will loom large in the century we are entering' (Kaplan 1994: 80). The form of Kaplan's essay is one of an aerial travelogue, looking down from an airplane window. Unlike the planners of US geostrategy in the 1940s and 1950s, whose vision was one of building and expanding, Kaplan's vision is declinist.

The 9/11 attack saw air travel itself becoming a vector of terror. However, the same imaginary had already been present in the declinist narratives of the coming pandemic. Perhaps more than any other research-related book that epitomized this change was Laurie Garrett's *The Coming Plague* (1994). The basic crux of Garrett's work was that exotic viruses were jumping out of their tropical habitats due to the developing global transportation networks that connected air routes to road building in the developing countries: local peripheries with fragile health-care sys-tems and their hitherto relatively isolated circulation of diseases were becoming fed into the global arteries through the hub-and-spoke infrastructures. Humanity was becoming more exposed as its links extended to tropical places and remoter global reaches became increasingly accessible. Kaplan and Garrett's influential works talked about the same alarming vision, the spreading of agents of regression. It is notable that the visions of global mobility turned into pessimism in the US, while in China, infrastructure was seen as key in competing with the US for global great power status. The Silk Road and, later, the BRI are aimed at pushing China's ambition to be at the centre of foreign policy efforts as well.

Power and mobility have an ever-tightening relationship. The control, secur-ing, and dominating of the architecture of hubs and spokes provide for rise or decline in the global power hierarchy. Urry (2009: 34) makes the case that aero-mobility is based on 'a dynamic and flexible systemic structure articulated horizon-tally across the globe'. This dynamic and flexible framework is in accordance with the contours of the existing assemblages of hegemonic governance and provides a major expression of what is meant by global interdependency (Hardt and Negri 2001: 13–14; Aaltola 2005: 268; Agambe 1998: 123; Dillon and Reid 2000: 117). From this bridgehead, the hub-and-spoke air mobility has become an increasingly important register of security and vulnerability (e.g. Crang 2002: 571; Dodge and Kitchin 2004: 195). It is notable that the post-9/11 air mobility scenario includes a marked dystopian element (e.g. Knox *et al.* 2007: 267). Dystopian declinism knits the scenarios of air mobility closely together with geopolitical and public health security scenarios. During the spring of 2003 and again during 2020–21, the idi-oms of terrorism, governmental secrecy, superspreaders, and reckless tourists led to flight disruptions, grounded flights, health screening, severing of connections, quarantined passengers, and even, in some cases, air travel coming to a standstill.

Without deeply taking into account this modality of the global power and disease vector, the understanding of conflicts and pandemics would be incomplete.

The scenario involved two types of actors: protagonists of humanity and antagonists of the *pandemos*. Besides key protagonist figures such as health-care workers doing their duty, the SARS scenario offered different actors opportunities to demonstrate their high degree of expertise and their diligent adherence to the practices of containment. Such rule ascertaining and following actions can be instrumental in conveying the political/governance health of the underlying political order and reassuring the public against the actual realization of worst-case scenarios. At the end, when the dust settled, the SARS emergency allowed for displays of new containment-oriented practices and pretension of more resilient global travel and health systems.

Yet the politicized figures of SARS also contained people who were vilified, turned into antagonists, a modern-day version of plague spreaders. Much of the suspicion was still connected to the figure of the terrorist or rogue state who could use air mobility as a weapon. Such antagonists of the *pandemos* were extremist figures constructed from the global spokes or peripheries. These 'politopaths' were seen as people with politically dangerous and suicidal disorders manifesting themselves in extreme political attitudes and violent behavioural tendencies and a lack of conscience. The antagonist figures challenged power because power ultimately is intimate and invides making it felt bodily through, for example, monopolies of force or, then, acts of violence, destruction, and disruption. And they can produce situations in which the prevailing legitimate power is not felt but is instead hijacked by them, and they are able to make their disorderly form of power felt bodily. Although the figures of the 'superspreader' and 'reckless person' in the pandemic frame do not possess as extreme characteristics as that of the terrorist, the location is the same, the global hub-and-spoke system. In the SARS scenario, for example, the figures of 'frequent traveller' and 'tourist' became signifiers of a possible horrible failure in the containment drama because some of them seemed to defy the usual notions of protective barriers and quarantines.

The containment measures tailored to air traffic seemed inadequate. For example, the screening measures, although widely used and highly publicized, proved to be insufficient. The WHO recommended that travellers be screened at airports for symptoms and signs of SARS, such as sneezing and fever. However, 'in spite of intensive screening, no SARS cases were detected by the border-authorities' (St John *et al.* 2006: 6). There was a sense of helplessness especially as the severing of connections did not seem to be an attractive option since air transportation can be seen as the modus operandi of the global order. Disrupting it would have resulted in economic harm. However, the pandemic emergency and scare led to the cutting down of flights and, more importantly, to a decrease in individuals' desire to fly. However, many were also trying to flee infected areas (Caballero 2005: 483), a scene repeated during the Spring of 2020, as lockdown and flight restrictions were preceded by rushes to fly out and leave containment zones through others means of transportation.

The chronology associates SARS with the global hub-and-spoke network of air transportation. This link with SARS is commonly made in research literature too: 'The analyses indicate that airline network accessibility was an especially influential variable' (Bowen and Laroe 2006: 130). The recent background for this link was provided by the popular pandemic imageries of the 1990s (e.g. Garrett 1994: 571). Thomas (2006: 918) compares SARS with the historical encounters with pandemics in this respect: 'The outbreak of Severe Acute Respiratory Syndrome (SARS) . . . showed how quickly regional and global connectivity could be subverted in the spread of infectious diseases beyond national borders'. Posner (2004: 21) points out this unintended consequence of modern technology: 'Modern transportation, especially by air, facilitates the rapid spread of new diseases'. Studies have repeatedly pointed out how the hub-and-spoke directionality of global travel links with the spread pattern of influenza pandemics (e.g. Ali and Keil 2006). Global air travel is based on a system of flows that increasingly interconnect the global metropolises—the hubs—to the spokes of the many global reaches. The differential flows create opportunities for disease pathogens, which favour spreading through the hubs more than reaching all the spokes (e.g. Hufnagel *et al.* 2004). Whereas some places are more likely to become conducive to a pandemic disease, there are some travellers who are more exposed as well as more likely to pass the disease on to others. Hollingsworth *et al.* (2007: 1288) stress that different travel profiles have differential effects on the spread of pandemic diseases. Especially conducive to disease spread are the so-called frequent fliers. These diseasing tendencies are among the many factors that gave SARS its avian modality and stressed the need to secure and contain global air traffic flows.

As people fly, power is on the move and can be seen as finding its expressive grammar in the regular tempos of the mobile bodies (Aaltola 2005). The humming regularity of the national, regional, and global aero-mobility systems is often used to constitute and signify the power of the respective 'movers' in global politics. The opposite is equally expressive: the regular disturbances—such as cancelled, late, or delayed flights—in the hub-and-spoke dynamics easily translate into imageries of decreasing or lack of power. In this way, the steady flows of moving bodies act as registers of the status and health of the present world order. This aspect of mobile embodied power is vital when one wants to shed light on how and why aero-mobility dynamics is so entangled with the trajectories of power politics. From this perspective, SARS' expressive characteristics had much to do with its actual and perceived ability to disrupt the air flows of people and goods and thereby interrupt the power anchored in regular global flows. Modern pandemic diseases readily interfere with the power and mobility nexus and thus gain an alarming characteristic. They can potentially change the relative power status of various places and people. During SARS, the status of the internal air mobility system was under intense scrutiny as people saw it as a sign of the devastation that the disease could bring in its wake. On the one hand, there were fears that air travel would collapse, leading to the regression of the global order so heavily based on it. Thus, apart from war, it seems that global air mobility is increasingly viewed as a disease amplifier because it too can move a vast number of people.

COVID-19 as a Geo-Pandemic Event

One sign of the changing times is that Thucydides' grand movement is back in vogue; however, he is also repeatedly mentioned as an analyst of the Plague of Athens in the commentaries concerning COVID-19 (Allison 2017; Zaretsky 2020). This is not surprising because he saw both weakening of order and appearance of pestilences as parts of the same regressive grand vortex. The concept of the Thucydidean Trap in particular is used to analyse the world-order dynamics between the existing global superpower, the US, and its rising rival, China. Thucydides seems to fit our times in the sense that the US is possibly facing its first peer competitor since the fall of the Soviet Union. The world-order drama has led to the popularity of Thucydides, who diagnosed the emergence of a hegemonic clash and provided a prognosis should such events happen again. He wrote his book for future generations as a diagnostic manual in order for them to see the early signs of overall regression—both domestic and international—and avoid conflict, or at least be better equipped to avoid or survive it. At the same time, Thucydides' description sees epidemics as one symptom of hegemonic rivalry.

In the context of great power competition and possible power transition, the 'plague', COVID-19, acquires additional characteristics. It becomes not only pandemic but also geo-pandemic. Geopolitics can be defined as a school of thought that analyses patterns of power related to and influenced by geographical factors and uneven distribution of strategic resources. Its modern extension, the geo-economy, refers to how economies, trade, and financial resources influence power bargaining and statecraft. However, pandemics have their own geopolitical extensions as has been argued in Chapter 4. When the pattern of power as an economic, resource, and geographical modality becomes influenced by spreading disease with an uneven disease burden, the situation can be said to be geo-pandemic, referring also to the Thucydidean framework. Moreover, the disease itself and immunity against it can find expression in the form of disease nationalism, vaccine herding, and diplomacy—and as the subject of intense major powers' status and blame games, the term seems even more justified.

The global system is also hierarchical in the sense of immunity creation and vaccine production. There are only about a dozen countries that have companies that can produce vaccines. The herding of vaccines, export restrictions, and putting one's own citizens first have been a marked feature of the fall 2020 and spring 2021 COVID-19 competition and controversies (e.g. Hafner *et al.* 2020). The hopes that were raised by the quick production of vaccines were dashed as it soon became clear that production could not keep up with the high demand and that the global vaccination efforts were lagging behind developed states' capabilities. Developed nations were vacuuming the vaccines from the global markets by ordering vaccines from different producers to the tune of four to five times their actual need.

This vaccine nationalism took place because the vaccine producers were not able to meet the demand due to scarcity of approved production sites and because of lack of the components necessary for production (Felter *et al.* 2021). The situation developed into one of geopolitical struggle over a scarce resource, and bitterness was a common feature with regard to the relative success of some states—such as Israel, the UK, and the US—in vaccinating their citizens.

Vaccines are not developed by states but by multinational companies with head-quarters in Europe, China, Russia, and, especially, the US. The key vaccine producers with their own relative independencies and mutual dependencies when it comes to production cycles, value chains, and component production are the so-called Club of 13: Argentina, Australia, Brazil, Canada, China, the EU, India, Japan, South Korea, the Russian Federation, Switzerland, the UK, and the US. Production of an effective vaccine in general needs about 20 components. Not all the members of the Club are equal in their ability to produce the components in their own states:

> The shares of imports of key ingredients from other vaccine producers as a group ranged from a low of 76.4% (India) to 98.7% (United Kingdom). In contrast, 68% of vaccine producers' imports of all goods came from the Vaccine Club. The two top exporters of key ingredients are the United States and the European Union, which accounted for half of total exports, followed by United Kingdom, Japan and China with significantly smaller shares.
>
> *(Evenett et al. 2020)*

The Club is in a league of its own, yet any export restrictions of vaccines or key components can significantly hamper the functioning of global vaccine production.

The security of the supply model in many fields, as also in vaccines, is based on the global mobility system. Transportation costs are low, and the idea is that the markets will be efficient in the distribution of critical materials and products. The efficiency of the global system has overwhelmed the more nationally based ideas of security of supply. Smaller countries cannot afford the costs of development of many of the critical products that their citizens depend on in their everyday life, let alone the supplies needed in emergency situations.

Already at the start of the COVID-19 outbreak in the spring of 2020, there was an acute scarcity of PPE such as high-quality masks. The main production sites in East Asia were swamped with orders, and the delivery times got longer and prices went up. Many countries, including the US and the EU member-states, did not have adequate production and stockpiles of their own. The levels of preparedness were low as was the kick-starting of own production; in addition, there were not enough certified testing sites for masks and other protective gear. Over-reliance on the global market-based supply security suddenly seemed a risky proposition (e.g. Mellish *et al.* 2020: 9). The national production of PPE in high labour cost countries requires state-level investments in the private sector and can even be illegal in some states because of the rules against unfair competition.

The scarcity of PPE and vaccines opened up space for corona or vaccine diplomacy. The term did not originally have the geopolitical and geo-pandemic connotations that it took on during the COVID-19 outbreak. For example, Bollyky (2021: 4–5) notes:

> All 39 countries to which China has donated vaccines are participants in its Belt and Road Initiative. . . . The manner in which these vaccine diplomacy efforts are being conducted suggest that they are more a means of cementing spheres of influence rather than advancing global health equity and bringing this pandemic under control as soon as possible.

Bollyky also points out that most donations for the global distribution effort are coming from autocratic countries. It was recommended that the US should also take part in vaccine diplomacy:

> The United States has historically been a leading proponent of vaccine diplomacy and equity and has significant interests in continuing to be a leader in this pandemic. Safe and effective vaccines can meaningfully alter the trajectory of this pandemic and lessen its economic and humanitarian consequences at home and abroad, but success depends on getting doses to vulnerable populations who can benefit from them the most. Yet, efforts to bridge the global gap between the vaccine-haves and the vaccine-have-nots have stalled as the United States and other nations grapple with the domestic threat of this deadly virus.
>
> (Bollyky 2021: 2)

The recommendation for the US to enter into vaccine diplomacy stems from two worries: first, that the US should make an actual contribution to the 'one world, one health' principle, and, second, that the US should counter the autocratic vaccine diplomacy with its own efforts or fail in status and reputation in countries where there is scarcity of resources and which are in danger of falling geostrategically into China's interest sphere.

Restricting production to one's own citizens and a containment approach can be seen as diplomatically more problematic than a more compassionate approach. However, the US, the UK, and the EU faced domestic political constraints in exporting a significant number of vaccines. The nearest-is-dearest approach seemed to be the more politically powerful sentiment in the COVID-19 scenario than compassion for the distant other, although there was a strong foreign policy interest in countering China's geo-pandemic campaign, which supported the more 'compassionate approach'. China was using a more calculated strategy in its approach than the universal principle of 'one world, one health' would suggest (Gyu 2021: 1). While the domestic imperative seemed to prevail over national geostrategic interests in the bigger Western democracies, in China, the domestic imperative was balanced with external interests.

The balance shifted rapidly as a function of the changing domestic pandemic situation and as the domestic vaccine programmes advanced. The US and the EU adopted policies that saw the possibility of starting vaccine exports once a satisfactory situation was achieved at home. The US started with smaller-scale exports to its neighbours, Mexico and Canada, in April 2021. However, in a summit meeting in March 2021 of the Quad countries (Quadrilateral Security Dialogue), India, the US, Japan, and Australia, it was decided that '[w]e will, therefore, collaborate to strengthen equitable vaccine access for the Indo-Pacific, with close coordination with multilateral organizations including the World Health Organization and COVAX' (White House 2021). Similarly, the EU promised exports to its Eastern European partners as well as to Africa. It is clear that the starting of the exports can be interpreted to have been an extension of the nearest-is-dearest approach, to regions nearby or to regions of vital geostrategic interest. Because of the near suffocation of the pandemic situation in China, it was better placed to start exports to countries in its strategic interest before the US and the EU.

Contemporary times are uncertain. Much seems to be in flux, and the flux has spread from the more peripheral areas to the heartland of the democratic West. The progressive narratives, expectations, and perhaps even somewhat naive wishes of the post–Cold War era are gradually receding to the background. Brute destabilizations and grim political disunity are spreading. At least for the time being, states are de-normalizing, democracy is no longer spreading, markets are not opening up, multilateralism is in trouble, and interdependencies can be used as power-political tools or weapons.[2]

During the SARS outbreak, the scenarios of conflict and pandemic overlapped only partially through two characteristics: they coincided with and further inflamed the sense of political anxiety during the build-up to and duration of the Iraq War, and, second, they challenged the sustainability of the key modality of the global order, air mobility, which is needed for the present global system to function and stands as a key signifier of the global order's operational efficiency. The emergence of COVID-19 did not tie into a war scenario, but it had consonancies with the increasing major power rivalry that was already present in the political interpretations of SARS. Power was seen to be on the move—a global power transition was speculated to be on its way. In this way, COVID-19 can be seen as emerging in a geopolitically charged situation, and it immediately led to interpretations concerning patterns of enmity between the great powers. First, the speculations concerned the role of China, its secrecy and ability to contain the disease domestically, and then, the attention turned to talk about global decoupling, economic disruption, and the failure of the US to contain the domestic spread of the disease.

If nothing else, 'hub-and-spoke' is an abstract designation for a multifaceted embodied transportation experience underlying the feeling of being global and of being part of a global flow. As already pointed out, the tight conceptual bridge between hegemonic governance structures and hub-and-spoke political architecture is often made in research literature. The best-known example of the hub and spoke as a political model involves the US imagery of the Pacific security system after World War II. The US power moves in the Persian Gulf have also been explicitly framed in terms of a hub-and-spoke system (Saab 2016). The model became popularly known in the 1980s as the hub-and-spoke alliance structure. It meant that the US (the hub) maintained a system of bilateral security arrangements with individual Pacific Rim states without a strong multilateral regime (the spokes) (Pyle 2007: 225). Similar to a system of airplane routing, all the arrangements were supposed to converge in a US 'hub' (Ikenberry 2009: 71). From an embodied perspective, one important reason for the rise of the hub-and-spoke system as an international relations cultural model was that those innovating and experimenting with extensive notions such as 'the Pacific security architecture' were among the foremost frequent fliers. Experts, university professors, decision makers, and politicians were all among the global elite who were able to live and prosper through the existence of the hub-and-spoke air mobility dynamics. For them, the system's physicality was tacit embodied knowledge. It seemed to reveal something worthy and significant with a single relatively self-evident schematic. The accompanying air travel imageries are not limited to how people feel when they fly though the global aviopolis. The sentiments of air mobility may be seen as ways of embodying global order based largely on air mobility flows. This power-related modality is especially vital for getting a fuller grip on how it is used to symbolize the architectures of global power. One might expect that the kinaesthetic cultural models making sense of (de)accelerations and stabilities are especially suited to shed light on the nexus between air mobility and power. This kinaesthetic approach turns the hub-and-spoke model into a multidimensional model in which sensory and emotional meanings easily interact and interlink with the political signifiers of the abstract architecture.

COVID-19 made its appearance as a major disruptive event in a world that was already experiencing growing tensions. Against the Thucydidean framework, this was not an unexpected turn of events. The global power system was in a constantly reactive mode of experiencing different types of 'shocks' ranging from tensions in the Middle East and the South China Sea to war in Ukraine. This growing constant shock syndrome signifies that power is on the move and perhaps in transition. In this context, COVID-19 was quickly geopoliticized and co-opted for power-political purposes in terms of blame games, propaganda, status shifts, and other familiar features of pandemic politics and was propelled by being connected to citizens' somatic worries.

The Overall Imageries of Dis-eased Interconnectedness

SARS and COVID-19 were alive and felt in their particular anxious political contexts. In the case of SARS, the suspicions over terror cells and allegedly evil nations like Iraq, so inhuman that they could use violent diseases such as WMDs, amplified the sense of dangerous incompatibility and alien foreignness. It is suggested that these fears were hyperbolized in the context of major wars. SARS was repeatedly used as a benchmark for what might happen if terrorists were to use WMDs: 'The SARS epidemic, while deadly, is simply a mild portent of what may be to come' (Hamilton 2004: 85). The images of SARS became associated with such types of dangerous contact across regions, which were at different stages of development, across ideological separations, and across West–East demarcations. The speculative stories about the origins of SARS often high-lighted the transgressed interspecies boundary in the 'hot' markets of Southern China—a theme prevalent also in the more recent pandemic scares. The 'fever' was associated with the feverish agitations of the global age and with its lowered and porous boundaries. The rapid transmission of SARS from Hong Kong to Toronto exemplified the dangers of air travel, as did the SARS-related alarms in many international airports. SARS was believed to spread rapidly to every place where the international hub-and-spoke network of airports spread. From this perspective, it was noteworthy that SARS did not afflict only people. It was also seen as afflicting the system of international travel and, through it, every-body. Flights were cancelled and re-routed, travel warnings were issued, airlines experienced financial hardships, and the tourism industry suffered. International travel turned into fears of people fleeing from the infected areas—in the SARS case, Hong Kong and Singapore. Flights are a constant fear during epidemics as people try to find places of safety and with effective medical care. SARS' con-tainment drama was clearly linked to globalization and to the disappearing of vast distances through the ease of flying and, incidentally, of flights from the perceived containment zones.

Using SARS as an example of what a biological terror attack might look like, Hamilton (2004: 85) calls for the US and the EU to heighten their preparedness. His arguments for the development of resilient societies are fairly representative of a trend in interpreting the lessons learnt from SARS and WMDs. Furthermore, Hamilton identifies the intersections of flows of people as the main focal points in such a creation of resilience:

> [I]t has become clear that controlling borders, operating ports, and manag-ing airports and train stations in the age of globalization involves a delicate balance of identifying and intercepting weapons and terrorists without exces-sively hindering trade, legal immigration, travel, and tourism—all aspects upon which European and US prosperity increasingly depend.
>
> *(Hamilton 2004: 85)*

This argument summarizes many points present in the SARS chronology. The measures implemented to fight SARS had the potential to adversely affect systemic-level networks. WHO had to balance its measures to control the international and intercontinental spread of the disease with the need to keep businesspeople and tourists on the move. However, the emphasis on resilient societies is not value free or politically inert. It can be seen as blending geopolitical speculation of where the threats are emanating from with the need to secure the global order against emergent challenges.

COVID-19 emerged in even more feverish geopolitical rivalry. It combined with aspects of the tense geopolitical competition. This was not surprising because influential relationships often emerge from two parallel processes: besides the fierce competition between disease agents and humans, an equally ferocious contention takes place between states (McNeill 1976: 1–10). Although COVID-19 was regarded as a dangerous threat, it was made to fit the large-scale patterns of world politics. In many places, the disease was identified with China or the ethnic Chinese in the popular media representations—a repeat of the SARS episode. Appearing amidst fierce international and regional competition, which is highly sensitive to rumours and suspicions, lethal epidemic diseases tend to blend the self-interest of power politics with honest and genuine willingness to prevent and stop human suffering. In some respects, all the actors had conflicting agendas. Judging from the history of disease encounters, the most often used means for fighting the negative power-political effects of epidemics are diversion, deception, and secrecy. These tendencies also gave substance to the COVID-19 scenarios and cascading effects. The cultural stereotypes that China and the Chinese were secretive, closed, and somehow suspect provided material for the understanding of the Chinese danger (e.g. Luckhurst 2020: 54). In the increasingly ideological competition between democratic and autocratic political systems, China's secretive political system was seen as one of the most important causative agents of COVID-19. This sentiment was already present in the case of SARS: 'In deciding to hush up the SARS outbreak in Guangdong province in 2002, the Chinese government gave the virus a head start and allowed it to spread globally' (Crawford 2007: 230). In the COVID-19 case, China was seen as having delayed the notification concerning the disease to the WHO and also as having failed to cut the international routes of transmission in time. China is still seen as an outsider in the international community—limited in its transparency, only partially reformed and unevenly developed.

Because China was increasingly a part of the global system, the 'errant' ways of the Chinese authorities and the closeness of the system were framed as a worldwide threat. The specifying of the people associated with 'China' as the most susceptible, and therefore the most threatening, group reinforced lingering politico-ethnic suspicions in many parts of the world. At the macro level, China and its systems were seen as dangerously diseasing. The micro-level attributions of blame reflected existing political animosities.

Although thoroughly interconnected, the global fabric space is not evenly spread out. It thickens near and gravitates towards the global hubs. The global air traffic embodies this uneven or lumpy pattern. At the same time, pandemic diseases—diseases affecting the whole of the *pandemos*—can embody and be used to narrate the different fears that this system might become conducive to regressive spiralling processes. While the global hub-and-spoke system is a signifier of globalization, pandemics register long-existing fears and worries that the rapid long-distance connections are dangerously dis-easing. To a large extent, SARS and COVID-19 came to be constructed as diseases of global networks. At the macro level, it was seen as having the capacity to force the closure of modern life's support systems and upset the polities that have become reliant on them. At the micro level, it meant actions such as the closure of schools; turning hotels, hospitals, and apartment complexes into containment zones; and paralysing cross-border movements. In a way, SARS and COVID-19 were interpreted to have come with an ominous message for political reform, global decoupling, and severing of interdependencies.

The two coronavirus pandemics seemed to demand the re-imagining of social organization, political authority, and expert governance and to hammer home the importance of resilience and preparedness as the key signifiers of future security. The official documents on SARS often highlighted the close connection between naturally occurring and intentionally caused outbreaks of disease. Moreover, it was perceived that the measures aimed against naturally occurring outbreaks offered a way to combat possible intentional outbreaks. The preparedness over naturally occurring diseases was seen as a testing ground for developing security in the case of biological warfare. This combined dynamics provided a powerful undercurrent to the term 'global health security'. It follows from the emphasis on readiness, preparedness, and resilience that there is a strategic interest involved in why societies readily turn into paranoid sites, 'where even an unsubstantiated claim about a threat to public health is likely be taken seriously' (Loosemore *et al.* 2006). The discourses of pandemics are likely to be used to create senses of security utterly unrelated to what pandemics as epidemiological phenomena are supposed to be.

Notes

1 Apart from lethal diseases, nuclear threats were also much in use. There was a general trope repeated, for example, by the then National Security Advisor Condoleezza Rice that the world could not afford to wait for the 'mushroom cloud' (CNN, 10 January 2003).
2 For more on this, see, for example, Freedom House (2019) and Linn (2018).

6

COVID-19 AS A CATALYSER OF GROWING ANXIETY, POLITICAL DISTANCING, AND GLOBAL DECOUPLING

Since late 2019, through waves of variants, the world has come to know and sought to respond to a pandemic of global significance and cascading consequences, the outbreak of coronavirus disease (COVID-19). After the first line of defence in Wuhan, China, failed, the response has been lacking global coordination and has been based on a patchwork of national responses. Lessons have been learnt from what is perhaps the worst calamity to hit the world since World War II. The initial response to COVID-19 was too slow and a precautionary approach—recognizing it as a possible pandemic outbreak based on the SARS-like nature of the disease agent—should have been used instead of the wait-and-watch attitude that was adopted in many places. Furthermore, COVID-19 has shown how diseases can be paralysing and catalysing in multifaceted psychological, social, political, and economic ways as they involve politosomatic anxieties that cause multifarious effects. This chapter overviews the (geo)politics of COVID-19 to examine the scope of its challenge to citizens, existing domestic orders, international actors, and the modus operandi of the present world order. The analysis is based on the assumption that contagious diseases should be treated as compound phenomena with various features—they are not reducible to biology alone. Precursor cases are used to shed light on the political aspects and tendencies of geographically extensive diseases. This review can be used to illuminate the longer-term consequences of the COVID-19 pandemic.

Vital to managing a pandemic outbreak are good governance and effective order maintained by responsible actors. However, there were significant weaknesses and vulnerabilities in the global governance system when COVID-19 hit the world. Pandemics usually hit at an inopportune time. Besides pointing to the fact that there never is a good time for a pandemic outbreak, the above statement also points to how regression of global multilevel governance structures opens up spaces for diseases to take hold and for the efforts to contain them to fail. Weak governance

DOI: 10.4324/9781003169147-6

structures produce opportunities for disease agents. Even though it was equipped with the International Health Regulations (IHR), which had been strengthened further post-SARS, the WHO found itself with no effective tools to coordinate the efforts against COVID-19, only a whole lot of norms and rules. The IHR was the only major international binding agreement on pandemic security. But it constrains rather than enables an effective response, especially in terms of rapid expansion of air travel, because it discourages travel restrictions and 'balances' economic justifications with the need to contain disease spread through the air travel vector:

> The bias of the current system of pandemic alert is towards inaction—steps may only be taken if the weight of evidence requires them. This bias should be reversed—precautionary action should be taken on a presumptive basis, unless evidence shows it is not necessary.
> *(The Independent Panel for Pandemic Preparedness and Response 2021: 51)*

The WHO's agenda and scope for action have been growing over time, but its tools and resources have remained weak. Small wonder then that in the COVID-19 pandemic situation, we are witnessing that Thucydides' basic point, reviewed in the first chapters of this book, is still valid: when the orderly political space with its governance structure weakens, the polity—whether the communal polity or the human polity—is left exposed to infighting, competition, and unforeseen events such as catastrophes and plagues. At the same time, COVID-19 has clashed with some of the basic elements of the present global political reality: the global political order based on mobility and infrastructure connecting markets with production regions as well as the intensifying great power rivalry using these very interdependencies as strategic weapons for clashes such as trade wars, sanctions, espionage, cyber-attacks, and infrastructure development. The focus was elsewhere and lacking. The WHO was underfunded as a large part of its funding comes from earmarked funding from its member-states. This fragments the funding and erodes the ability to put together coherent programmes. It also turns a multilateral institution into a strained organization where the secretariat managed, at bilateral directly through a member-state-by-member-states way, the coordination of its activities.

On the other hand, COVID-19 has brought with it a set of memories as well as practices of the lessons learnt from previous uncontained spreads. For example, forgotten pandemics like the Spanish Flu were suddenly recalled and analysed in detail in media and expert commentaries. The lessons learnt from past epidemic and pandemic challenges reveal how the interaction between diseases and people has affected political struggles for power and how the diseases themselves have had an impact on these power struggles. COVID-19's cascading havoc also shows how notable contagious diseases are invariably more than mere biological and epidemiological phenomena. To make sense of them, one needs to recognize their strong social, economic, and political reactivity and their relatively well-trodden historical paths. Because of this, they cannot be eradicated or controlled by epidemiological efforts alone—governance and politics are always key parts of the mixture, whether for good or bad.

The most important precursor disease of COVID-19, the SARS of 2003, raised suspicions that China was not only acting as a dishonest stakeholder in the world but also that as a country, it was incompatible with the mobile interdependent world order. The failure to disclose the outbreak of the virus and the inadequate management of the initial response to it were also present more recently in the crucial onset phase of COVID-19. The blame game here has been similar to that during the SARS outbreak. Since COVID-19 is a more widespread disease than SARS, with outbreaks in multiple continents and almost all countries, it will likely act as a strong precursor case for the next contagion. To this effect, COVID-19 has already (re)created more instinctive rationalizations for (poorly) responding to a health crisis both domestically and internationally. These include holding back knowledge about disease outbreaks as the consequences can be dangerously far-reaching, acting in ways that can hinder response efforts but quell the public demand to do something, implementing measures which deviate from any human rights norms and basing actions on highly stereotypic and xenophobic reasoning (e.g. Pillinger 2020).

Seven years after SARS, the world is even more feverishly interconnected but also more suspicious and strategically competitive. COVID-19 reveals a much larger challenge to the underlying principles of the world order at a time when its underpinnings are actively undermined by great power contestations, trade wars, and rising political and economic neo-nationalism in the US and China. As a result of the transformed atmosphere, as COVID-19 has turned into a feared global pandemic, it is likely to trigger lasting and lingering changes. It accentuates the themes of political distancing and economic decoupling that are already strong tendencies. It can also create a strong linkage between individual anxieties and patterns of enmity that seem to fit those fears, thereby heightening hostilities and legitimizing stereotypical understanding that translates disease maps into geopolitical 'realities'.

Politics and Geopolitics Cast a Long Shadow on Pandemic Control

Although expertise-based logic resists the idea of explicit politics in pandemic security, the allocation of resources to experts is already a political decision. Thus, political mobilization is needed to allocate resources and enable expertise in fights against pandemics. At the same time, contagious diseases interact with and strongly contest the basic characteristics of the political order in which they occur. COVID-19, in particular, initially challenged China both domestically because its response was spectated by citizens, dissidents, and commentators and internationally because its global trust levels decreased significantly. Similarly, the actions taken by the US were seen as inadequate. It was missing in action quite literally before the large-scale vaccination programme started in the spring of 2021, and it changed its policy concerning the intellectual property rights of the major vaccine-producing companies.

While the main players suffered politically or were missing in action, COVID-19 roamed free and reshaped the global order and its status hierarchy by triggering further distancing between the major actors and strengthening the calls for economic decoupling. International public health governance, led by the WHO, may also become partly delegitimized as the COVID-19 outbreak has brought to light the lack of harmony between local, national, and global efforts. The failure of the IHR to stop the disease was clearly visible, and it was seen as hampering rather than enabling mitigation; efforts have now been launched to reform the IHR (e.g. The Independent Panel for Pandemic Preparedness and Response 2021).

The prevailing understanding of global health as a functional realm of expertise has led to a relatively technocratic and narrow definition of 'politics' in global health governance. Legitimate politics is defined as an enabler of the efficient functioning of expertise, enactor of health institutions, and mobilizer of adequate resources (e.g. Siddiqi 1995: 170). Politics plays a supporting role in providing funding for the building of offices and laboratories and the financing of health programmes. The role of politics is not seen as harmful when it results in relatively minor disagreements as long as they do not result in the paralysis of the underlying mission and method. Perceived harmless disagreements include 'competition' between states over the right to host health institutions, for example. There is also the politics of expert debates over the most effective policies and optimization of those policies with funding requirements.

However, the line between legitimate politics and negative politics is seen as crossed when politics does not enable the functional field but co-opts it for other purposes. This happened, for example, when vaccine exports were being directed by state-based strategic reasons (e.g. Gyu 2021; Wen 2021). The general opinion seems to be that such co-option leads to less effective health policies and that it reflects badly on the perceived legitimacy of global health policies and institutions. That said, it should be noted that any political co-option relies on the existence of effective and legitimate public health functions in the first place. Considering this fundamental need, even negative politicization and co-option can lead to a relatively horizontal, 'partnership' kind of collaboration between those professing the modern global health perspective and those with other more political agendas. This can be seen in resource allocation as the political objective is clear. For example, the large-scale travel restrictions implemented during the COVID-19 outbreak are scientifically debatable, but for politicians, doing nothing was not an option. The apparent protection of health was seen as a vital driver for public health policy. At the same time, partnership was needed for the WHO to have at least a degree of access and collaboration with the Chinese authorities. Thus, the WHO was left in a difficult position with regard to achieving a balance between its mission and the need to have partners in the containment efforts. This equation led to reluctant WHO approval of large-scale travel restrictions. Such loose partnerships tend to reaffirm and re-establish the underlying legitimacy of the public health perspective while, at the same time, opening up opportunities for serving additional political goals and facilitating political co-option of pandemic security governance.

For example, a co-optive relationship may be based on a hierarchical situation in which global health is directly subordinated to other goals, such as a strong vision of national security interests. Health becomes defined as one front in the wider struggle towards a preferred goal. In this spirit, the US' HIV- and AIDS-related PEPFAR programmes explicitly aimed at preventing state failures and spread of terrorism through effective health programmes. It was not so much a fight against a disease but a co-option of health programmes to fight radicalization (e.g. Mojola 2017). This perhaps less harmful co-option means that global health also becomes one element in a larger bundle of activities with at least a modest degree of benefit in the sense of global health.

The third co-optive arrangement involves actors who purposefully resign from the modern public health paradigm in the interests of their state. Health expertise ceases to be the driver or even part of a package. China was accused of this during the 2003 SARS, avian flu, and now the COVID-19 outbreaks. Secrecy and tightly controlled and selective information flows have been relatively usual in pandemic situations. But China's stance was seen as directly hindering global public health efforts and, thereby, as directly associated with the causation of an epidemic disease. Time is essential for effective pandemic containment, and secrecy and hesitation in revealing the true nature of the challenge at the global level can be a direct causal factor in the spread of disease agents. However, the deeply sedimented histories of plague and people have other co-optive patterns as well. Diseases and immunities matter: since they are seen as signifiers of political weakness and crumbling of power, they can be used in propaganda, information about them can cause disruptions and disorder, and they can provide effective excuses for actions with other motivations. For example, after the 9/11 attacks, the capturing of Osama bin Laden was a priority for the US. In order to locate him, the US began a polio vaccination campaign in Pakistan (e.g. Gostin 2014). This led to problems in later vaccination campaigns in Pakistan as the locals became suspicious about the ultimate goals of international vaccination programmes (e.g. Gulland 2012).

Thus, the modern, functional, expertise-focused approach—for example, in the form of the 'one world, one health' approach—sheds inadequate light on the actual overall relationship between politics and epidemic diseases, which hampers deeper analysis of the current COVID-19 scenario. The political significance has to do with the fact that contagious diseases, and especially pandemics, have the potential to redefine the patterns of human political affinities. As the underlying politosomatic scenario suggests, diseases enact immediate sentiments of hostile and threatening surroundings. Pandemics can change the overall balance of solidarity against people, governments, and other entities that are perceived as carriers or facilitators of the contagion. The connections felt towards locations and groups of people are redefined accordingly. The global hierarchy of political health is redivided according to the perceived and felt patterns and geographies of disease burden. The deliberation over commonality is displaced by the policies and practices of separation, isolation, containment, and cordoning, and political rhetoric changes accordingly. The scenario is traditionally about the rediscovery of the areas and limits of political persuasibility. Under pandemic conditions, the persuasion is less inclined towards strong bias against connections with the perceived places and people of a contagion. As a result, the global community is reimagined in rapid sequence as a place that needs to be cured but also secured, the emphasis being strongly on re/establishing the conditions for one's immediate group's securability with methods that are in direct contradiction with the mobility paradigm that prevailed before COVID-19.

An overview of the politically reactive characteristics of COVID-19 has to examine the scope of its challenge to the existing domestic orders, to international actors, and to the modus operandi of the present global order. Contagious diseases should be treated as relatively open-ended bundles of biological and political features. They readily combine with their own contemporary trends and features. They trigger and catalyse. However, the underlying logic of 'combinatorics' is not random or only non-linear. The logic of how diseases react is a relatively well-trodden path formed through previous encounters with 'plagues' of different types. Keeping this sedimented history in mind, precursor diseases can be a useful tool in reviewing and shedding light on the political tendencies of COVID-19 and on its political reactivity. A review of these cases can be used to illuminate the possible political courses the COVID-19 emergency could take and their consequences.

COVID-19's Precursor Diseases

COVID-19 brought with it a package of lessons learnt from historical precursor contagions. At the same time, it has reacted radically with the basic ingredients of the present global political conditions—that is, with the global political order based on mobility and infrastructure connecting markets with production regions as well as on great power rivalry. The havoc wreaked by COVID-19 also shows how notable contagious diseases are invariably more extensive and go well beyond the biological and epidemiological spheres. They are dynamic scenarios with strong social, economic, and political characteristics. Because of this, they cannot be eradicated or controlled only by epidemiological efforts. Political mobilization is needed to allocate resources and enable expertise. At the same time, diseases react with and strongly contest the basic characteristics of the political order in which they occur. The challenges posed by COVID-19 are likely to reshape the global system by triggering further distancing between the major actors and economic decoupling. It also poses a major potential for the delegitimization of the WHO's international health efforts as it has brought to light the cleavages between the local, national, and global levels of health governance.

The most important precursor disease of COVID-19 was the SARS outbreak of 2003. It raised suspicions that China was not acting in good faith. The COVID-19 blame game has also been similar to that of SARS. Since COVID-19 is more widespread with outbreaks around the globe, it will likely act as a strongly paradigm for what kind of future pandemics might be coming next. After the first wave which hit China and the EU very hard, followed closely by the US, the second and third waves have been particularly devastating in places like Brazil and India. With multiple waves hitting all around the world, the disease has already killed 4 million people as of July 2021.

The other important precursor disease to COVID-19 was avian flu. I will review it in more detail because SARS has already been extensively examined, and, more so, because avian flu reveals many of the politosomatic tendencies that are at play during the COVID-19 pandemic. Avian influenza, also called bird flu, is a viral infection that affects birds mostly, but also humans. Its most serious variants are H5N1, which can affect humans and other animals, and H7N9, which can affect humans.

Avian flu is caused by viruses adapted to birds. In poultry, it may rapidly kill up to 90% of a flock in a very short time. Most alarmingly, the causative agents can, in rare cases, spread to humans although no human-to-human transmission is yet to be widely evidenced. However, the mere possibility of mutation into a human form allowed for media, states, and international organizations to speculate about the disease's movement across species and regions. Relative to the fatalities of COVID-19, avian flu was more of a scare than a real pandemic encounter. However, it allowed for political imaginaries of global space where differential spread of vulnerabilities emerged from the myriad of speculative scenarios concerning national preparedness and resilience. Such imaginaries of the pandemic threat as well as national immunity offer insights into how diseases are still used to contain and border in an age of vanishing boundaries and interconnected global reaches. Its trajectory of public attention turned it from an ordinary livestock disease into a hyperbolic mutable 'killer disease'—the coming plague.

Speculative worst-case scenarios were a prominent element of the avian flu scare. The starting hypothesis was that the media's epidemiological speculation served a primary political purpose. The disease provided the means to build scenarios of high national preparedness and underlying communal health. At the same time, avian flu provided opportunities for the narration of the dangers stemming from faraway places and their cultures in the seamless avian globality. In this respect, the scare was set in motion by the historically conditioned representational potentials inherent in the interfaces of contact and contagion between distinct politico-cultural entities, for example, states, regions, cultures, and civilization.

Domestic audiences turned avian flu's perceived pattern of spread into politically meaningful stories according to their own sensitivities. On the other hand, the overall form of a pandemic outbreak was becoming globally shared and synchronized (Price-Smith 2009: 192–6). Articles in *NYT* illustrate the contemporary US, and also a more global, construction of threat images and legitimate political authority. The central guiding questions of the analysis are these: What are the means by which avian flu was synced with and co-opted by the historically conditioned public sensitivities? What and whose political purposes did avian flu serve and what stereotypical constructions were used to nationalize, or Americanize, the avian flu narrative? I reviewed *NYT*'s news stories on avian flu from 1983 to 2005. The first stories appeared much before the pandemic scare that brought the disease into intense focus in 2004. The idea was that these stories would shed light on how the disease developed into the cultural construct that it was during the peak of the avian flu scare.

The first avian flu–related news story was printed on 13 December 1983. It was a short piece that briefly overviewed the containment and quarantine policies that were believed would stop the spread of the 'deadly' disease of birds in Pennsylvania and New Jersey in the US. The variant was left out as the attention was not on mutability and different variants as it is today. The spread of avian flu to domestic and wild birds was actively followed during the winter of 1983–84 mainly because of the economic implications. In a story published on 26 February 1984, the disease was claimed to have killed some 75% of the chickens in the US and left the rest of the birds unprofitable because of strong market reactions. It was pointed out that the disease was so virulent that once it was noticed, all the birds in a flock had to be immediately culled and carefully buried to stop contagion spread.

Back then, no one seemed too worried about the disease crossing the interspecies boundary to humans. Because there was no speculation concerning the human variant, there was no fear of consumer panic in the *NYT* stories. The contemporary security-related conceptual bridges between food production and illnesses had not yet been formed. These conceptual connections started to develop only during the late 1980s. The first hint of such a discursive combination was the worry over the mutability of the flu in birds. The first news story in *NYT* that highlighted such mutability as a worrying aspect was published on 23 February 1986. The story pointed out how the disease had mutated into a form that could kill about 10% of a flock in a single day. Avian flu was thus reframed as a disease that had mutated into a more dangerous form and might continue to do so in the future. The last *NYT* news story concerning the disease for 10 years was published on 16 August 1987. The story on that day overviewed the disease's mutability and its pattern of spread on the East coast of the US from 1983 to 1984, during which period millions of birds were 'destroyed'.

The news stories changed dramatically in the 1990s as the coming plague genre took hold with its fundamental notion of mutability of disease agents. The next *NYT* news story about avian flu was dated 21 December 1997. It was an interview with two specialists on the issue, Kennedy F. Shortridge, a microbiologist at the University of Hong Kong, and Dr Daniel Lavanchy, the head of the WHO's influenza programme. This story managed to capture many new conceptual combinations and bridges on avian flu. It is worth reviewing in detail. The domestic focus had changed here into a global one. The headline emphasized that China was seen as the centre point of the disease as it spread. The news story started with the following graphic statement: 'A violent-yellow sign stencilled with interlocking black rings and a single word hangs over Kennedy F. Shortridge's laboratory: "Biohazard"'. The hyperbole was new and probably a hybrid of the coming plague scenarios of the 1990s. The end of the Cold War era made pandemics a comprehensible global threat scenario as they connected well with the underlying global order based on interdependency and mobility systems crossing vast distances. Intercontinental disease agents were seen as a key enemy of the order.

Media stories echoed the then recent experiences with Ebola in Zaire during the spring of 1995. Ebola was connected with the eating of badly cooked monkey meat. The Ebola scare highlighted the vulnerability of the global community to fast-spreading contagion via the transportation infrastructure, the hubs being connected to ever remoter spokes. The word 'pandemic' had also emerged into global awareness by the 1990s. It had started to be a marker of great anxiety and worry as the success of much of the twentieth century's work against epidemic diseases was brought to a halt by the emergence of HIV and AIDS in the 1980s.

Another important template for the changed understanding of avian flu was the experience in 1996 with another potential food-borne scare, BSE or mad cow disease. BSE changed the way in which animal-borne diseases were understood. BSE was connected with economic disturbances and market reactions; it was mystified into a complex fed by rumours, lack of information, and the presence of a novel disease agent, a prion; it was turned into a myriad of new administrative practices such as obligatory marking of the origin of bovine products. It conveyed a tangible sense of anxiety over the dangers inherent in modern industrial food production; it was politicized and localized when many cautionary measures were directed against the UK. The continued reframing of avian flu combined with these other strains of pandemic discourses.

Avian flu was thus deeply entangled with the politico-medical landscape of the late 1990s. Another new element in the stories was the foresight aspect of the containment drama, which was connected to the perceived mutability. Although the disease had not yet become a significant threat, according to the story, it could turn into a lethal epidemic disease in the future. Because of this ominous mutability, the 'seeds' of a future pandemic needed to be handled extremely carefully. The great concern felt over the handling of the disease in the story reinforced military metaphors. The containment had to be done by the most modern weapons in the arsenal of the global health community. These biocontainment, protective gear, and disease warrior tropes were widespread in the epochal works of popular culture. Pandemic movies such as *The Outbreak* brought to people's attention certain ways of talking about a pandemic disease. Many works in non-fiction further induced curiosity and anxiety. These works also reinforced certain expectations, which had to be taken into account by *NYT* and also by the global public health community. Pandemic diseases interested people and brought into prominence new fields of authority and expertise.

However, the focus on China reiterated that there were some weak spots in the preparedness to fight disease, and these spots on the globe could turn into disease hotspots. The use of the words 'a violent yellow sign' was polysemous enough to allow for the connection with the US discourse of the 'yellow danger'. China was turned into a new danger because of its 'teeming' cities and different ideological system, and its veil of secrecy was seen as being conducive to the emergence of pandemic threats. The story claimed that the disease jumped from animals to humans for the first time in China and, because of this, China could provide the location for such jumps in the future too. The story explained its reasoning through references to the ancient agricultural practices in China. The combination of premodern and modern practices prevalent there seemed to make China the ideal 'incubator' for avian flu: [T]he emergence of a new influenza virus, while not necessarily this particular one, seemed inevitable, given both ancient agricultural practices in China and the current system of farming in Guangdong province, the source of much of Hong Kong's food'. While China as a whole was seen as the main reservoir of the disease, southern China was described as the disease hub: " 'China is the principal reservoir for influenza," [Mr Shortridge] said, "and southern China is the influenza epicenter"'. China was admittedly a modern economic juggernaut; however, within China, there were dangerous premodern practices that were now seen as being too intimately connected with the rest of the globe. The story went on to explain how the mixing of practices and humans with animals in China was a cause for worry: 'And because in most southern Chinese villages, ducks and chickens and pigs and people all live in very close contact, often with the animals next to or even in houses, influenza viruses moved into pigs and then to humans'. Through the act of localization and nationalization, China itself was turned into a suspect element.

The next stories were published in 2003: there were several news stories dealing with diseases in the SARS context. These stories differed in their affective climate from the stories of 1997. They did not speculate as much as they refocused on the domestic context of avian flu. However, it seems that the domestic disease was not as interesting as the disease in China. It could be that the elliptic treatment of avian flu in the US was partially caused by the saturation of the collective psyche with SARS stories. Pandemic scares seem to allow for public focus in only one place at a time. The SARS stories also focused much attention on China. Because of the association of SARS with China, the spread of avian flu in the US was not considered that eventful. During the first part of 2004, there were news stories on the occurrence of avian flu in East Asia and Northeast Asia. The role of China was pushed to the background, and it was referred to in passing when the discussion turned to the perceived origin of the disease. Moreover, these stories brought out a new theme in which the spread of the disease in wild birds provided the main eye-catching element.

On 27 January 2004, *NYT* published a story on how the pattern of spread was closely connected with migratory wild birds. This novel emphasis created new alarm and worry that went beyond farming and culling. Now wild birds became the target of the containment drama. The movement of diseased birds around the world was tracked continuously. Cases were reported around Asia and increasingly close to the West. This conceptual development heightened the sense of fear exponentially.

Another notable feature of these news stories was the focus on efforts by public health authorities to defeat the potential pandemic. In the beginning of 2004, *NYT* focused on the efforts of the WHO and Centers for Disease Control and

Prevention (CDC), together with the pharmaceutical industry, to develop new drugs and vaccines. For example, on 5 February 2004, the paper reported on the progress of the development of a vaccine for avian flu. At the same time, the news story stated that the disease was not likely to spread in the US because the farms there were being monitored carefully and because important bans had been implemented. The fuss about avian flu died down early in the summer of 2004, although many stories warned that the nation should be prepared for a re-emergence of the disease.

During the fall of 2004, the stories focused on preparing for another outbreak. International measures and cooperation were reviewed in the context of vaccine development. On 12 September 2004, *NYT* carried the following headline: 'A War and a Mystery: Confronting Avian Flu'. Attention was directed to the occasional bits of news on the various outbreaks of avian flu in Asia. During the following year, *NYT* concentrated on worries over lagging efforts to fight the disease, as in the headline of 9 September 2005: 'The Frontlines in the Battle against Avian Flu are Running Short of Money'. At the same time, there was a lot of focus on medical advances against avian flu. On 5 April 2004, the newspaper reported on a new drug, Tamiflu: 'Should We All Be Stocking Tamiflu?' At this point, it seems that there were concrete policies that could be taken up to raise national resilience and preparedness. The US government's efforts to stock Tamiflu and other medications were reported. The stories highlighted the opportunities opening up in the fight against the potential disease. At the same time, the news stories pointed out the inequalities in the global public health efforts: some governments were seen as not doing enough, while some were seen as too mismanaged and poor. These deficiencies in the global effort were seen as risking failure in the fight against avian flu.

Although thoroughly interconnected, the global space fabric is not evenly spread. It thickens near and gravitates towards the global hubs. The global air traffic embodies this uneven or lumpy pattern that points out remoteness as a signifier and cause of vulnerability. At the same time, pandemic diseases can embody and be used to narrate the different fears that this system might become conducive to regressive circulatory and downward spiralling processes. While the global hub-and-spoke system is a signifier of modern progress, pandemics register long-existing fears and worries that the rapid long-distance connections are dangerously dis-easing. The resilient global order highlighted in the SARS and avian flu spectacles seemed to demand the re-imagining of social organization, political authority, and expert governance and to hammer home the importance of resilience and preparedness as the key signifiers of future security.

Multidimensional Enmities Accentuated by COVID-19

The COVID-19 scenario has included all the elements of the immediate precursor imaginaries: China, human–animal relationship, mutability, and biohazards. It has accentuated enmities that have political relevance. However, the geopolitical situation has shifted from the times of the precursor diseases. Scepticism about the sustainability of the global order has increased among its key stakeholders, and major power competition is out in the open. The politics of co-opting the disease was no longer so much about legitimate and safe belonging to the global order but increasingly about one's rightful place on the top of the hierarchy and having one's own hub-and-spoke system rather than belonging to one prevalent version of it, the so-called liberal rule-based world order. China had become more assertive, and the Donald Trump administration in the US was openly challenging the 'liberal' characteristics of the global order.

The politics of contagious diseases is not only about intercommunal relations, competition, and conflicts. Pandemics highlight the hostility and incompatibility between natural and human-made environments. Although the transmission of dangerous influenzas to humans usually takes place through domesticated intermediary species, much of the global attention has been focused on the diseases of wild animals, from the HIV of monkeys and the avian flu of birds to the SARS of bats and the COVID-19 of bats and/or snakes. This highlights one of the most persistent themes or thresholds of recent pandemic scares: humanity's sustainable relationship with nature, or the nature–human boundary, which is also much emphasized because of global climate change. Many of the recent health scares translate into crossing of the species barrier dramas. The common socially interpreted theme seems to be that a border that should not have been violated has been transgressed with the result that nature has turned hostile to human ways. Although the nature–human relationship is often deemed tense and hostile in modern interpretations of pandemics, the most consequential part of the overall sense of enmity is the hostility that pandemics accentuate within the international community. In pandemic situations, the multidimensional frictions that run across humanity become acute when the outbreaks receive their communal interpretation.

Like the COVID-19 epidemic, SARS was easily perceived to be associated with China or with people of ethnic Chinese origin. To a degree, the pervasive images of China as a secretive, closed, and corrupt country contributed to this association. China was still an outsider in the 'modern' international community and seen as a country with limited transparency, partial reform, and uneven development. Thus, arguably, epidemics and pandemics of violent influenzas come with a political message. They can tell 'stories' of the incompatibility of certain states with the overall international order, or they can contain a message concerning the 'unnatural' nature of the whole system, the system based on globalized flows. Today, this kind of critique is already being presented in neo-nationalistic rhetoric, for example, by the past Trump administration. In China's version, the disease somehow originated from outside of China, perhaps through frozen food products from South America. This theory, although unlikely, was also put forth in the preliminary report by the WHO:

> SARS-CoV-2 has been found to persist in conditions found in frozen food, packaging and cold-chain products. Index cases in recent outbreaks in China have been linked to the cold chain; the virus has been found on packages and

products from other countries that supply China with cold-chain products, indicating that it can be carried long distances on cold-chain products.

(WHO 2021a: 8)

This theory was later downplayed and refuted as unlikely. However, it revealed how out of sync the different national assumptions were concerning the origin of the disease. It also showed how reliant the WHO was on its partnerships with the key member-states. Why were the origin 'theories' important? Because the point of origin had consequences for the geopolitically laden status games and blame games that were being played out in the global arena. The point of origin was co-opted for political purposes in ways that could be managed easily by the slowly gathering scholarly evidence. Strategic use of knowledge can manipulate and over-whelm the processing of scientific evidence too (e.g. Farkas and Schou 2020). For China, the key COVID-19 challenge was to control and counter the message of its possible incompatibility with the relatively borderless global order. This bat-tle for status was demanding in two ways: on the one hand, it had to demonstrate through its actions its compatibility to and trustworthiness with regard to an order on which it was economically dependent. In this respect, it had to appear to be an effective and legitimate stakeholder of the global order. This meant China had to contribute to the global effort to contain the disease. China offered what it saw as help in delivering PPE and, later, vaccines to the rest of the world, albeit, as pointed out in Chapter 5, in highly selective ways. At the same time, China was directly challenging narratives which put the blame on China. This was done through counter-propaganda and disinformation campaigns and also through other means such as cyber espionage operations aiming to catch up with vaccine production, to spy and also to influence (Bolder 2020; Thomas *et al.* 2020). From the point of view of international relations, the external challenge was tricky yet vital. China's position in the global value and security of supply chains is fundamental to its eco-nomic and political model. Its trustworthiness is often debated. In addition, many of the emerging influenzas of the past decades have originated from China. China's reputation as a source of global vulnerability and exposure highlighted arguments that were counterproductive to its attempts to portray itself as a benign yet rising major power that also had the legitimate right to be assertive when it came to its core interests.

On the other hand, the Chinese political system had to demonstrate its health and legitimacy to its own citizens who were getting increasingly anxious about the viability of the Chinese domestic order. Domestically, China moved towards con-taining the epidemic and achieved good results. Thus, China was at the same time a global failure as also a success story.

As evidenced by China's struggle for internal and external legitimacy, pandemic situations involve scenarios in which political legitimacy contains strong moral, shame, and guilt-based messages. These legitimacy dramas, if dealt with success-fully, can be used to reaffirm or reinvent national ethos and purpose (Lindenbaum 2001: 264)—they act as signifiers of communal values and beliefs (e.g. Turner

1957: 107). Legitimacy dramas tend to have a plot: they involve a fight by the presumed protagonist—often taking the guise of the whole nation or even humanity—against the bad elements of a perceived chaos or hostility. The protagonists of morality plays include such stock figures as watchful authorities, proactive doctors, efficient national, international and transnational health agencies, and politically accountable politicians. The disease and disease-causing agents, on the other hand, become easily associated with some ethnically, nationally, or ideologically defined group or minority. Examples include casting the blame on the gay community in the case of HIV and AIDS, on the primitive habits of West Africans in the case of Ebola, or on China in the case of SARS. The COVID-19 blame game pointed a finger at China. In China, it led to xenophobia against foreigners and in particular against people of African origin. In India, people of the north-eastern border regions were blamed because of their proximity and association with China. It seems that each national location had its own enmity hierarchies at which blame could be targeted. These agents of disease find their historical equivalents in the older collective memories about polluters, untouchables, plague spreaders, and well poisoners. These two extreme types in the dramatic plot define the end points in a continuum along which there exists a whole variety of other types: for example, emigrants, tourists, drug addicts, air travellers, truck drivers, prostitutes, food production industries, greedy politicians, and so on.

COVID-19 is no exception. It can be understood as a drama that has included the domestic, regional, and global stages, each with its own unique features. COVID-19's multiple dramas for political legitimacy have been about passing communal verdicts: a judgement is passed about the status of those involved, whether at the national level in China and more widely at the different national levels or at the global level. One interesting feature was the 'rally round the flag' phenomenon. The communal verdicts put the limelight on actors' values, accountability, and their ability to make the correct choices. During the COVID-19 outbreak, there was a huge initial demand for leadership. In a way, this demand fuelled the popularity of any action taken. Only later was the verdict passed on the leadership, based on actual delivered results. The arrival of COVID-19 was a diversion from politics as usual. It originated from outside all the other states, except for China. It offered governments—political in-groups and elites—the opportunity to manage the status quo by declaring an emergency over foreign danger. This created a 'rally round the flag' effect that offered solutions to fix existing domestic tensions. In the democratic world, in particular, the favourability numbers of incumbent leaders went up as a result of the danger and resulting emergency measures (e.g. Kishi *et al.* 2021).

Especially during the initial wave, there was much demand for action and political accountability. Any ameliorative action was warmly welcomed by the publics. During the first wave, support of governments went up in democratic countries and presumably also elsewhere. People projected their deeply embodied anxieties of being globally exposed to the administration in power and expected results (Schraff 2020). If the demand was met with demonstrable actions and effects—such as declining infection numbers—the support was sustained. However, in many cases, in Europe and the US, the situation worsened and political leaders were criticized.

It is clear that the pandemic influenced as well the US presidential election in November 2020 (e.g. Maizland 2020). President Trump had downplayed the significance of the disease in the US and tried to cast the blame on China using terms such as 'China virus'. The voting turnout for the election was the largest in decades because of the heavy polarization and also because of the heavy stakes in terms of pandemic accountability. The politosomatic effect was in full play. Fear of COVID-19 made people politically mobile because it had become clear to them that politics does have consequences. The Trump administration's COVID-19 approach had been patchy. The pandemic thus had a clear impact on deciding who would be the president of the world's leading power: 'We find that COVID-19 cases negatively affected Trump's vote share. The estimated effect appears strongest in urban counties, in states without stay-at-home orders, in swing states, and in states that Trump won in 2016' (Baccini *et al.* 2021: 739). Pandemics do not only act as non-linear drivers or catalysts, they also have direct trust, accountability and legitimacy-related political consequences.

This continual drama of passing verdict adds to the overall political pressures and, if the cumulative pressures are high enough, perhaps triggers political change or adds to causes of unrest. The waves of the public drama did to a degree correspond to the actual COVID-19 waves. However, in many countries, the communal drama put pressure on politicians to lift lockdown measures more quickly than was reasonable. The disharmony between the two patterns of waves—of the disease and of political gain—threw up challenges for the effective containment of the disease and led to the evaporation of the 'rally round the flag' effect. The primary question boiled down to how well the main actors chose at the onset, during and at the conclusion of the pandemic's trajectory in a way that caused unnecessary actions to be taken and led to unintended consequences. For example, the Trump administration's decision to cut transatlantic flights late in the spring of 2020 led to crowded airports and long lines that probably fed the arrival of the first wave in the US. The pressure to implement reasonable disease control measures on the one hand, and the pressure to demonstrate that something was being done on the other, led easily to paradoxical outcomes.

The legitimacy plays happened at the global level as well as in states that experienced COVID-19 outbreaks. The main actors, whose decisions (or indecision), reactions, and actions were being evaluated actively, were China, the WHO, and major states such as the US. For these actors, doing nothing was not a viable option. This also led to fumbling actions that fed the global blame game, resulting in hasty tactical moves. The multilevel domestic and international legitimacy plays meant that particular resolutions of the situation in specific domestic contexts were done in complex interactions with others' legitimacy plays. One sign of this multifaceted coupling between local, national, regional, and global was China's criticism of states that had implemented travel restrictions on flights to and from China.

As a result of the fast-worsening situation, and as the first line of defence against the COVID-19 outbreak had clearly failed in Wuhan, travel restrictions were imposed by multiple states towards the end of January 2020. On 1 February 2020, the WHO decided to give COVID-19 the status of a 'Public Health Emergency of International Concern', marking just the sixth time it had done this. The designation meant that COVID-19 represented a potential public health risk to other states, and the situation required a coordinated international response. In the COVID-19 case, the WHO had failed to reach the required conclusion multiple times. Furthermore, it seems that anxieties about the economic and political consequences led the WHO to delay an explicit declaration. On 11 March 2020, instead of 'declaring', the WHO 'characterized' COVID-19 as a pandemic: 'We have therefore made the assessment that COVID-19 can be characterized as a pandemic' (WHO 2020b). This wording gave countries much leeway in their response. The WHO made it clear that '[d]escribing the situation as a pandemic does not change WHO's assessment of the threat posed by this virus. It doesn't change what WHO is doing, and it doesn't change what countries should do'. On the basis of the same scientific information, different countries advised by their respective health authorities reacted differently. This exemplifies how ambiguity and leeway change the pattern whereby political leadership interacts with health expertise. At the global level, many states had prepared specific plans involving relatively draconian measures in the event of a pandemic. These plans would be triggered if (and when) the WHO explicitly declared a pandemic emergency. Besides having significant economic and societal ramifications, the declaration could also lead to the implementation of the wrong type of plan, which did not fit the specific requirements of the COVID-19 situation. A further factor behind the WHO's second-guessing might have been concern about its own reputation in having failed to control the morphing of a localized outbreak into a global pandemic. The WHO's actions were late and inadequate, mostly for reasons of lack of authority, the need to maintain sustainable partnerships with major members, and scarce resources that were spread too thinly.

When the pandemic emergency was declared, the WHO did not recommend travel restrictions. Yet connections were being cut. Furthermore, many states took the decision to restrict the entry of Chinese nationals and people who had been on the Chinese mainland to their respective territories.[1] The travel restrictions and subsequent criticism by China were painful, especially to states that had tight economic and trade relations with it. For China, what was at play was its position and trustworthiness. It argued that the drastic and unprecedented actions that it had taken should have been enough and the other states should have waited. As the episode with the flight restrictions demonstrates, the pandemic legitimacy drama manifested itself in spectacular acts of being on guard and in control, of sounding alarm and conducting surveillance. In these plays, the sense of legitimacy derives from the ability to maintain critical societal functions (at least) at a certain level throughout the episode—that is, to maintain a relatively orderly situation and a sense of eventual restoration of normalcy.

The attention is on active and proactive measures and how well they can slow down or seem to contain the spread, if not actually preventing the spread of the disease. The judgement, a key aspect of political significance in the drama, is based on a stern, much-needed lesson about the disastrous consequences of lax-ness and lack of vigilance.

Avoiding and diverting blame was a clear characteristic of COVID-19 from the very beginning. The first novel COVID-19 cases were already seen in December 2019. However, it took until 20 January 2020 for the outbreak situation to be fully clarified and acknowledged to the international community. Already back in December 2019, reports had started to emanate from Wuhan, the capital of Hubei province in China, that an unknown disease was spreading. According to publicly available information, it seems that the early outbreak was connected to a seafood market in Wuhan. While this may indicate animal-to-human transmission at the outset, the disease soon started to spread from human to human. After a crucial time gap, the WHO's country office in China took action on 31 December 2019 and notified the mother organization based on newspaper and other reports. By 3 January 2020, 44 cases had been reported. A causal disease agent was reported to the WHO on 7 January 2020 by the National Health Commission of China although the human-to-human transmission was not clearly spelt out at that point. Precautionary measures should have been applied at a much earlier stage. Yet this was not done mostly due to reasons stemming from the politics of disease that have long historical roots.

The blame for this time gap was placed on the local authorities in Wuhan. Key party officials in the Hubei province were fired from their posts for their ineffec-tive response. However, there are clear signs that knowledge of the outbreak had reached Beijing:

> The central government is not entirely exempt from blame. Online discus-sions on the outbreak were silenced on December 8, when eight people from Wuhan were reporting a "mysterious virus" that hospitalised many. The trending #WuhanSARS hashtag was closed down on Weibo (a Chinese social media platform similar to Twitter), which is unlikely to have been done at the request of local authorities.
>
> (NYT 2020a)

And Beijing's own investigation had reported on 11 January 2020 that the situa-tion was under control. According to NYT (2020b), it was only after Hong Kong reported cases of COVID-19 that Beijing acknowledged the outbreak and ceased to downplay the epidemic as a local problem—'a chain of events eerily reminiscent of the SARS outbreak' (The Diplomat 2020). The situation held similarities to China's months-long silence on SARS in 2003. However, this time, the Chinese government seemed more transparent on the reasons for the time gap and dem-onstrated at least a degree of accountability by firing local officials and placing the blame on the local-level administration.

As evidenced by the growing alarm, the onset phase of COVID-19 had already launched the judgemental blame game that is part of the long-standing pattern of disease politics. The onset phase lasted from the starting of rumours in January 2020 to about mid-March 2020 by when the disease had hit Italy and spread to many countries in Europe. The first line of defence had clearly been defeated by the virus, and with that, the whole world was open for its spread. The tipping point was reached in mid-March in Europe. This tipping point can be defined in two ways: the clear exponential rise in the number of cases, and the pandemic overwhelming most if not all other topics in public discussions (Aaltola *et al.* 2021). In the US, the case load started to increase significantly in April, especially in New York City. The increase continued with wider geographical spread in August and started to decline only in January 2021 once the vaccination programme was under way. Vaccination programmes became another political stress point in many Western democracies because they proceeded at different speeds. This fed further the circles of the overall blame game and the spread of mistrust. In the EU, the member-states blamed the EU governance, and the EU institutions blamed the multinational vaccine companies. At the same time, developing nations alleged that the developed parts of the world were practising vaccine nationalism and herding vaccines for their own use.

Historical Patterns of Pandemic Politics

Contagious diseases and political bordered actors—states—are closely intertwined both conceptually and historically as reviewed in the previous chapters. When one considers the potential scenarios that epidemics can effect in politics, it is useful to first review the specific history of human reactions to epidemics that cross political boundaries (Aaltola 1999, 2012a). Although much of the interplay between lethal epidemics and the realm of state interaction is contingent upon specific circumstances, some general, recurring, and conventional themes and combinations can be detected:

1 *Imbalance of disease burden:* The uneven distribution of the burden of disease among states can cause direct shifts in the prevailing balance of power and distribution of capabilities.
2 *Status signifier:* Epidemics are evidence of mismanagement and bad governance, which can be read as a sign of overall weakness, and dent the status and respect of a state associated with a disease as well as lower the levels of trust.
3 *Disease diplomacy, propaganda, and blame game:* Lethal epidemic diseases can offer effective propaganda tools for eroding perceptions about one's competitors or enemies. Effective propaganda can heighten the domestic 'rally round the flag' effect and cement enemy images.
4 *Political co-option and tactical opportunism:* A state can use the outbreak of a lethal infectious disease as an excuse for politically motivated actions such as a military manoeuvre or economic sanctions.

5 *Scare factor and disinformation:* Epidemics cause panic and drastic reactions which can cause economic hardships (e.g. in the shape of market failures and loss of tourism). It can erode trust levels in a particular country and thereby offer opportunities for further heightening fear through misinformation and disinformation.

6 *Burst of civil religiosity and moral panics:* Diseases feed a sense of contamination by disease agents and carriers associated with dis-easing lifestyles and cultural habits. This stereotype reflects a community's attempt to guard its moral boundaries as a ritualistic way of getting rid of carriers and to gain immunity.

Besides these, there are other tendencies, such as a disease striking an individual statesperson and causing power vacuums, internal squabbling, periods of indecision, and increasing uncertainty, that also have significance in some cases (e.g. Aaltola 2012a).

The aforementioned five-point list of notable themes can be further elaborated in the following manner:

1 *Imbalance or the asymmetrical effect of lethal epidemic diseases:* 'Plagues' usually afflict some states disproportionately. This uneven or lopsided spread constitutes an important way in which epidemics can react with international relations (Robins 1981: 76). In a general sense, disease maps can be used to perceive who is who on the map of power when it comes to supposed efficiency and capabilities. Besides the level of impressions, in more specific cases, asymmetry affects the outcomes of specific turns of events, for example, military campaigns.[2] Historical examples abound. Asymmetry affected the lopsided military outcome of the contact between the Spaniards and the Native Americans in the case of the Aztec and Inca empires. Another example is the fate of Napoleon's Grand Armée in Russia. Again, the waves of Spanish Flu influenced the war efforts on both sides during World War I. However, it seems to have had a more significant effect on the US efforts:

> The virus traveled with military personnel from camp to camp and across the Atlantic, and at the height of the American military involvement in the war, September through November 1918, influenza and pneumonia sickened 20% to 40% of U.S. Army and Navy personnel. These high morbidity rates interfered with induction and training schedules in the United States and rendered hundreds of thousands of military personnel non-effective. During the American Expeditionary Forces' campaign at Meuse-Argonne, the epidemic diverted urgently needed resources from combat support to transporting and caring for the sick and the dead. Influenza and pneumonia killed more American soldiers and sailors during the war than did enemy weapons. (Byerly 2010: 82)

Besides the incapacitating and slowing down of military operations, the lopsided effect of the disease burden can influence economies and investment flows. A more recent example is that of the very uneven HIV and AIDS burden. Developing countries, especially in southern Africa, faced a relative disadvantage as compared to the developed north. Thus, sharp asymmetries in the distribution of the disease burden can result in shifts in the distribution of power. Moreover, the uneven distribution turns easily into disempowering stereotypes and corresponding biases. The pattern of spread attracts culturally meaningful explanations. It can cause emotional storms as sometimes rash and irrational actions are taken to fight a disease or maintain relative immunity from it. The 'innate' tendency of states to derive legitimacy from a certain sense of physical and moral superiority with respect to other states can lead to the common belief and resultant practices that other states or groups of states are more prone to the horrors of epidemics. Every time an epidemic struck somewhere else, the state's legitimacy as a secure, privileged, inimitable, and exemplary entity, predestined and chosen for sovereignty, was reinforced. Epidemics can thus foster nationalist and exclusionist identities and support accordingly elite factions and political parties.

In terms of the geographical spread of the burden, COVID-19's dynamic was clearly uneven. The initial phase affected China, thereby slowing down its economy. It originated in a Chinese city and was confined in the beginning to a few provinces of China. The draconian efforts to contain it led to a widespread imposition of quarantine and isolation that hit the Chinese economy and global supply chains, as, for example, in the supply of PPE. Trade was hampered and the economy slowed down in and around China. However, as in the case of SARS, the Chinese economy was able to bounce back in a few months. The next epicentres of the disease were in the developed West—in the EU and the US. The US was particularly hard hit. Its economy sank and unemployment rose. In relative terms, the Chinese economy was already recovering and production levels were on the rise. Although the pandemic did not significantly change the underlying distribution of its military capabilities in the short term, it did give a jolt to China in economic terms. The US has been boosting its economy with massive economic packages, and the expectation is that the US economy will recover. At the same time, COVID-19's unevenly distributed waves have had an overall impact whereby US–China relations have become much more distant politically, and international cooperation much weaker.

2 *Signifier of legitimacy:* Public health is not important only in the direct material and physical sense; it also proves to be an invaluable instrument in establishing one's status among other states as a legitimate and respected actor. Legitimacy can depend on the ability of states to provide for well-being and to contribute to domestic and international public health. A rampant lethal epidemic disease can easily be read as a strong signifier of governance failure—as a sign of decline in the global hierarchy of power. A rampant epidemic disease becomes easily

associated with other symptoms of a more acute and dangerous 'political disease' such as corruption, secrecy, mismanagement, and bad governance. From this perspective, the historically well-established attempts to hide a disease can be motivated by the logic that transparency concerning a disease outbreak can automatically downgrade a state's standing and appeal in the eyes of others as well as those of its own citizens. For example, when the bubonic plague hit the Indian city of Surat in 1994, concern over the international repercussions led initially to attempts to hide the problem and, when that became impossible, at downplaying the seriousness of the outbreak (e.g. Sharat 1995: 2912; Catanach 2001: 131). The Indian government tried persistently to rid itself of the image that Western countries often associate with post-colonial, developing countries—that they are uncivilized, weak, and chaotic second-rate states inherently incapable of taking care of their own citizens. This Western view translates into India's lack of political and economic influence, which does not befit the world's most populous democracy. What made the outbreak of bubonic plague an even more embarrassing and conspicuous sign of incapability was the fact that the knowledge of how it spreads and how it can be cured and eradicated has been around for a full century. In political power games, an outbreak of this type was a 'euphemism to embarrass a less developed country in the hopes of making the more developed look better and safer' (Sharat 1995: 2913). Similar fears led the Gabonese government to try and hide an outbreak of Ebola in 1996 and to confiscate blood samples from international health workers (Troy 1996: 22). A further example of attempts to conceal an epidemic disease is provided by Thailand's efforts to conceal an outbreak of cholera in 1997 by calling it 'severe diarrhea'. This tendency to hide diseases in an attempt to avoid international embarrassment, which could potentially harm the state's political and economic interests, can be witnessed all over the world. As the UK's failed attempts to hide BSE in 1996 demonstrated, states are rarely totally open about the outbreak of a potentially serious epidemic disease. They are aware that they have too much to lose in terms of respect, legitimacy, and status. On the other hand, it is clear that it is becoming harder to conceal serious outbreaks as information travels faster today and global health monitoring systems have become more efficient (e.g. Mykhalovskiy and Weir 2006: 42). Getting caught hiding an outbreak can cause even more serious reputational damage.

We now know that the different central and local authorities in China tried to downplay and cover up the initial spread of COVID-19 in December 2019 and January 2020. The reasons for this, at least in part, had to do with worry over the consequences of an outbreak for China's modern status and its hopes to contain the outbreak locally. Irrespective of the motives, China became a repeat offender as it was once again seen as intentionally hiding the facts as it had done during the 2003 SARS outbreak. In the COVID-19 case, the likely presumption is that China's initial management of the disease has been at least partly affected by the need to safeguard perceptions. Similarly, in the US, the

Trump administration tried to downplay the significance of COVID-19 during the initial phase, which led to much criticism of its inaction. The concern is that status-related worries and fears can lead states to hide or downplay the actual number of cases and deaths and inability or unwillingness to respond adequately. Cover-ups for status purposes can hamper containment efforts quite drastically.

One other front where status has played a role in the COVID-19 outbreak is vaccine nationalism and diplomacy. The main vaccine-producing regions were able to produce effective vaccines in a short period of time. However, their global solidarity was fairly limited and based on a 'nearest is dearest' approach—vaccinating one's own citizens first and then moving on to more politically and culturally important partners. Compared to other types of emergencies, pandemics are in a league of their own. One key characteristic of a pandemic emergency is the anxiety connected to the processes of contagion, infection, and spread. The term 'pandemic' signifies that the first line of defence at the local level has failed, as happened in the initial stages of COVID-19. Whereas natural catastrophes are usually locally contained without additional concerns stemming from the fear of spread, pandemics are, to a degree, anti-humanitarian by their very nature. They usually lead to a knee-jerk reaction to step back and buffer oneself to prevent the harm from spreading. From this perspective, pandemic solidarity is far more limited and qualitatively different. Instead of compassion for distant others, a 'nearest is dearest' approach is adopted. In the case of COVID-19, the global vaccine efforts lacked funds until the spring of 2021. The main players in the vaccine diplomacy were China and Russia, which began exporting vaccines to like-minded nations. Vaccine diplomacy is an effective form of aid in the sense that it tells the citizens of the recipient countries that their health is being guaranteed by certain outside actors. This can shift loyalties in the longer term similar to the delivery of food aid in cases of famine (e.g. Aaltola 1999: 371).

The status games of COVID-19 are still being played out. However, the tactical posturing, secrecy, nationalism, and vaccine diplomacy indicate two contemporary patterns. On the one hand, disease still matters when it comes to a state's internal standing and external status. The long history of disease and its patterns lingers on during contemporary times. On the other hand, very open status games also indicate the eradication of the common interest of all states. The WHO's performance was hampered by the member-states' lack of commitment to the common effort. Much of the WHO's budget is earmarked for the pet projects of individual funders. The WHO's secretariat spends much time, resources, and effort on bilateral negotiations with members of the supposedly multilateral organization. The wheeling and dealing on matters relevant to global pandemic security clearly demonstrates a lack of overall responsibility. In this atmosphere of regressing governance, diseases become nationalized and are used for purposes of national interest.

3   *Disease diplomacy, propaganda, and blame game*: Diseases have always called for a socially and politically understandable explanation. During the centuries of plague in Europe, the pestilence was interpreted as a divine punishment for sin and moral corruption. Not surprisingly, for a short moment when the plague epidemic struck, city-states and other localities became citadels of righteousness. However, as time passed and people grew more accustomed to the disease and to the fact that it killed both the righteous and the corrupt in equal numbers, the divine origin of plague had to give way to more mundane explanations. The various ways in which the people of the time viewed plague outbreaks were closely interwoven with the existing political conditions. In many cases, political expediency played a role in the societal effects of epidemics: the alleged disease spreaders became enemies of the people, and people's enemies, whether domestic or foreign, were easily presented as related to the spread of the epidemic. These foreign elements and states, which were already viewed in negative terms, were not hard to come by for purposes of apportioning blame and distributing propaganda.

The stock narrative of an epidemic thus contains a well-established narrative dynamic that easily leads to the attribution of contagious disease to foreign sources and political adversaries. This tendency has been particularly pronounced during periods of heightened interstate conflict and world-order tensions. For example, the spread of HIV and AIDS in the early 1980s was soon adopted for politically advantageous purposes. The Soviet authorities, in their propaganda, falsely insisted that HIV was the outcome of a US military experiment that had gone wrong (Nelkin and Gilman 1991: 39). The aim was to point out that the US was a vicious, perverse, underhanded superpower that could not be trusted. At the same time, for the Soviet Union, the syndrome offered an opportunity to point out that it was free from HIV and AIDS and that it had no minorities as the homosexual community in the 'over-liberal' West.

COVID-19 was instantly turned into a public diplomacy and propaganda drama in which the narratives of its origin mattered. China was keen on showing that the disease came to Wuhan from somewhere outside of its borders. The Chinese authorities stressed the frozen food theory of causation. The US authorities have been suggesting that the point of origin could have been the Wuhan Institute of Virology. Misinformation and conspiracy theories were widely circulated in the context of state-sponsored 'theories' of origin that rightly or wrongly made it to the WHO's reports as well (e.g. Alaszewski 2021: 74). The general confusion over fact evaluation was made further worse by the social media platforms on which many people get their news. The transnational sites circulated many fake news on COVID-19 quite independently from the state-sponsored efforts, and the confusion itself affected mainly the democratic digitalized polities (Aaltola 2020: 4–10). China, for example, has state-controlled traditional as well as social media. The domestic information environment in autocracies is tightly controlled, thereby creating incentives to add to the confusion in the democratic world through misinformation campaigns targeted at undermining the levels of trust and legitimacy (e.g. *The Guardian* 2021).

4 *Political co-option and tactical opportunism*: By assigning the role of plague spreaders, well poisoners, and conspirators to some external enemy, such as Catholics, Protestants, or other states, or to conspicuous internal groups such as Jews, young women, and other perceived enemies of the state, a state could both divert people's anxiety and frustrations away from its own actions and also justify its actions against these perceived enemies. It was not unusual for hospitals set up for patients during an epidemic to be full of political opponents and dissidents, nor is it extraordinary in modern times for politically unwanted elements to find themselves in quarantine or isolation in one form or another for reasons of public hygiene. Such manipulation and trickery have not been confined to the abuse of internal enemy images—they have been extended to the level of international interaction, too.

The management of epidemics can be an act put on deliberately to divert attention or to legitimize actions that would have been otherwise unjustifiable. Declarations of intent by states are often deceptive and misleading. Throughout the history of states' interactions with epidemics, it has been very difficult to distinguish between genuine efforts to minimize the health implications of epidemics and opportunistic attempts to gain political benefits from an outbreak. States have been well placed to take advantage of the mystery surrounding such diseases as plague in the seventeenth century; cholera in the nineteenth century; and BSE, SARS, and avian flu in the twentieth century. Moreover, the character of this manipulation is entirely dependent on one's position in international interactions. The truth-value of different points of view is notoriously difficult to ascertain. However, mere appearances and suspicions are enormously compelling reasons for taking conventionally appropriate actions in international relations, which means that propaganda and prestige are of immense importance and have to be taken into account in managing epidemics. International relations have witnessed some attempts to use epidemics as a pretence for military or strategic gain. States have used regulations whose original purpose was to stop the spread of epidemics by containment to 'reap political benefit' (Delaporte 1986: 142). For instance, states have long used epidemics as an excuse to declare a *cordon sanitaires* against their neighbours and perceived enemies. The US government considered the term 'blockade' to be too strong during the 1962 Cuban missile crisis. Instead, the US imposed a quarantine, which carried at least some sense of international legitimacy. Furthermore, disease-related practices provided ways of legitimizing otherwise politically impossible decisions, which were primarily motivated by economic and political self-interest, ruthless ambition, and power politics. In many respects, the German ban on US pork products in 1880 offers an example of the relative ease with which real health concerns are intertwined with economic protectionism and political interests:

> The German ban has proved the most interesting animal product ban of the era because it was clearly argued on sanitary grounds, but was consistently tinged with a very different motive, namely, the protection of domestic livestock producers in particular and economic nationalism in general. (Hoy and Nuget 1989: 199)

The health scare was based on the discovery that meat infected with *Trichinella spiralis* could kill humans. Regardless of the 'true' motives for the ban, it is clear that the dispute had much to do with protectionism, because the ban benefited Germany's own pork industry.

The worst pandemic since the Spanish Flu, COVID-19 has brought with it intense political co-option. Much of this is related to status and blame games. However, COVID-19 has also been an excuse for other political motivations. For example, arrested opposition members have been denied access to proper legal procedures using COVID-19 as an excuse or they have intentionally not been protected from the disease in overcrowded prisons, as, for example, in Belarus. The opportunistic co-option of COVID-19 for political purposes was rampant as the attention shifted to containment measures against the pandemic: 'Governments must cease using the pandemic as a pretext to crack down on dissent, rein in police overreach, ensure accountability for misconduct, and stop the slide into surveillance states' (Amnesty International 2021: 43). Crackdowns on opposition movements took place in autocracies such as Hong Kong, Belarus and Russia as COVID-19 measures were used to contain people's movements as well as to prohibit gatherings of the opposition. For example, the Belarus regime enacted new travel regulations denying the right of its citizens who did not have permanent foreign residency permits to leave the country. COVID-19 was touted as the reason, but the more likely reason was to prevent people from leaving the country, especially the members of the opposition.

COVID-19 itself fed major power competition as it was used in propaganda. Overall, it was often seen as an opportunity for weakening competitors and sowing seeds of domestic discord. It was also used to implement different types of export and travel restrictions that were overtly justified on health security grounds but were, at the same time, clearly politically motivated. For example, the Chinese government ruled that only Chinese vaccines would be approved and implemented an entry requirement to that effect to make the point that China saw its own measures as qualitatively better than those in the West.

5   *Scare factor, panics, and disinformation*: One of the most common narrative paths of the recent epidemic-related reactions has involved predictable market reactions and seemingly irrational actions from the public. For example, when an epidemic disease (re)emerges, reactions almost automatically lead to havoc in

the financial markets and in consumer behaviour. The markets panic, and the economy suffers when there are sharp changes in consumption patterns, or trade barriers are established between states. In the globalizing world, scare-based reactions are one of the most common ways to express the deep anxieties provoked by pandemic diseases. The societal pandemic expressions can at times be only loosely connected with facts and reality. For example, during the first wave of COVID-19, one of the expressive reactions was people buying up toilet paper in large quantities, which led to shops running out of this vital product. Mimicking and model learning can start to circulate with the effect that the supply chain becomes overburdened, and the product goes out of stock, thereby further feeding the frenzy. The action becomes a self-fulfilling prophecy that cannot be contained by facts as, increasingly, people become stimulated by the behaviour of others. Lack of trust also plays a role because people are aware that the authorities might try to calm them down in order to avoid public health harm. At an individual level, people can start to be sceptical of the health information put out by the authorities and see it as propaganda meant to calm them down. Even worse, in low-trust pandemic environments, public health information can cause scepticism about any facts offered by the authorities or established media. This can agitate the situation and promote conspiratorial attitudes such as corona denialism and vaccine scepticism that are mainly organic, an expression of low trust levels in a society. The mistrust easily finds its expressive channel in scepticism towards official measures and in various conspiratorial attitudes.

The first wave of COVID-19 also spread panic in the global financial markets. However, this was soon calmed through central bank measures that infused large quantities of money into the markets. The fears also found their expression through regionally directed lockdown and containment measures inside countries. These measures indirectly revealed local groups of people that had high infection rates and thereby fed situational scenarios wherein certain localities and the people there were seen in a negative light. There is a close relationship between air travel and microbial traffic (Ali and Keil 2006: 30). The rapid spread of a contagion can be associated with intercontinental flight connections; however, they also became associated with domestic connections. The disease hit large cities particularly hard, while more scarcely populated places had relatively lower infection rates. This could match dormant identity signifiers and differences reinforcing social psychological boundaries between population groups in ways that were politically significant.

6 *Burst of civil religiosity and moral panics*: A contagion puts the focus on the methods of spread as well as the people who are seen as spreaders and carriers. Epidemic diseases heighten the sense of contamination by foreign and domestic actors that are associated with dis-easing lifestyles and cultural habits. Minorities have often been singled out as suspicious 'spreaders'. For example, in the US, hate crimes against Asian Americans increased during the waves of COVID-19. This stereotype reflects the community's attempt to guard its

moral boundaries as a ritualistic way of getting rid of carriers and its efforts to gain immunity. These bursts can have a political effect as they can catalyse already existing patterns of xenophobic behaviour or discrimination, which can be co-opted by populist movements and politicians.

COVID-19 as a Spectre of Past Epidemics

The rapid increase in anxiety and fears over COVID-19 did not happen out of the blue. They were part of the expressive language, the origin of which has to be located within the recent sequence of pandemic emergencies and scares. However, the perception of a contagion adapts not only to local memories and practices concerning contagions but also to the wider surroundings such as global power hierarchies and domestic political order. In the case of pandemics, this environment is not only local but also national and global. For example, the responses of the wider international community to avian flu were commonly based on a practical logic that brought together existing stereotypes, media representations, government information campaigns, and popular rumours (Padmawati and Nichter 2008: 31). However, in most studies on lethal epidemic diseases, this wider socio-political aspect is missing or only implicitly recognized. I will next examine the political characteristics of what are arguably the most important precursor epidemics to COVID-19. The precursor sequence contains the relevant memories and modes of representation which render the scenario of COVID-19 meaningful by emphasizing its 'key' characteristics while making other features of the past cases recede to the background. Out of the recent pandemic scares, SARS and avian flu are the best descriptive of COVID-19's dynamics. Yet the oft-repeated fear over the so-called Disease X also needs to be considered as it contains the synthesis of the worst-case scenario. Each of these precursors provides different aspects of the COVID-19 discourse: for example, tuberculosis provides the background frame for flu-like pandemics, while SARS provides for an exceptional sense of emergency.

SARS

The primary manifestations of SARS were fever that lasted three to seven days, followed by chest pain and breathing problems. The mortality rate was alarmingly high, around 5% according to WHO statistics (WHO 2003). The SARS pandemic struck during the spring of 2003 and was first registered by the WHO in February that year. In March, there were already several hundred reported infections in Hong Kong, Singapore, Toronto, and Taiwan. During April, the media coverage of the outbreak peaked, and by summer, around 800 people had died.

The public imagination of SARS focused on fast global links that crossed continental divides in hours. The imagery of SARS also consisted of people being screened, profiled, and quarantined at airports. SARS was often associated with the feverish agitation of the globalizing world, which was seen as reaching dangerous levels. The rapid transmission from Hong Kong to Vancouver was used to represent the dangers of rapid intercontinental air travel. SARS seemed to be able to spread everywhere that the international hub-and-spoke network of airports extended.

The sudden outbreak of SARS in 2003 resonated with existing patterns of hostility within humanity. The political variant of SARS, which was regarded as a novel and dangerous threat, was made to fit existing patterns in contemporary world politics. In many places, the disease was associated with China or with the ethnic Chinese. The idea that China and the Chinese were secretive, closed, incompetent, and somehow corrupt provided material for this stereotyping interpretation. China was often seen as an outsider by the international community—limited in its transparency, only partially reformed, and unevenly developed. The lack of transparency in China was attributed to the existence and operation of the closed one-party political system. It can be argued that the message of SARS was clear: the disease was interpreted as a call for domestic political reform in China before the country could be safely allowed into the mobility-based global system.

Avian Flu

The spread of H5N1, a subtype of influenza A virus, in birds was considered in 2004 as a huge epidemic threat. The major outbreaks happened in Vietnam and Thailand in January 2004 and spread from there to many neighbouring countries. The fear was that avian flu could jump from birds to humans. In the end, avian flu, despite all the fears, killed only about 50 people, mostly children. One curious aspect of the avian flu scare was that though there were strong beliefs about the low probability of the worst-case scenario, public attention was very much focused on rehearsing just that. The media proceeded on the assumption that the risks involved were of such magnitude that preparations had to be undertaken—the precautionary principle. The creative energies seemed to require constant innovativeness in maintaining a sense of drama and finding new ways of being concerned about the potentially deadly disease (Aaltola 2012a). It was as if the public wanted to relive the disease scare and, through it, how something could be done to alleviate extreme bodily harm in the case of some other future pandemic. The global response could be characterized as a drill for the worst-case scenario—and for COVID-19. However, the lesson learnt highlighted the need for a calm approach and discounted the need for any hype. Thus, avian flu, similar to the Zika virus in 2009, came to mark an overreaction. As precursors to COVID-19, these two pandemic scares led to doubts concerning the need to immediately declare pandemic emergencies. They might have fed the relatively reluctant attitude towards understanding the global threat present in the Wuhan outbreak by offering calming reminders of past 'overreactions' to apparently pandemic situations. These hyped situations led to hesitation on how strongly to approach the developing COVID-19 situation.

It is clear that proceeding on the basis of the worst-case scenario can serve more than health-related functions. The gearing up of preparedness can heighten the restaging of communal constituents and the sense of national cohesion that are seen as desirable for other motives. Many seem to be highly anxious about the sustainability of the world order. In this sense, ulterior motives stemming from the need to secure the world order and one's position in it might provide a better answer to the question why pandemics are restaged in the current form irrespective of their status as mere scares or actual 'plagues'. Pandemic scares can offer material for 'global order drills'. These pedagogic scares may be extremely effective in narrating what is at stake and what must be done to secure the situation. At the end, the recurring pandemic spectacles channel concerns, worries, and fears about the sustainability of the modern global way of life into a form that is reasonably manageable. In this way, avian flu and the Zika virus were necessary drills for mobilizing resources and preparedness planning. At the same time, they proved to be much tamer diseases than first imagined. As such, they built expectations that COVID-19 would also be manageable and containable.

Spanish Flu

The literature on pandemics often refers to the 1918–20 Spanish Flu as a benchmark outbreak. The outbreak infected about a quarter of the global population. In many ways, the Spanish Flu comes closest to describing the biological antagonism inherent in COVID-19. The mortality rate was high, about 10 to 20 times higher than in a generic influenza pandemic. The mortality and virulence appear to be a close match to COVID-19 based on the current information, although both diseases, for different reasons, are yet to be fully understood (e.g. *NYT* 2020b). The Spanish Flu began by spreading among the British forces in Spain, which is how it got its name, although the first cases were reported in the US, from where it spread aided by the movement of troops. It caused much havoc in the military operations as it hit, in particular, people in the 20–40 years' age group (Martini *et al.* 2019). In Europe, the disease spread through France, Great Britain, Italy, and Spain, causing havoc in the World War I military operations. Three-quarters of the French troops and more than half of the British troops fell ill in the spring of 1918 complicating the war efforts. During the Meuse-Argonne operation, more than 1 million men fell ill. Although the Spanish Flu is sometimes called the forgotten epidemic since it was overshadowed by the calamity of the war, it still had political consequences. For example, it was immediately used in war propaganda in a predictable way to highlight the maliciousness of the enemy and the resilience and stoicism of the home front. Stories started to circulate that the disease was a product of an enemy warfare experiment (Honingsbaum 2013: 165). Interestingly, this dated idea has resurfaced in the recent COVID-19 disinformation.

Disease X

Besides the concrete pandemic cases, it is almost impossible to understand COVID-19 without reference to the much-feared 'Disease X'. On the one hand, the speculative Disease X encapsulates the age-old fears and memories concerning the plague and other killer diseases, while, on the other hand, Disease X is a function of the contemporary world order based on rule-based logistics and standardized flows and movements between the global market and production sites that are geographically dislocated. The WHO listed Disease X among the known serious contagious diseases requiring urgent action, including, for example, the Crimean-Congo haemorrhagic fever, the Ebola and Marburg virus diseases, Lassa fever, Middle East respiratory syndrome coronavirus (MERS-CoV), SARS, Nipah and henipaviral diseases, Rift Valley Fever (RVF), and Zika (WHO 2015). The WHO website also refers to a future potential source of urgent action with the name Disease X:

> Disease X represents the knowledge that a serious international epidemic could be caused by a pathogen currently unknown to cause human disease, and so the R&D Blueprint explicitly seeks to enable cross-cutting R&D preparedness that is also relevant for an unknown 'Disease X' as far as possible.
>
> *(WHO 2018)*

This potentially (re)emerging disease would be accorded priority due to its high human-to-human transmissibility, case fatality rate, spillover potential, evolutionary potential, and risk of international spread. Furthermore, Disease X would be difficult to detect and control, it would occur in areas where public health would not be at a satisfactory level, and it would potentially also have a high social impact.

When, in late February 2020, COVID-19 cases were reported in South Korea and Italy, speculation about a potential Disease X started in the media:

> Unlike SARS, its viral cousin, the Covid-19 virus replicates at high concentrations in the nose and throat akin to the common cold, and appears capable of spreading from those who show no, or mild, symptoms. That makes it impossible to control using the fever-checking measures that helped stop SARS 17 years ago.
>
> *(Bloomberg 2020)*

This speculation itself was a sign of the socially and politically disruptive character of the virus. The root vision is based on the idea of a feverishly connected world which is extraordinarily vulnerable to rapidly adapting and mutating disease agents. The fast connections and Third World urbanization, together with secretive governments and patchy levels of health care, create evolutionary niches for pandemic influenza in a way that is unmatched by the development of the epidemic surveillance and control systems.

Conclusion

Modern societies which are compatible with the world order characterized by mobility and cross-border flows are seen as forming the safe, secure, and sanitary top of the global hierarchy. China found itself in a disadvantageous position in this hierarchy at the onset of the COVID-19 outbreak because it had been associated with multiple pandemic outbreaks in recent times. Its place as a legitimate core member of the global club of nations with an adequate, functioning governance and political system came under increasing doubt, and not only because of the cases of pandemic disease. Much of the early commentary on COVID-19 and China focused on domestic political challenges. For example, there has been speculation that by centralizing all power in its top leadership, China has stumbled into a situation in which, in the case of perceived failure, all responsibility is centralized as well. Some argue that change can sometimes happen in a revolutionary manner, that it can be produced by sudden unconventional triggers, as in the case of the Arab Spring or the Soviet collapse in the aftermath of the Chernobyl nuclear accident (e.g. Anderlini 2020). Other commentators were right to be more nuanced. However, even they saw that there was potential for a more nuanced change, towards a form of autocratic rule that is more open to less coercive methods of governance (e.g. Truex 2020). Overall, in the early spring of 2020, COVID-19 was read as a challenge to China and also in the political sense. It was geographically localized, and, reading through the early commentaries, there is a feeling that the pandemic was not global but China's national issue. This could have been due to the precursor implications of earlier pandemic scares. It took a while to understand the true global meanings of COVID-19 and their possible feedback loops to China from where the disease originated.

At the same time, the early epidemic situation in China further reinforced coercive authoritarian tendencies instead of being a driver for more democratic change. China has developed increasingly pervasive forms of surveillance. At the same time, its external policies have hardened after 1 year of the pandemic. This is not surprising because historically serious infectious diseases have led into the pursuit of further purity and civil religious adherence to norms and virtues that are associated with getting out of harm's way. China's reaction to the COVID-19 outbreak was to blame the local authorities in Wuhan and Hubei province for trying to hide it for too long. This attribution of causality also indicates stricter centralization in the future, depending on how the situation proceeds. Furthermore, the speculation about the ramifications of the disease in China did not take into account the fact that—irrespective of actual culpability—COVID-19 was rapidly becoming a global disease that had an impact not only domestically and societally but, more profoundly, globally in a way that also influenced China's position in the global order. I now examine some of these impacts.

1   *Global decoupling is gaining traction after COVID-19*: At the global level, disruption caused by an epidemic disease provides one more reminder of the risks posed by the efficient yet inflexible global system. The system's resilience was stress-tested by COVID-19, and the result(s) might accentuate the ongoing decoupling process. Multinational companies are reconsidering the long-term implications of investing too much in China. They have already started to shift their production to other countries in an attempt to save money as well

as to become less reliant on China due to the US–China trade tensions and, more recently, the growing risks brought about by the COVID-19 outbreak.[3] COVID-19 has suddenly decreased the production in China as large quarantines and travel restrictions have been put in place. As such, COVID-19 can be read as a sign of the times, leading to further decoupling.

2 *Contagious diseases are political:* During modern times, contagious diseases have become a part of the language of health governance. The idea has been to separate health governance as a functional field of expertise from the politics of diseases. With this in mind, the modern understanding of governance sees politics, at best, as counterproductive and, at worst, as detrimental to the expertise-based international health activities. COVID-19, together with its precursors, clearly points out that any widespread epidemic is, from the onset, always political in ways that the modern global health paradigm cannot make sense of or cope with. Patterns of politicization should be recognized, and governance activity should try to mitigate their impact on the actual pandemic preparedness and control.

3 *Trust in global health governance is declining:* The WHO was seen in an almost heroic light after its successful management of the SARS epidemic. Avian flu and the Zika virus posed more confusing cases, and the WHO's reputation suffered when it was seen as taking too hasty steps in declaring a global pandemic emergency. Instead of being too proactive, the COVID-19 case has led to the questioning of the (WHO) defence of China's draconian efforts as measures that provided the outside world crucial time to prepare. The praising of the Chinese way of handling the situation seems to have simply ignored Beijing's initial inability to control the disease and its attempts to hide it. It was in the first few weeks of December 2019 that the broader outbreak of COVID-19 could have been avoided and managed (within China). Also, it took the WHO several weeks to negotiate access to China. The weak WHO response put China in the driver's seat in the control efforts. Now that COVID-19 has turned into a widespread global pandemic, trust in health authorities and health governance at the global level will inevitably decline.

4 *Large-scale restrictive practices are gaining ground:* Measures that aim at restricting movement on a large scale, such as quarantines and *cordons sanitaires*, were thought to be relatively clumsy and even counterproductive responses. At best, they were seen as delaying the spread of the disease but not actually affecting the cumulative impact over time. Modern best practices have emphasized the need to act quickly in detecting chains of contagion and isolating all exposed people so that no large-scale policies need to be implemented. Large-scale quarantines could also be harmful for the much-needed meticulous detective work, as panic would likely start spreading and people seek to escape the hot zones. However, social isolation (locally), large-scale quarantines (regionally), and travel restrictions (internationally) became the 'best practices' as COVID-19 spread in China (and subsequently elsewhere), potentially legitimizing such measures also in future epidemic situations.

5   *Lack of trust in governance between the local, national, and international levels is grow-ing:* The seams of global multilevel governance, considered here with regard to health, seem to have been strained from the very beginning of the COVID-19 outbreak. China's central government blamed it on the authorities at the local and provincial levels. At the same time, many states were suspicious of China, including its response and reporting of infections and casualties, and they imposed travel restrictions despite Beijing's protests. The WHO was also criticized by many commentators for its praise of China's approach to the outbreak. On the whole, the blame game gave the impression that the governance system as a whole was not optimally synchronized. On the basis of COVID-19's political history till the time of going to press, the more general historical disease patterns, and the precursor diseases, there are going to be more lasting impacts of the Chinese status and internal development.

6   *China's status and legitimacy are increasingly in doubt:* Modern societies that are supposed to be compatible with the world order, which is characterized by mobility and cross-border flows, are seen as forming the safe, secure, and sanitary top level of the global hierarchy. This world-order pattern puts China in a disadvantageous position as it has been associated with multiple pandemic outbreaks in recent times. Its place as a legitimate core member of the global club of nations with an adequate, functioning governance and political system is coming increasingly under doubt.

7   *Western powers on both sides of the Atlantic were the epicentres of COVID-19:* During the first year of COVID-19, the US was largely missing in action and did not assume its expected global leadership role. Similarly, the EU was also a key epicentre of the pandemic. After the election of Joe Biden as president of the US, the transatlantic community's ability to set the agenda has increased. However, the guardianship of the global order remains in doubt, and COVID-19 seems to have driven the regressive processes forward as great power rivalry was accentuated rather than revealing any sense of coming together as a well-governed unit working for the common good.

Notes

1   More on this, see, for example, *The Wall Street Journal* (6 February 2020).
2   For example, the brutal fate of Napoleon's Grande Armée provides a case in point of the lopsided and decisive effects of lethal epidemics (Marshall-Cornwall 1967: 1; Robins 1981: 77).
3   For example, *The Financial Times* (23 February 2020). Coronavirus is speeding up the decoupling of the global economies. www.ft.com/content/5cfea02e-549f-11ea-90ad-25e377c0ee1f

7

DYNAMICS OF AN EPIDEMIC OF INTERNATIONAL AND NATIONAL ORIGIN_

Cases of Haiti Cholera and the Mad Cow Disease

Besides being a biological entity, a serious lethal epidemic disease always results in individual anxieties, political stir, domestic hatemongering, and international opprobrium. It accentuates existing insecurities, enmities, and catalyses societal cleavages. The key question from the Thucydidean politosomatic aspect is the nature of the context in which an epidemic disease emerges and spreads. What other regressive processes co-occur that a disease can bind and combine with? This chapter draws lessons from two very different cases: Cholera epidemic that engulfed Haiti starting in 2010 and the mad cow disease (BSE) of 1996 concentrating mainly in the UK. The idea is to further examine the local and international dynamics fed by the heightened sense of somatic insecurity—how the local, national, and international levels interact in shifting and attributing the blame. As has already been reviewed, politosomatics has tendencies such as bursts of civil religiosity, status and blame games, scares, ethnicization, and sexualization. Yet they can also be localized/nationalized and internationalized. In the case study of Haiti, the focus is on internationalization and, in the case of BSE, it is on nationalization of a disease.

Haiti Cholera 2010

Haiti has had a difficult history, with calamities—both natural and political—occurring at regular intervals. Torn societies and weak governments are full of valencies and possible opportunities for binding with other negative factors. The political troubles in the 1990s brought in interventions by the US and the UN Peacekeeping force. Then, in January 2010, a devastating earthquake hit Haiti. It can be suggested that the cholera epidemic arrived 10 months later at a very inopportune time as the situation was ripe for downwards spiralling negative processes.

The causal relationship between the epidemiological and political characteristics is non-linear and entangled and offers a difficult subject for strict analytical

DOI: 10.4324/9781003169147-7

dissection (e.g. Tuite, Tien, Eisenberg, et al. 2011). For example, it is generally felt that COVID-19 and its management had a notable political impact on the US presidential election in 2020. That said, it is difficult to clearly spell out in what ways and to what degree the impact was felt. Similarly, the disease agitated polities, and the effects were seen in the streets of many countries. Yet its role in political unrest, as, for example, in the streets of Belarus and Russia, cannot be easily analysed using a reductive analytic model. The case of cholera in Haiti 2010 onwards gives us an important case in point regarding the ways in which a national-level epidemic outbreak can politically stir and agitate (e.g Cravioto *et al.* 2011). This case study can also enlighten us on the qualitative impact of a disease as an enmity catalyser.

As pointed out in the beginning chapters, Thomas Hobbes' translation of Thucydides' work provides a useful bridgehead into the underlying issue of disease as an agent for spreading political anger and hate. Hobbes, who observed plague in his own day, translates the key meaning of the Plague of Athens to focus on two readings of justice:

> Neither the fear of the gods, nor laws of men, awed any man: not the former, because they concluded it was alike to worship or not worship, from seeing that alike they all perished: nor the latter, because no man expected that lives would last till he received punishment of his crimes by judgment.
>
> *(Thucydides, The Thomas Hobbes Translation 1959)*

First, justice was not seen in the general randomness or perceived patterns of how people were inflicted with the disease or how they died. The fears and actual occurrences of untimely and unusual deaths left people distrusting the usual civil religious understandings of the role of death as a sacrifice of some sort. A horrible disease simply offered no way of 'dying well' as it was conventionally and traditionally understood. Second, judgement, as a judicial (trials and punishments) and social (shame and guilt) process, was no longer fully effective as political institutions, civil religiosity, and social customs had all but collapsed under the crush of the plague. The constitutive element of political friendship between citizens dissolved to an alarming degree.

The guardianship of Haiti's governance was placed largely in the hands of the UN Peacekeeping force which were already in the country helping to deal with the political unrest initially and then with the aftermath of the earthquake. The particular enmity-breeding aspect of the cholera epidemic that followed the earthquake was, first, the result of the overall combined calamities and, second, the fact that the disease was brought to Haiti by the supposed guardians, the UN Peacekeeping force. The overall sense of lacking meaningful explanations and the prevailing injustice found specific outlets in riots and demonstrations against the UN and the international humanitarian efforts. The proto-conceptualization of old themes about a 'foreign' dis-easing presence and the negative consequences of 'foreign' elements was easily triggered in the atmosphere of overall distrust and paranoia. Moreover, the repeated denials by the UN and its vague responses, even when the causation of the disease was clear, did not help in calming the anger but aided a sense of justice not having been served (e.g. *The Lancet* 2010).

This chapter deals with the domestic consequences of a situation in which the political leadership was dispersed and seen as unaccountable and where international crisis management efforts were seen as acting as an epidemic vector. It is a case study of factors that might also influence the pandemic containment efforts in pandemic outbreaks where different domestic contexts experience the situation in varying ways, depending on the local characteristics and specific patterns of political authority and governance. One of the clear challenges for the global polity's pandemic security is the lack of effective cooperation and collaboration between the key global organizations and the individual states. The global ownership of the containment along the various contagion routes/vectors seems to be far too dispersed, even largely missing in parts. For example, the way in which WHO managed the outbreak of COVID-19 in Wuhan, China, has been much criticized but also defended. International organizations that are supposed to act as the guardians of global health can fail for several reasons. They can be victims of major states' failure to cooperate in full. Their own wide mandate, scarcity of resources, and bureaucratic politics can put constraints on their effective performance in time-critical situations. However, international organizations are also single unitary actors to a degree. They can also be unintentional instigators of an emergency and then try to cover up their actions to sustain their own legitimacy. These factors came into play in the tense situation of the cholera outbreak in Haiti.

Politosomatics of the Double Calamity in Haiti

Haiti was dealt a double blow in 2010: first, a massive earthquake in January and then, in its wake in October, a nationwide cholera epidemic (e.g. Carlowe 2010: 19). As of January 2012, the number of cumulative cholera cases had overrun the local government's health-care capacity and had emerged as a key fear factor for the Haitians who had survived the earthquake, which had killed between 100,000 and 160,000 of the population.[1] By 2020, around 9,000 people had died of cholera, and the disease had afflicted about one-tenth of the Haitians. The epidemic also spread to the neighbouring Dominican Republic resulting in 500 deaths, and there were also reports of cases in Venezuela and Cuba. In this context, the world order and its governance directly translated into local vulnerabilities, into a Haitian configuration of differentially exposed bodies. Besides the cholera revealing the differential vulnerability, the massive earthquake had already shown how one's position in the development hierarchy determines to a large extent the consequences of disasters. During the same time period, earthquakes of similar magnitude hit three countries. In New Zealand in 2011, around 200 people were killed, while in Chile in 2010, 500 people were killed. Of course, it is difficult to compare the varying characteristics of different earthquakes. However, the less-prepared governance and underdevelopment clearly contributed to the high death toll in Haiti.

In epidemic emergencies, a state's location in the lower levels of the global hier-archy translates into somatic-level stress and vulnerability as well as anxiety, panic, fear, changing social expressions, and other types of disease-related behaviour. The ensuing paranoia is further fuelled when the exact nature of what has happened is kept hidden. Finally, after years of deep suspicions concerning the role of the UN-led operation in the outbreak of cholera in Haiti, the UN finally acknowledged the high likelihood of this on 25 October 2016:

> Exactly six years ago, United Nations peacekeepers brought cholera to Haiti for the first time in that country's history. Soon, 10,000 people will have died as a result, and 800,000 will have been infected. Eight per cent of Haiti's total population has thus been affected.

The sad saga from suspicion to admission is illustrative of the role of epidemics in politics (OHCHR 2016). In a statement on 19 August 2016, the spokesperson of the UN secretary-general took 'moral responsibility' for the situation although the wording was crafted in such a way that no official declaration of responsibility and direct liability was made:

> The Secretary-General deeply regrets the terrible suffering the people of Haiti have endured as a result of the cholera epidemic. The United Nations has a moral responsibility to the victims of the cholera epidemic and for sup-porting Haiti in overcoming the epidemic and building sound water, sanita-tion and health systems.
>
> *(UN Secretary-General 2016)*

The origins of the disease had received scientific attention, and there were convinc-ing studies that established the highly probable origin of the outbreak (e.g. Houston 2017). Still, even by 2021, no compensation has been paid to the epidemic victims, while, at the same time, funding for the aid effort has been on the decline.

In 2010, the legitimacy of the 'rule', 'order', and 'power' of the UN operation in Haiti was suddenly and unexpectedly challenged by cholera. The epidemic and the denials over its origin led to decreasing trust in the UN-led overall humanitar-ian effort. The epidemic made many Haitians realize their disadvantaged position as lower-rank members of the international community and also gave them a rea-son to suspect the authority of the UN in the longer term.

The ensuing scenario was acutely politosomatic. The politicization of the role of the supposed helpers and the increasing scepticism towards the UN led to a political shake-up in Haiti and to the dis-easing of the overall situation in the multilevel global governance system. The more encompassing political embodi-ments, such as a sense of an ordered world, a secure state, or an organized local community, were felt not only to be under pressure and duress but also as sources of local and national-level suffering. This perceived regressive influence between the micro and macro level of political bonds and the expectation of major disruption in the wider extensions of one's situatedness did cause worries and anxieties that were lived through somatic worries and expressive disease behaviour, such as contagion-related suspicions, and encapsulated into the ways in which actual physical symptoms found their public expressions in demonstrations and riots. In Haiti, the cholera epidemic was earth-shaking. It caused the reversal of the role of the supposed do-gooders into that of suspected disease spreaders. This role reversal was potentially perilous to the UN operation in Haiti and to the UN's reputation there.

Even before the earthquake, Haiti was seen by many outsiders, and by Haitians themselves, as a suffering society and a failing state (e.g. Torgman 2012). It is argued that the suffering because of the cholera changed and concentrated, for the moment, the public expressions of this wider political pain as it acquired a shared expressive language accentuated by the perception that outsiders had brought the disease to Haiti. At the same time, the expressive language of suffering from the cholera changed in both the cognitive and emotional senses. In this way, the use of politosomatics as an analytic frame helps in discerning the important dynamics between the different forms of 'bodily' pain and embodying and directing the political suffering in Haiti.

An overview of the cholera epidemic in Haiti and among Haitians reveals the tensions it opened up between Haitians and the representatives of the international community and the anxieties it caused in the international community over its own perceived governance failure and the tarnishing of its self-image. Multiple scenarios meshed together after the earthquake in Haiti: First, the tradition of a dis-eased community interacted with compassion for the suffering other because the earthquake killed tens of thousands of people. The international community rushed in and brought cholera with it to Haiti. The politico-somatics relationship disrupted the first coupling—between the suffering community and the helping international community—and produced further telling complications about the dynamics of politico-somatics in a situation where regressions— political crisis, bad governance, and susceptibility to natural disasters—tend to group together.

Trust or lack of it became a key characteristic of the scenario. The helpers—the international community with a myriad of organizations—were suddenly seen in a negative light, as a 'foreign' element that had exposed Haiti to a deadly exogenous epidemic. Another key characteristic was secrecy, which is a common attribute of epidemic outbreaks; however, it is not commonly associated with actors that advocate good governance and the rule of law. The cholera outbreak allowed for the politicization of the situation by the local Haitian political forces thereby changing the balance of situational dynamics in favour of those advocating more traditional, nationalistic, populist, and xenophobic politics. The dynamics need to be mapped out in detail because they bear a close family resemblance to other outbreak situations, and they also reveal patterns common to COVID-19 but from a different situation and point of view in the global hierarchy.

The Politics of Cholera

From the Haitian Red Cross' interviews with Haitians, it was learnt that they commonly believed that the locals had been so exposed to different diseases that they had become immune to them (Petit-Goâve *et al.* 2010). The decades-long absence of cholera lent some support to this belief. The belief contributed to the popular account due to which the 2010 cholera outbreak stood out and could be regarded with deep suspicion. The Haitian Red Cross report contained representative quotes from the interviews: 'We have been living in these conditions for many years and we did not get cholera' (Petit-Goâve *et al.* 2010). The disease scenario saw the spread of the cholera epidemic as proof of more ominous background influences. Other quotes in the Haitian Red Cross report are these: 'It is a poison brought by foreigners to divide us'; 'It is a disease brought by foreigners to exterminate us and take our land'; 'It is a disease brought by NGOs in order to get more money'; and 'It is another divine sign (after the earthquake) that the end of the world will come soon'. Besides these interpretations, the theme of 'foreignness' and of the foreign origin of the disease is repeated often. The attribute of 'foreignness' is an important signifier of cholera's embodiedness. As a modality of knowledge, it conveys an outside point of origin for the disease: the emotive and sense-related modalities of a 'foreigner's disease' can be seen as influencing the ways in which the disease was feared, its suffering was expressed, and how the sufferer was understood in their community. The fear of cholera got its more specific situated scenario when it blended with anti-foreign feelings, genocidal colonial experiences, and national helplessness in the face of multiple catastrophes.

The sources of the politosomatic anxieties stemming from the cholera epidemic were multiple. First, cholera stood out because it was a novel threat for the Haitians. Cholera epidemics have not been recorded in Haiti in the last 80 years at least (e.g. Piarroux *et al.* 2011). Second, the origin of the cholera was mysterious, controversial, and ominous. Epidemiological research, which strongly suggested that the *Vibrio cholerae* was introduced in Haiti in one event and spread from a point source (e.g. Dowell and Braden 2011: 1299; Ali *et al.* 2011: 699). Piarroux *et al.* (2011: 1162), lent scientific support to the prevalent suspicions and rumours by pointing to the presence of the Nepalese peacekeepers in the United Nations Stabilization Mission in Haiti (MINUSTAH)[2] camp in the temporal and geographical epicentre of the cholera epidemic just above a stream flowing into the Artibonite river: 'Haitian epidemiologists observed sanitary deficiencies, including a pipe discharging sewage from the camp into the river. Villagers used water from this stream for cooking and drinking'. Third, the origin was at first actively covered up by the UN, thereby directing much of the public anger to the representatives of the international community. The overall effect of the cover-up in the face of scientific evidence was a heavy blow to UN respect and legitimacy (e.g. Frerichs 2016: 149).

Categorical denial was the UN's first reaction to the spreading rumours concerning the cholera and its origin—the UN mission spokesperson in Haiti denied the suspicions and allegations concerning the peacekeepers' role in the outbreak. A WHO spokesperson equally played down the importance of finding the cause of the disease, saying it was 'not important'. The suspicions concerning the origin of the disease and the disgust over the cover-up reinforced the practice of embodying the disease as an outsider's—a foreigner's—disease, a disease which was 'international' in origin. Fourth, the proliferating meanings could be co-opted by Haiti's politicians to express genuine worry or to score political points as the country geared up for its presidential elections. The local politicians reacted to the spreading news in the heightened affective climate of the approaching presidential elections. Already on 10 November, Haiti's senior health official had said that the outbreak was 'no longer a simple emergency, it's now a matter of national security'. The health minister of Haiti stated that the nation was suffering from an 'imported disease'. Fifth, the outbreak was seen as an embarrassment for the UN, which had struggled to govern and control Haiti after the earthquake. The UN authorities tried to fight off their failures and their clear lack of preparedness by stating that they had adhered fully to all possible standards and procedures.[3] The situation soon worsened and started to complicate the public health efforts. During the following months, riots broke out in several places across Haiti. Suddenly, the stakes became very high. The credibility and legitimacy of all of the UN were suddenly at stake in Haiti. The cholera turned into a political variant that quickly spread within the Haitian society. This political variant contained the message of failure, not of Haiti, which had already failed, but of the global governance that was supposed to provide it relief and aid in its recovery, but which had instead caused the epidemic outbreak, either unintentionally or through bad governance.

Arguably, the internationalized governance of Haiti had gained legitimacy from administrative practices and from keeping day-to-day services running in difficult conditions. However, the international machinery apoliticized individual Haitians, displacing them from their own polity or polities, as pointed out in Chapter 2. It is significant that the places where these acts were carried out were the camps built for people displaced by the earthquake. The UN-led humanitarian intervention to help Haitians produced an archipelago of camps, first for displaced people and then for the cholera patients. Still in the spring of 2012, more than 600,000 Haitians were living in close to 900 camps set up and administered by the 'international humanitarian partners' (e.g. Ramadan 2013).

Besides these camps for the Haitians, there were a large number of camps for the aid workers and for the international peacekeepers. Those living outside of the mosaic of camps were also in many ways subject to the governance emanating from them. The key to the understanding of Haiti and Haitians as objects of international governance in the system of camps is the individualization of the sufferer in humanitarian spectacles. This common 'zooming-in' to the individual allows for the construction of the epicentre of suffering, where the voiceless sufferer—one of supposed quiet humility—communicates only through the visual language of a body in pain and its expressed needs instead of through lived-life injustices and historical grievances. This production of political quietness is achieved by stripping the sufferer of the essential characteristics of a citizen of a polity and placing the politically disembodied figure into a refugee camp (Malkki 1996: 380). It seems that for a sufferer to become a legitimate recipient of international aid, they are denied membership of other more narrow local or national political communities. A sufferer to become the target of humanitarian motivated applications of technical solutions. Understood in this way, international governance refers to a repertoire of established and well-rehearsed 'solutions' (Agambe 1998: 132; Malkki 2002: 353; Rozakou 2012: 562).[4]

Moreover, Haiti itself could be considered a largely cordoned-off site— a non-polity—legitimized by the cholera outbreak and patrolled by the US Navy and Coast Guard to stop refugee flows (McKinley and James 2010). It should be noted that 'cordoning-off' was among the most immediate 'humanitarian' reactions to the earthquake. US troops in Haiti handed out tens of thousands of battery-, hand-crank-, and solar-operated portable radios. This provided Haitians some means of communication because much of the country's electric grid was down and many radio stations destroyed (McKingley 2010). The US Air Force then used military planes to transmit Voice of America's news and call-in programmes to the Haitians. The radio transmissions included constant messages aimed at stopping the feared mass migration of Haitians.[5] It appears that some of the US' emergency response activities were first and foremost aimed at containing migratory flows and stopping people from becoming mobile. Evidently, the goal of checking the spread of a perceived problem by containing people's movements was a modus operandi of the humanitarian operation (Donini 2010: 224).[6] The Haitians' resistance to this ethos of containing, cordoning-off, and fencing-in was at first low because of the desperation and paralysis caused by the earthquake. However, the epidemic-containment frame of the cholera outbreak revealed the camps in the light of quarantine and *cordon sanitaire* measures, thereby increasing the direct stakes of being encamped and heightening the health-related risks. The cholera outbreak might have accentuated the sudden reaction against the UN governance. On the one hand, the stringent health security scenario hyperbolized the tendency to contain, cordon, and quarantine. This reframed the idea of camps and medical centres. At the same time, the specifics of the outbreak—such as its imported origin, the cover-up, the building of fenced cholera treatment centres—accentuated a sense that the UN efforts were illegitimate and a cause of actual bodily suffering. Contrary to the desires of the international agencies administering their lives, many Haitians started to press their self-understanding of the situation, highlight their national suffering, and resist their humanitarian designations. In this way, the cholera outbreak challenged the apolitical appearance of the internationalized governance by briefly producing loud sufferers with political understandings who expressed their dissent through riots and stopped playing their usual voiceless part in the humanitarian spectacle.

UN Attempts to Prevent Internationalizing the Cholera Epidemic

Recent pandemic emergencies have led to the emergence of global public awareness over the worst-case scenarios of 'the coming plague' and 'blow against civilization' imageries. These imageries have been spread effectively by works of popular culture and popularized accounts of global health security since the mid-1990s. The UN and its sub-organizations exist as the predominant global authorities expected to manage pandemic emergencies. On the basis of its unique role, it is possible to claim that the UN's conception of epidemic diseases is to a high degree conditioned by these popular accounts and expectations, which it has to satisfy. Keeping this in mind, the claims in Haiti that the UN had directly caused an epidemic disease were anything but insignificant. They were in conflict with the UN's authority and its messaging and led to a conflicted self-understanding with regard to the global 'placedness' of both Haiti and the Haitians. The UN's desire to save face and maintain a sense of authority was tied to its role in the pandemic scenarios of global health security. These are similar to the more local Haitian understanding of the cholera epidemic. However, there are some differences between the local epidemic and global pandemic scenarios. Many Haitians chose to interpret the cholera nationalistically. The epidemic involved one nation, and it did not spread to its neighbouring states. To a degree, the cholera signified the negative influences of the international presence in the country. In this connection, it should be noted that this diseasing movement suggests any 'curative' action to be the reversal of leaking boundaries: the reversing of the foreign element seems to require restoration of the polity's boundedness so as to keep the foreign element out. In contrast to this, the global pandemic scenario is, right from the beginning, based on the impossibility of bordering since globality is conceptually synonymous with connectedness and interdependence.

When, in the summer of 2011, the UN released the Independent Report by experts on the cholera outbreak in Haiti, the contradictory tendencies between the local epidemic and global pandemic scenarios were at play. The report on the cholera in Haiti was written by an independent commission hired by the UN. The executive summary of the report placed the cholera in the context of the devastating earthquake: 'Ten months after the devastating earthquake of January 12, 2010, cholera appeared in Haiti for the first time in nearly a century'. This opening sentence seems to be aimed at putting things back in their 'real' context. However, the first paragraph also states the reason for the Independent Report: 'The source of the cholera has been controversial'. The report goes on to state three alternative hypotheses for the origin of the outbreak:

- Cholera 'arrived into Haiti from the Gulf of Mexico due to tectonic shifts resulting from the earthquake';
- it 'evolved into disease-causing strains from non-pathogenic strains naturally present in Haiti'; and
- it 'originated from a human host who inadvertently introduced the strain into the Haitian environment'.

Since much of the political speculation and rumours favoured the third option, the opening paragraph goes on to explain it further: 'A specific form of the third hypothesis, that soldiers deployed from a cholera-endemic country to the Mirebalais camp of the United Nations Stabilization Mission in Haiti (MINUSTAH) were the source of the cholera, is a commonly held belief in Haiti'. The report emphasizes that its authority is based on it being an independent report compiled by experts on the issue. From the beginning, it is evident that the independence of the report has one major caveat: it has been authorized by the secretary-general of the UN. This same organization is implicated by the third hypothesis since the MINUSTAH operation was run by the UN.

The summary ends with the following clear statement: '[T]he Haitian cholera bacteria did not originate from the native environs of Haiti'. The single location for the outbreak is clearly established in the report, although it does not explicate the source in a straightforward manner. However, although the purpose of the report was to investigate the origin, it puts much emphasis on the reasons for the 'explosive' spread:

> The introduction of this cholera strain as a result of environmental contamination with feces could not have been the source of such an outbreak without simultaneous water and sanitation and health care system deficiencies. These deficiencies, coupled with conducive environmental and epidemiological conditions, allowed the spread of the *Vibrio cholerae* organism in the environment, from which a large number of people became infected.

The evidence indicates that the outbreak spread 'along the Artibonite River'. The sanitary conditions at the MINUSTAH camp were deemed to be insufficient to prevent the disease agent from spreading to the river. In this context, the report states that 'MINUSTAH contracts with an outside contractor to handle human fecal waste'. This statement reminds the reader that the placing of the blame is complicated even if the facts of the case seem to point at the peacekeepers. The report indicates that a review of the hospital records indicates that the baseline rate of the cases of severe diarrhoea lasted till 20 October, when a clear—'explosive'—outbreak occurred. The area hospitals were ill-equipped to deal with the outbreak: 'Hospital staff reported walking on feces in cholera units'. It is pointed out that intra-hospital transmission contributed to the spread. Poor sanitary conditions in different places along the river are highlighted in the report: 'There is significant human activity along [the Meye Tributary System], with women washing, people bathing, people collecting water for drinking, and children playing'. These highly embodied signifiers of people urinating and defecating and also washing and eating close by convey a reservoir of regressive meanings concerning the Haitians. Besides these references, the report indicates failures at various levels in the Haiti infrastructure and governance. The overall impression is that the disease was able to spread rapidly because of local failures and low standards. The report implies that the locals were involved in several ways in the spread of the disease.

The report concludes that the epidemic was caused by a 'confluence of circumstances'. Rather than assigning blame, the report states that the cholera epidemic is not reducible to any single factor and 'was not the fault of, or deliberate action of, a group or individual'. The technical approach taken does not address the underlying controversy. It points out that the true origin was an emergent unforeseen property: the underlying 'cause' was a huge network of potential and actual actions that took place in highly particularized contexts with intertwined relational linkages that emerge from factors residing within the local context. Thus, the UN-sponsored report largely bypasses and merely wiggles around the obvious—the fact that cholera was introduced in Haiti by its peacekeepers. Arguably, the political function of the 'confluence of circumstances' phrase was to construct the cholera in a way that fitted the overall political objectives. To a degree, this meant allowing the international community and its various representatives to continue their work for the Haitians and against the cholera. However, from a more encompassing perspective, the phrase was meant to save the humanitarian legitimacy of the UN effort and the prestige of its agents not only in Haiti but in many other places around the world and in the future.

In their recommendations, the panel points out how the recurrence of such a complex 'confluence' might be stopped in the future. The first recommendation addresses the probable reason why the bacteria came to Haiti:

> To prevent introduction of cholera into non-endemic countries, United Nations personnel and emergency responders traveling from cholera endemic areas should either receive a prophylactic dose of appropriate antibiotics before departure or be screened with a sensitive method to confirm absence of asymptomatic carriage of *Vibrio cholerae*, or both.

At this point, the underlying sequence of events—as opposed to the confluence—is referred to in this recommendation. However, the recommendation is in a context of signifiers referring to the complexities of the earthquake catastrophe. One should also note that the recommendation's point about emergency respondents can lead to a mix-up concerning the role of the peacekeeping operation in Haiti. This may be misleading since the MINUSTAH operations were already established in June 2004. The peacekeepers' mission was to maintain security, rather than being quickly recruited emergency responders.

Thus, the main performative of the report seems to be to point out and remind us that the cholera took place at a precise instant in time because everything was right for the outbreak to occur. The report gives the impression of something happening by coincidence, something simply happening. If anything had been missing from the required parameters, the outbreak would not have occurred. In this way, the role of the peacekeepers was reduced to just one condition among many; it was not the precipitating event that was turned into the outbreak by the real driving force, the confluence of circumstances inherently unforeseen at the time. The series of events were only understood as contributing factors afterwards when they could be seen as errors and mistakes, which were magnified, so the reports claim, by the confluence of circumstances. Significantly, Latour (1993: 21) refers to the nineteenth-century doctrine of 'morbid spontaneity':

> This doctrine . . . corresponded perfectly to the style, mode of action, and facts, since disease appeared sometimes here, sometimes there; sometimes at one season, sometimes at another; sometimes responding to a remedy, sometimes spreading, only to disappear as suddenly.

The complexities of individual outbreaks puzzled people and, consequently, the simple sounding theories of external causes in different disease agents did not at first appear credible. The mass of details in every particular case seemed to overrule the possibility of any one concentrated place—a bottleneck—or point where the disease could have been easily stopped. Morbid spontaneity considered human bodies in their milieus, where complex, harmful, disease-catalysing, and unhygienic stimuli interacted with agents of hygiene and health (Barnes 1995: 43). The coming about of the Pasteurian hygienist movement proceeded to bypass the mass of factors by the simple sequential—as opposed to confluence-based—method of following the microbial thread to its source: 'There is a specific microorganism: it does not jump from one place to another; we must follow the thread' (Latour 1993: 45). One could argue that the report's 'confluence of circumstances' is a modern version of morbid spontaneity. The talk about gutters, overflowing septic systems, poor sanitation, Hurricane Thomas, the massive earthquake, and so on formed a system that all the participants could recognize and could as such attribute as circumstances quite likely related to the spread of cholera. Most strikingly, the 'confluence of circumstances' approach contradicted the UN's work in successfully fighting pandemic threats, which have been based on the diligent following of the 'contagious thread'.

The Independent Report's cholera narrative has to be contextualized among other narratives dealing with epidemic diseases to see how local epidemic disease comprehension differs from a more global pandemic stock story. One point of contrast with the report is the WHO's chronology for the SARS outbreak in 2006. SARS was of pandemic relevance. It was often linked with the increasingly tight-knit fabric of global interdependency. The differences in the accounts about the SARS outbreak and Haiti's cholera outbreak are immediately obvious. The SARS chronology pays attention to the global patterns of spread, suspect types, and clear causal relations. The invisible world of viruses is made culturally comprehensible using very different methods from those used in the cholera report. The confluence of circumstances trope is not used. The air mobility-related hubs-and-spokes of SARS had a clear regional pattern. The spread is analysed methodically without any polysemous metaphors. The SARS chronology accounts for the progressively more diligent tracing and containment of the superspreaders—the index cases—as the epidemic spread. The SARS story is given a narrative form that refers to specific people, places, and the directional pattern of spread. This directionality is largely absent in the Haiti report, which does not account for the global interlocational city-hopping patterns of cholera, although it does say that the Haiti outbreak was part of an ongoing cholera pandemic. The Haiti cholera is conceptually contained in a local phenomenon. The systematic and methodological approach used in the SARS chronology is absent from the cholera report. The cholera report does not use tropes and codes to signify the ways in which the disease spread. The role of the Nepalese peacekeepers and their practices are not used to convey a sense of why the spread happened. The thread between the various people, their role, status, and mobility is not followed because, as the cholera report explicates, there are only random accidental patterns. Although much diligent and good work must have been done by the many people fighting the disease in Haiti, the cholera report is clearly written with other goals in mind. It tries to fight the contagious idea that the UN and the global community were and can be sources of suffering. The report does this even at the cost of a stereotypical portrayal of Haiti as a place where epidemics emerge spontaneously. SARS was a success story for the global public health organizations and, through the politico-somatic connection, for the legitimacy of the encompassing global embodiments. Haiti's cholera report had to be written to hide the more regressive nature of global connections even when they are made for ethical reasons. The report's confluence statement was a supposedly noble humanitarian untruth.

Embodied Epidemics

The Haiti cholera outbreak's trajectory of politicization fitted with the cross-cutting themes in the history of 'plagues and people', and it should have been anticipated by any politically aware and sensitive health governance. I will next review these historical patterns of politicization to see how basic disease schematics may be used to convey political meanings. This overview of historical tendencies can be used to understand how the Haitians' somatic fears and anxieties suddenly became registers of political dynamics.[7]

A national 'epidemic' and its global derivative, 'pandemic', can be seen as providing an overall embodied object world. Its processes of contagion illuminate the dynamic relations between the key objects—'I' extends to 'we', and both stand in opposition to 'them' and 'a foreign element' through a dynamic characteristic of contagion. More specifically, a Haitian feels the local interconnectedness within a national we-community, and this we-community stands in a particular cholera-determined outer or inner relationship to the clear in-group, the UN, to troop-sending foreign powers, to the international aid community, and to the peacekeepers from 'Nepal'. These international groups were signifiers of the collapsing distances as compared to the earlier situation. This distance-crossing relationship was a commonplace occurrence in Haiti's history. Yet the emerging contagious disease had the potential of reframing these relationships between outer and inner into dangerous liaisons between local and foreign/far-off interconnections. Awareness of this potentiality could have been one of the motivating factors behind the UN's decision to downplay the question of the epidemic's origin (e.g. WHO 2021b).

The embodied epidemic object world also presents a politico-somatic scenario: the somatic-level sensations and anxieties stem from individuals' sensing, through the networks of their local and global connectedness, a harmful, uncontained, and contagious spread. From this perspective, the relationship between 'health threats' and 'effective governance' can turn political legitimacy, trust, and accountability into central characteristics. The perceived 'health risks' easily unravel the political legitimacies as people shift their political loyalties up or down in the global multilevel governance based on the perceived 'curative' or 'dis-easing' (in)capacity of the organizations and actors. As people bodily sense their wider surroundings as embodiments, any 'spreads' or 'contagions' on these wider 'skins' are acutely sensed and worried about, thereby changing the worth and value of the wider embodiments ranging around them. In the case of the Haiti cholera, the spread of the epidemic disease translated into dramatized geographies of fear within Haiti and among Haitians, yet the contagion was also a signifier for Haitians about the ambiguities of and changes in the status/legitimacy of others, such as the UN and NGOs. In this context, it becomes understandable that the language of fear and suffering derived from cholera found its political expression in riots against the UN and, to a degree, into hesitation towards and avoidance of Western medical expertise.

Many Haitians knew how health worries limit personal agency. The conflicted cholera subjectivities were deeply felt as the Haitians were forced to renegotiate their local vulnerability based on perceived and actual contact with the contagion's directionality. The historically sedimented cross-cutting epidemic reflexes were thus anything but distant or abstract (e.g. Aaltola 1999). First, a scenario of an uneven disease spread referred to a spread where the disease influences one state, region, or distinctive group of people disproportionately. Generally, in such situations, the unevenness in the spread tends to highlight cleavages and tensions within the key actors. Any outbreak's local meanings are crucially influenced by the perceived origin and the supposed direction of its spread. It is the movement and directionality that tend to determine the outbreak's interpretative implications (Lee 1998: 675). The uneven impact of the cholera in Haiti was obvious to all.

The disease initially affected remote locations, leading to some internal tensions within Haiti. Another factor of unevenness followed soon after as the Haitians fell ill and the international workers remained disease-free due to better availability of medicines and higher levels of sanitation.[8] This tendency implicates a second historically conditioned disease characteristic: diseases easily turn into signifiers of illegitimate governance and into a pattern that accentuates patterns of hostility and enmity within and between localities and groups. Haiti as a polity had suffered from a chronic state failure, and its governance had been effectively internationalized since the mid-1990s. Because it was already a failed polity, the cholera could not reveal images of bad governance by the traditional political elites and in-groups. Instead, it started to act as a register of the failure of international governance—and the high likelihood in the past and in the future of such failures.

Second, perhaps the most politically relevant dynamic of an epidemic object world is externalization. Epidemic situations result in diverse containment-oriented tendencies aimed at various out-groups. The epidemic scenario usually involves a tendency to externalize the perceived 'evils' of the situation into a complex disease construct that is distinct from and outside of the supposed pure forms of being a local. The externalized disease entity can then be further associated with a distinct group of people (Sontag 2001: 63). The overall scenario tends to become a register of political hostilities and enmities that lay dormant before the outbreak (Tuan 1979: 87). The tendency to externalize means that any notable disease is prone to be territorialized, nationalized, ethnicized, racialized, sexualized, and, in the case of Haiti, internationalized.[9] When the suspicions concerning the role of the Nepalese UN peacekeepers became stronger, the pattern of spread as well as its directionality triggered the reflexive externalization of blame and danger into a foreign embodiment with nuanced yet xenophobic characteristics. The Haitians started to talk about the 'foreign' nature of the cholera. The foreigner's disease was seen as having been exported to Haiti by the UN either on purpose or through negligence.

Third, since diseases easily signify failing polities and failures by governance bodies, they can be used effectively as propaganda weapons. Many of Haiti's presidential candidates used the cholera outbreak to show their patriotism and willingness to stand up against the international presence in their country. They effectively synchronized and morphed the outbreak with their diverse political goals. The cholera could be used to build up and re-arrange national we-communal sentiments by demonizing the perceived sources of and groups associated with the origin of the outbreak. This also allowed for competition over who and what type of elements are included in the transforming in-group of Haiti. Fourth, there is an inherent tendency to try to conceal epidemic outbreaks as the various authorities worry about the negative impact that public awareness could cause in terms of power, economy, and prestige. This tendency to hide diseases in an attempt to avoid international embarrassment, which could potentially harm the state's political and economic interests, can be witnessed all over the world. In Haiti, the UN tried to cover up the cholera outbreak for many years; it was only when its likely role in the outbreak was widely publicized by the international media that it became interested in investigating the true origin of the disease.

Fifth, the scenario of co-option has a rich history as actors struggle to use epidemic disease as a pretext for politically or economically motivated actions ranging from *cordons sanitaires* to military manoeuvres to embargoes. In Haiti, the co-option involved the local politicians' efforts to use the UN secrecy and failure as a demonstration of the legitimacy of their own efforts to secure Haiti's national honour. The local politicians participated, partly due to the impending elections, in the inflaming of the popular interpretations of why the disease spread the way it did. Similarly, the international authorities could further justify the continued existence of a massive mosaic of camps on the grounds of public health. The sixth interrelated repercussion is fear and panic as epidemics cause impulsive actions and drastic reactions such as social disruptions. In Haiti, the scare led to brief yet widespread politically expressive rioting and unrest against the UN and NGO efforts to establish fenced-off camps. The scare aspect was also reflected in the fear of the locals to take the medicines distributed by the international agencies because they believed them to be poisonous.

The aforementioned recurring and persistent dynamics provided the power-related situational characteristics for the Haiti epidemic scenario. These historically conditioned tendencies mean that any notable epidemic outbreak is likely to become politically expressive very rapidly and almost instinctually. Moreover, these cross-cutting dynamics should be seen as broad interlinking nexuses that overlap and flow smoothly from one to the other and back. Keeping this in mind, it is important to note that the cholera's object world contained visually, kinaesthetically, and emotionally charged schematics that captured this temporal and situation-specific morphing between the different characteristics. In this way, the externalization of the threat to foreign sources—to the UN and to the Nepalese peacekeepers—opens up possibilities for the local politicians to co-opt the disease in order to play up Haiti's insecurity and their ability to deliver political health. This move in the social cognition directly reinforced the idea that the disease burden was somehow purposefully uneven. This schematic also cast in a negative light the efforts by the various aid agencies to distribute medicines and establish cholera camps. It can be suggested that the political tendencies inherent in the disease scenarios started to provide reinterpretations of the core relational positions of the key actors and embodiments. This transformation drew material from the popular cognitions about epidemics and from the concrete specifics of the cholera in Haiti and abstracted from them a situational scenario concerning Haiti's security and Haiti's vulnerable locatedness within the wider world.

Thus, the underlying object world of an epidemic outbreak should be seen as inherently dynamic. An epidemic scenario contains strong kinaesthetic—that is, downwards spiralling, regressive circulatory—meanings such as infection, spread, and contagion that can easily be used to animate the relationships between key embodied objects in a way that accentuates dis-easing influences: Who are those around me and, by extension, Haiti, possibly endangering me or my community?

From whom could I or those associated with me get the disease? How does it feel to get an infection and what are the consequences when some members of my community become 'infected'? What happens to me when I am one of the infected? Should I or my relatives go to the UN clinic to get treatment or should I remain in my home and use local remedies? The mental projections of lived-life considerations such as these onto the different scenarios existing in the political realm were the key mobilizing factors in Haiti's cholera unrest and riots. They are also memorable and stick as mnemonic images strung together in the minds of many Haitians. In a sense, the cholera heightened the stakes for everybody involved because it brought out powerful and concrete bodily modalities.

The cholera contained combinatorial possibility. It suddenly turned into a sub-narrative reinforcing a more general stock narrative. From this perspective, the spread of cholera to Haiti and among the Haitians was bound to cause sensitivity to other types of regressive influences. It produced a gaze, a particular way of looking at interacting individual and collective bodies. This might have further framed the UN as a negative political influence in Haiti, and it could have fed the media image that rioting and unrest were spreading in Haiti. On the other hand, it should be noted that the animation of the political world in terms of disease kinaesthetics simultaneously changes the way in which diseases are experienced and expressed. The severity, for example, of contagion is continuously being reimagined and re-evaluated when it is seen as spreading across and afflicting different social and political bodies. It can be suggested that it was a different experience for an individual Haitian to suffer or die of a 'foreigner's disease' than of some other disease.[10] One additional characteristic is that fear and anxiety grow as the disease becomes a more hyperbolic phenomenon in public life and media. One's own horror of eventual infection might be amplified when there have been graphic public displays in the media of how horrible it is to die of cholera.

Drawing Lessons from Domestic Epidemic-Related Dis-ease

The Haiti cholera seems to have had a certain political agency. For example, it challenged the UN governance, showed it in a non-apolitical light, and politicized the practice of containing people in camps and centres. It embodied loud protesters with strong political claims. Latour's (1993) way of collapsing the dichotomy between nature—science and nurture—society can shed some light on the agentic capacity of politico-somatic relationships. Instead of being pure and above politics, scientific ways of seeing are implicated in the intricate complexities of power—for example, through UN sponsorship of the scientific research as detailed in the Independent Report. What is seen through the archetypical eye of a scientific instrument might appear as a disease agent; however, at the same time, the observation inevitably embodies, reflects, and projects political power. Latour illustrates his case through a narrative of Pasteur's hygienist battle in nineteenth-century France. Latour shows how Pasteur ceases to be an individual genius and takes on the role of an embodiment. He is, in Latour's language, an actant, a hybrid of an agent, and an actor who is devoid of typical individual human qualities. As 'he' blows ahead with the army of hygienists, 'Pasteur' desperately needs allies in diseases and fearful people. To achieve them, the invisible world of disease agents is framed in a way that it is visibly worrying, compelling, and mobilizing. As diseases became allies in a societal reform process, they turned into agents or actants in their own right. They extended the state's power and reach to previously private and unregulated realms. The Haiti cholera was allied to different parties in the absence of effective state and as the UN had brought it into the country. It did work when it briefly unravelled and confused the UN-led international governance system in Haiti. Because of this, the mobilizing power of the cholera needed to be neutralized. To achieve this end, the term 'confluence of circumstances' was invented since it diffused the blame and produced a gaze that showed a scenario in which the UN was doing its usual good work under the extreme conditions of complex emergencies.

As the Independent Report implies, cholera was brought to Haiti by the very people who came there to help the Haitians. The compassionate rushing in to help was followed by a containment failure because peacekeepers from countries where cholera is endemic were part of the mobilization. This was done in full knowledge of the fact that post-earthquake environments are especially susceptible to cholera. A clear breach of the 'do no harm' principle had occurred (Piarroux *et al.* 2011: 1167). It is this embarrassing yet deadly failure that the UN investigated in the Independent Report it commissioned. It is possible to suggest that it is because of this that the report is not written in the usual genre of diligent epidemiological investigation. It does not trace index cases, and it does not follow contacts. No background story is given to how the cholera was brought from Nepal to Haiti.

For the most part, the report uses the term 'confluence of circumstances' to bury the paradox of helpers becoming a source of extreme danger to public health. A reader of the UN report is left with the sense that a more detailed probe could have had a detrimental effect not only on UN work in Haiti and other places around the world but also on the future legitimacy of its efforts in the eyes of the locals and the global viewing public. This leads to the question: What lessons, if any, were learnt from Haiti? At the end, one is left with a sense that Haiti was treated as an anomaly that could and should be bypassed. In the end, the Independent Report was an exercise in crisis communication. It was not a genuine effort to reflect on the UN's multiple roles, tendencies to fail, and lessons to be learnt. The Haiti cholera outbreak demonstrates how much can be at stake in local epidemic situations and how much is at stake that may complicate the attempts at diligent and vigilant public health work. The cholera outbreak ceased to be a merely physical fact; it got turned into a politosomatic entity, an embodied signifier of blame, shame, marginalization, and disempowerment. The unevenly distributed markers of perceived contagion and seeming immunity were juxtaposed with the historical record of perceived power disparities (e.g. Fidler and Gostin 2008: 170). This composite image of 'cholera' produced brief but strong local reactions, which affected the authority and legitimacy of the various actors.

Thus, the cholera outbreak turned, to use Sontag's (2001) notion, into an ideally comprehensive entity in its own time and place. Cholera and its imagined regressive trajectory served to crystallize momentary individual and political fears and worst-case scenarios. This insight can be used to argue that the reason why the cholera epidemic in Haiti became hyperbolically feared was a blend of local historically conditioned political sensibilities and insecurities. The cholera blended different scenarios of situational knowledge that had gripped Haiti historically and after the earthquake. The central cross-cutting issue in these schema-imageries was that the interaction between the different perceived crisis factors and dynamics—as, for example, the massive earthquake, historical destitution, sense of being colonized and abused, political corruption, and being at the mercy of the aid agencies, foreign militaries and NGOs—further induced the particular way in which the cholera was sensed, felt, and understood. It brought with it a particular ideal comprehensibility of the cholera outbreak as well as induced fear of it and created a particular type of bodily suffering and emotionality, such as shame, victimhood, blame, and expressions of pain. Besides fear of foreign influences, the cholera brought with it a specific type of shame. This ranged from the more encompassing shame of the infected communities to the private shame of being a carrier of a foreigner's disease and of embodying foreignness though the disease. These politico-somatic senses fed back to the abstract cartography of locations and locatedness and undermined the legitimacy of those in Haiti who represented foreigners. It is possible to hypothesize that the myths and feelings associated with the nature and origin of the disease started to embody 'foreigners' with disease-causing attributes. According to the Haitian Red Cross report, these beliefs concerning the disease 'mixed with the disappointment of the international aid response to the earthquake which has generated a lot of distrust, scepticism and suspicion toward the international organizations' (Petit-Goâve et al. 2010). The Haitian Red Cross report further states that the widespread popular belief among the Haitians was that the cholera was a 'political disease' connected with the massive foreign presence in the country.

In Haiti, 'foreign' influences became politicized. This was further fuelled as people's somatic sensations, fears, and anxieties were reframed when global embodiments and their local influences turned into uncontained and dis-eased ones. The more intimate this process got, the more acute the worry and its manifestations became. The outward expressions changed and became increasingly all-encompassing after 2010. Furthermore, disease scenarios involve processes of politicization: they are traditionally ethnicized, sexualized, culturalized, and geopoliticized; are used in enemy image construction; and possess political ramifications. In the case of Haiti, the epidemic was also internationalized to particular UN bodies and their activities. The Haiti cholera showed clearly how perceived disease origin mattered as did the felt unevenness of the cholera disease burden. All of this translated into giving it a political meaning and the means to express this.

It can be argued that politico-somatics has a long cultural history. These histories vary in different places, yet they have an impact on the situational scenario that takes place in the case of an actual or seeming epidemic outbreak. In the case of

Haiti, the main ingredients had to do with long years of bad governance nationally and breakdowns in the rule of law. It also had to do with the long history of colonial presence and that of the international community in later years, and the perceived regressive international influences. The Haitian sensitivities and charged debates during the cholera outbreak did not happen by accident, although they were relatively instinctive. Furthermore, these historically conditioned sensitivities were not elicited solely by the specific characteristics of an observable disease agent. Rather, they linked up with a larger category of 'regressions' and 'disruptions'. The regressions lumped together disease contagions and other types of disruptions such as wars and conflicts.[11] The imageries of lethal cholera circulations were anything but intense. The cholera reactions lead to expectations of corresponding pains in the local and national Haitian embodiments. The fear of the 'foreign' and 'international' could also be used in politics to intensify fears that 'feel' somatically and can be seen in the others that are given the 'stigma' of being 'foreign' or 'international'.

The Trajectory of Mad Cow Disease as a UK Issue in European Politics

Bovine spongiform encephalopathy (BSE), aptly called mad cow disease, brought to the foreground public anxieties about potentially serious diseases crossing the animal-human barrier in early 1996. Beginning of the chapter dealt with the domestic-level contestations and their internalization to UN and global humanitarian efforts in the aftermath of the cholera outbreak in Haiti. The case of BSE continues with the theme of domestic versus international but also points out the containment failures at the interspecies barrier—with the constant theme of pandemic emergencies, that is, speciation, which is understood here as politicization of the animal origin of human disease and the breaking of the interspecies barrier—which appear as a fairly constant feature in the blame game that arises from a pandemic emergency along with nationalization, internationalization, ethnicization, and sexualization. The last part of this chapter also contributes to the understanding of disease emergencies as a temporal process with an onset point as well as a point when public interest wanes: the sense of a unifying emergency with everyone rallying round the decision makers gradually changes into acrimony and disagreements before the public loses interest in the emergency scenario.

The Thucydidean framework used to analyse politosomatic emergencies starts from the fundamental question: What other regressive and grander or more limited downwards sloping characteristics, besides an epidemic, exist that can form consonantial or combinatorial relationships with a health crisis? It is clear that the relationship between the UK and the EU had always been cautious, and in the mid-1990s they were taking a turn for the worse as the EU's deepening integration and enlargement that was feeding migration to the UK became heated topics. Brexit, the UK's decision to leave the EU, was a long time in coming, and some of the negative trends were briefly catalysed by the BSE crisis, even though the 1997 election produced a new vision for a new Europe with the UK at its heart (e.g.

Westlake 2020: 191; Daddow 2012: 1219; Hardt-Mautner 1995: 177). Popular opinion during the BSE crisis increased the support for the 'leave' opinion concerning membership of the European Community. BSE has to be seen in the light of this long and contentious relationship with the EU and concerns about British sovereignty.

During the BSE outbreak, the televised images were all about sick and stumbling cows. The focus was on bovine products that could lead to a variant of the deadly CJD, called vCJD, which results in a transmissible type of brain disease called spongiform encephalopathy. Around 180 people have died of this disease in the UK since the BSE outbreak in the 1990s. The air was heightened with fear and uncertainties as nobody knew the true extent of the risk to humans, for example, through eating hamburgers. There was a sense of an unnatural situation that could spin dangerously out of control. As is usual with high-public attention zootic epidemics, the BSE drama embodied the fears and anxieties of multiple broken boundaries: the sense of a perversely industrial pattern of food production, the British countryside somehow becoming more unnatural, the strains on British society associated with the deregulation of the Margaret Thatcher years, the Europe-wide concerns over the EU integration, the worries over British sovereignty, and the contested state of European politics. The BSE tremors were seen as a highly comprehensible reflection of the political climate and the cleavages therein. Many bewildering developments were condensed into a hyperbolic form in the politico-somatic drama that took place during March–April 1996. Anyone who had eaten any cattle products in the UK was thought to be in danger. The harrowing images of the brain-degenerating vCJD disease were deeply felt and feared by many. It can be suggested that unknown to them, they suffered mostly from a somatized impact of the political anxieties of their time.

The political drama found its most headline arousing modality in the contestation between the UK government and the EU institutions over the cordon imposed on British bovine products, including the UK's retaliatory decision to boycott the EU decision which briefly paralysed EU decision-making and the ongoing Intergovernmental Conference, one of the most sacrosanct institutions of the EU. These interventions and counter-interventions were all done in the name of public health and scientific evidence. However, the seemingly public health-related, yet fundamentally diversionary actions and counter-actions, as well as the political co-option of underlying evidence can be seen as stemming naturally from the political ontology of the concerned states, as the result of a bargaining process between the various groups, their interests, and citizens. The health spectacles thrown up by BSE can be seen as expressions of an in-group contestation in some states or in-group conflicts in a more transnational sense—between the elites of the EU.

In contrast to the cholera outbreak in Haiti where the epidemic originated from the presence of an international body, the BSE emergency provided an example of a member-state of a supranational community being seen as a public health worry. Furthermore, BSE provides a case of a scare of a serious epidemic occurring in a Western European country which was then a member-state of the EU. It also provides a case in which interventions such as embargoes justified by public health concerns targeted the UK, an advanced Western actor. Moreover, these interventions were, after a brief onset phase, the subject of intense politicization and controversy: the scare reshaped political arrangements and the character of interstate relations at the EU level for a few months. The emergency scenario had direct but brief ramifications for the functioning of the EU as the British launched a boycott of the former's intergovernmental processes, thereby drawing them to a halt. At the same time, the BSE scare caused widespread market panic and consumer reactions as the consumption of bovine products plunged for a while (e.g. Barbarossa 2018).

The BSE scare provides a case in point of the ways in which pandemics interact with the political dynamics of their time. The BSE incident's political language revolved around the UK's relationship with the EU. It became politicized as a contest between the two, as a domestic-level issue in the UK where the blame was quickly internationalized to the EU. The dynamics of the BSE situation posited the UK's Eurosceptic stance against the integrationist stance of the other European member-states and the European Commission (EC) and probably contributed to some degree to the UK's decision to leave the EU some two decades later. The more entrenched images of enmity also synced with the measures taken to fight BSE. For example, the British press displayed anti-German and anti-EU headlines during the crisis. The ways in which BSE was politicized reflect the underlying close connection between lethal epidemic diseases and enmity. As was pointed out in the earlier chapters, the general form of a disease emergency tends to be in sync with the existing patterns of political enmity and the beliefs concerning the power hierarchies that separate the different actors. In this, the BSE crisis illustrated the general dynamics of plagues and politics. Second, it provided an important precursor case for the understanding of the political modalities of later disease emergencies, as, for example, in the sense of inflaming the interspecies boundary. Third, it provides additional elements to the ways in which certain political dynamics could interact with other contemporary political dynamics. Fourth, it demonstrated a pattern that is key to most hyperbolized contagions: a fast rise to attention, followed by a politicization, and then a gradual receding to the background and fading away from the media.

Sick, Jerking, Stumbling Cows

The sick, jerking, stumbling cows of the UK came to define European politics in the spring of 1996. BSE rose to international prominence amidst a myriad domestic contentions between the UK and the EU. Studies that demonstrated that BSE in cows was the likely cause of an emerging variant of the human CJD, called the vCJD, were beginning to proliferate by late 1995 and early 1996. Most of these studies were dismissed by the UK government as dubious scaremongering.[12] However, a scientific study by the UK Government Surveillance Unit specializing in CJD showed clearly that BSE was the source in at least some cases of human CJD. Because of the growing public outcry over the perceived government secrecy and anxiety over health, on 20 March 1996, the British secretary of state for health, Stephen Dorell, was forced to announce the possible link in a statement in the House of Commons:

> There remains no scientific proof that BSE can be transmitted to man by beef, but the Committee has concluded that the most likely explanation at present is that these cases are linked to exposure to BSE before the introduction of the specified bovine offal ban in 1989. Against the background of this new finding, the Committee has today agreed to the series of recommendations which the government is making public this afternoon.

Immediately after the British announcement, the EU introduced a ban on British beef and bovine products:

> Following statements by the United Kingdom Government concerning a possible link between bovine spongiform encephalopathy and the appearance of a number of cases of Creutzfeldt-Jacob disease in that Member State, a meeting of experts on the Scientific Veterinary Committee was held in Brussels on 22 March, the result of which formed the basis of discussions in the Standing Veterinary Committee on 25 and 26 March. In accordance with this Committee's opinion, the Commission adopted a series of temporary measures to protect against BSE.

The emerging drama gravitated towards taking into account the welfare and confidence of individuals defined in terms of scientific certainty, instead of the usual political expediency. However, the political controversy was immediate. Although the EC openly recognized that the primary problem was not a real widespread threat to public health but the widespread public perception of an immediate threat, it grounded its primary argument for the imposition of a ban on British beef on caution based on scientific advice and evidence. As later epidemic emergencies have shown, the science behind pandemic scenarios is complex and leads to multiple different policy applications that can balance the underlying elements—for example, state public health.

How did the emerging evidence that the animal disease, BSE, was linked with the degenerative vCJD provide a context for playing out national and supranational interests and goals? The concept of the morality play, as a further characteristic of an emergency scenario, is introduced to point out the importance of public health issues from the perspective of political legitimacy. Furthermore, the emergency trajectory—its sharp ebb and gradual waning dynamics—is used as an analytic device to point to the different phases of a typical health emergency crisis: the kinaesthetic experience of accelerated ebbing with heightened drama followed by the relative waning of the public focus. This wave-like pattern has been present in many epidemic and pandemic emergencies. In COVID-19, it has been tangibly demonstrated by the perceived waves of actual cases, and also in the governance pattern of emergency lockdowns followed by loosening of restrictions, a pattern that can be seen as facilitating the underlying contagion flows. Thus, epidemiologically and politically, diseases come in waves. Sometimes, these two wave patterns correspond with each other, sometimes not.

The BSE-related morality play ebbed and reached a tipping point relatively rapidly; the initial phase was defined by a sense of scientific uncertainty: a lot of research needed to be done and research projects sometimes take years to complete although the public outcry for certainty was immediate and policy response was critical. However, soon it became clear that the scientific community could not provide any certain and quick answers to the problem. Political considerations naturally came to prevail and were influenced by citizens and consumer rights groups till, in the summer of 1996, the issue lost its political relevance. However, the BSE incident had more lasting consequences from the perspective of how later pandemic emergencies came to be construed. It also showcases the ways in which diseases are nationalized and also internationalized, as the UK government saw quite soon that the EU measures, which it had accepted at first, were unjustified and politically motivated.

Epidemic diseases are often treated as afflicting populations that exist in a confined geographical space. From this perspective, the history of lethal epidemic diseases is often treated in terms of blows against populations in terms of density, distribution, and lethality. For example, it is fairly common to examine how human behavioural patterns, such as the human relationship with domestic animals, affect disease emergence and spread. However, diseases also afflict political communities and how specific political communities mould the way in which diseases are interpreted. Rather than accepting the customary human as animal framework inherent in the concept of population, the starting point here will be the Aristotelian notion of the human as a political animal (e.g. Abbate 2016). This politically aware understanding sheds light on how the appearance of the serious epidemic disease associated with BSE reflected the underlying nature of the European political order and the course of the politicized 'variant' of BSE.

The BSE crisis of 1996 is interpreted in the guise of a political morality play. In general, morality plays involve a fight by the protagonist—often assuming the guise of all polity from local, national, regional, or human embodiments—against the bad elements, the type of which is inherently connected with a specific political context. Who were the actors who took the role of the protagonist in the BSE morality play? Who gave the appearance of representing national or European general interests? Who were the deviant and antagonist elements?

In answering these questions, it is important to realize that the European political order is constantly shifting and varying. The macro-level movements hide more fleeting rearrangements which, nevertheless, are more tangible signifiers of what is going on at the more general level (e.g. Pijpers 2006). The levels interact, and, as such, any micro-level dynamics are a matter of intense interest for the actors involved. The temporal morality plays are framed in terms of the rhythmic ebbing and waning of different issues and the consonancies between different issue-specific dynamics. Accentuated by the unexpected appearance of BSE, European politics demonstrated a rhythmic, pulsing movement in international relations. This ebbing and waning initiated attention-catching events, which finally faded into political obscurity in a matter of months. Various contingent and instantaneous stipulations of shared standards of interpretation convey a sense of rhythmic political order. Such a pulse, at its zenith, is extremely compelling. The actors see in it their relative (dis)-empowered positions. The accentuated, situated scenarios which were brought into focus by the unexpected and unconventional emergence of BSE were used as a momentary criterion or standard against which the morality and legitimacy of the various actors and their actions were examined and evaluated. It can be argued that the failure to tap into such a rhythm translated into a deficiency in fulfilling the perceived obligations and accountabilities that are essential for membership and the consequent rights of the European society of states. Having a sense of international rhythm, therefore, can be essential to enjoying societal rights, such as the right to be treated with respect in the same way as the other states. The accentuated 'peculiarities', such as the BSE drama, give prominence to actions that are in step with one another simply because going against a current translates into a sense of either crafty strategic thinking or, far more probably and dangerously, into unwise insensitivity and inflexibility in the face of decisive events.[13] Any more 'real' concerns over general public health based on scientific understanding are easily of secondary importance for the pandemic-related public drama's ebbing and waning trajectory. What is prudent has its momentary context with specific situational requirements.

The politically constructed practices of societal responsibility, obligation, credibility, and duty were clear in the rhythmic flow of international interactions during the initial phases of the BSE crisis in the winter of 1995–96. Not surprisingly, then, the specific content of the BSE affair centred on competition over who had most meticulously and fully adhered to the perceived public health standpoint, irrespective of the cost to narrowly perceived national self-interest. However, the public health paradigm soon lost its ability to offer an unproblematic solution and to point to an obvious way of proceeding. As the weeks went by, more leeway opened up for political diversion and co-option of the affair. It can be argued that the accented public health paradigm lost it cohesion-creating character mainly because of increasing repetition and familiarity with the issues involved. Learning, awareness, and familiarity with the BSE scenario and its characteristics grew, greatly increasing the efficiency and skill with which these scenarios were used as political instruments in creating the desired effects by the various interest groups. The former deviant actors, such as the various national governments and especially the UK, gained ground at the expense of the initial protagonists of public health, such as the EC. The participants of the morality play started to gain ever greater skill and control instead of being exceedingly constrained by the original sense of the compelling rhythmic spirit of the times. The pulse that had originally emphasized the European public health authorities over the respective national governments gradually started to embody the interests of the member-states.

The rhythmic transformation that took place in the BSE morality play involved a gradual loss of perception of the supposed extraordinary nature of the situation. There was a distinct movement away from the BSE as a public health scenario to normal and routine political wheeling and dealing between governments. Instead of the emergency scenario being a contextual driver of the situation, it turned into one characteristic in a much wider political scenario. As the driving force of the whole transformation, the BSE morality play also involved politically innovative language games.[14] The coming into being of the BSE emphasis in the middle of March 1996 entailed a corresponding move of BSE from a national and functional issue to an entity at the supranational European level. In other words, the coming into being of BSE as an international relations entity initiated an epidemic play that was characterized by both unconventional initial actions and the eventual normalization of affairs. The rumours and claims about the BSE threat started to circulate in earnest in the winter of 1995. The uncertainty peaked in the decision to ban British beef in March 1996, which represented not only a reaction to factors external to the usual politics, but also a conceptual innovation in that BSE was made to look like an acute health threat emanating from the UK. The EC and some EU member-states argued that the threat could not be generalized to include European beef production as such. Rather, the health issues were connected with particular British policies, which involved lax oversight and deregulation.

The attempts by the EC and the EU member-states to see the BSE scare as a British problem followed the age-old pattern of blame-fixing when faced with dangerous epidemic diseases by nationalizing the disease and its characteristics. The most common way of making sense of an unknown killer disease has always been localization where the stereotypical patterns associated with the particular region are somehow seen in an adverse light and having at least an associative relationship with the disease causation. The pattern of blame revolves easily around questions concerning the disease's perceived origin and epicentre. In political terms, this means that epidemics are instinctively territorialized, nationalized, racialized, sexualized and, as in the case of Haiti, internationalized. In this way, the problems of UK farming and food production were attributed to the problems and lack of soundness of UK governance. The national dimension of the blame game was further highlighted by the fact that scientific knowledge about the aetiology of the disease was almost non-existent initially. Therefore, there were no historical benchmarks for understanding the disease as a separate apolitical phenomenon.

The EU concentrated its efforts on confining the BSE-related problems at both the physical and psychological levels by the extraordinary decision to ban British beef and beef products from the Common Market. Once BSE got alarmingly out of control, the mitigation of its ramifications became the top priority. It can be argued that for the EU, the substance of its decisions centred on making the disease geographically and conceptually analogous with the UK and its policies. In other words, the policies aimed at controlling BSE consisted almost exclusively of measures imposed on and required from the UK. The containment of the BSE crisis comprised checking the UK as the source of the outbreak. Two factors were emphasized here: the majority of the BSE cases had occurred in the UK and the information concerning the link between BSE and vCJD was made public in the UK. Thus, the BSE problem was made into a British problem. The control of the disease and its effects required clear concessions from the UK.

The policy of non-cooperation towards the EU adopted by the UK as it attempted to gain control over the situation framed the flow of events in a more nationally advantageous way. The British view was that the disease could have originated anywhere and, therefore, singling out the British was unfair and not a sign of European solidarity. After a brief initial hesitation, the interventionist measures by the EU were shown to be repositioning the disease as an infringement of British sovereignty. The UK represented BSE as a general scientific and medical problem, which, according to the UK, was unjustly made to appear as an exclusively British problem. Thus, instead of being fixed, the meanings of the actions of the various actors continued to evolve in the overall context of the gradual fading of the initially emphasized sense. At first, BSE was perceived as something that had clear and legitimate implications for European politics; then as an event, the requirements and implications of which were contested; and, finally, as something overwhelmed by other emerging issues and baseline political issues. The instantaneous transformation of order led to the eventual disappearance of the BSE-related public drama from the agenda of high politics and to the usual scientific compartmentalization into a functional expert issue area.

The emphasis in the BSE morality play rose to international prominence from out of several domestic and European political issues. In crossing the threshold, BSE momentarily coloured its surroundings with attention-catching and compelling features, briefly bringing about a sense of a distinctive meaning. Thus, the appearance of BSE entailed an attention-catching and accentuated event with a compelling sense of direction. The acute and overriding need to stabilize the situation by measures aimed at assuring people about the safety of their food was instrumental in crystallizing the spirit of the time in a specific way. BSE momentarily gave a fixed sense of what was taking place now and would take place in the imminent future.

The accentuated nature of the BSE epidemic derived from five primary sources. First, the disease brought the relationship between the different levels of European governance into the limelight. Europe lacked a genuine multilevel governance system in health and food safety issues. Because of this, the BSE drama highlighted the relations between the various existing, emerging, and lacking layers of the governance. There was a strong sense that the national governance had failed in the UK in ways that were counterproductive for the general interests of European citizens. One of the main concerns was that the various institutions had failed to take into account proper scientific evidence. However, public health was and still is handled mostly at the member-state level. In that scenario, whose research should be taken into consideration and by what entities?

Second, BSE had crossed the species barrier. Food-borne diseases may be regarded as especially marked signifiers of the perceived underlying wrongs and perversions when it comes to the human–animal relationship (Mahy and Brown 2000). Third, the disease agent involved in BSE and vCJD was a new one: a prion. What prions were stimulated much scientific debate and led to a short-lived burst of public curiosity (e.g. Collinge 2012: 411). Fourth, the 'madness' of the disease was associated with the uncontrolled food industry, which, out of narrow economic interests, used unsound industrial food production methods (Shaoul 1997). Fifth, the specific impacts of BSE were associated with a modern risk-sensitive society and hysteria-prone Western European public culture (Jasanoff 1997).

The initial announcement by the EU of the ban on British beef and beef products shifted the emphasis away from the usual European political wheeling and dealing to a more unconventional order characterized by the public health drama and shaken consumer confidence. The BSE crisis had been lingering for many years as the growing evidence for the link was hidden by the local and national authorities in the UK. However, the row was started by Stephen Dorell's official announcement on 20 March 1996 about the finding of a new CJD variant quite probably linked to people eating BSE contaminated food. The announcement revealed the possible link with BSE contaminated meat. The resulting market panic and health scare focused on beef products and particularly on beef imported from the UK. The EU announcement introducing the ban on British beef and related products (EC/96/239) set the tone for subsequent international interactions by referring to considerations conventionally beyond the scope of European high politics. The way in which BSE as a public health threat accentuated and saturated European politics became increasingly distinct when the European actions were reciprocated by the UK. The European governance quite openly recognized that the primary problem was not the real threat to public health but the perception of a threat. The grounds for policy action were still primarily referring to scientific advice and evidence. Similarly, the UK government, openly critical of what it considered to be the unscientific approach taken by the EU, still full-heartedly endorsed that all decisions should be based on public health considerations defined by the best scientific evidence. After initially agreeing with the decision to impose the ban on its own exports, the UK government started to openly disagree on the grounds that the European actions were based on perceptions rather than on available scientific evidence. Thus, all the actors involved emphasized that any actions taken had to be based on the best available scientific evidence though all parties were fully aware that there was a significant lack of such hard evidence. Although public health experts did not have conclusive evidence on the nature of the threat, they supported the use of tried and tested public health measures such as isolation and cordoning. The public health and scientific BSE language emphasized and aimed at the prevention of disease and the promotion of people's well-being on the basis of the idea that the disease was caused by minute biological agents and could be eradicated by checking the spread of these agents. The prevalent public health perspective narrows and contains the agenda according to which emergency management ideally proceeds to purely medical considerations in an effort to not dilute and weaken the response to the crisis by other 'extraneous' political issues. Furthermore, the modern public health perspective deals with immediate health crises by applying to them what has been learnt from past incidents: 'surveillance, education of the susceptible, and simple isolation procedures with infectives' (Benini and Bradford 1995). Public health language derives much of its power from the concepts of progress, reason, and enlightenment, which highlight the idea of individuality rather than nationality, and the concepts of globality, humanity, and universality rather than the state as a primary agent.

As an epistemic community, the public health perspective offers the technical skills and know-how required of governments or international organizations to efficiently manage emerging health hazards. However, the epistemic community is not only in a subservient role vis-à-vis politics. The European and worldwide community of medical scientists, public health specialists, epidemiologists, and scientists in other related areas constitute a network of power which bears major influence on how epidemic diseases are handled (e.g. Princen 2007: 13). Because of the transnational nature of the scientific community, it cannot be totally controlled by a single actor's political considerations. A case in point is offered by the ultimate inability of the UK government to discourage and prevent the publication of information hinting at a link between BSE and vCJD, the BSE-related variant of CJD. The transnational character of the scientific community can be a source of possible political tension, which is further reinforced by the prevalent scholarly notion that infectious diseases should be managed in a borderless global context since political borders are porous to the causative agents of diseases—'one world, one health'.[15]

Within the EU there existed in 1996 a wide range of institutionalized scientific bodies of both a permanent and more ad hoc nature, which, as sources of expert opinion, influenced various political decision makers. The rhythmic movements of the BSE drama brought to the fore such institutions as the EU's Standing Veterinary Committee and Scientific Committee and the UK's Spongiform Encephalopathy Advisory Committee. In addition to these institutional bodies, the scientific public health language was shared by and diffused over diverse institutes, universities, research centres, and laboratories, which were united by similar procedures and research methods. These research networks were relatively independent of any explicit state and regional political entities, with the result that their interactions were not totally contained within the European context. However, the intergovernmental and governmental bodies could exert effective pressure on many institutions relying on governmental sources for funding, as is made clear by the history of the BSE-related secrecy and even misinformation both in the UK and in the EC. Apart from the research networks directly linked with the scientific and medical approach, a wide array of public advocates, community-based organizations, NGOs, and consumer groups highlighted the need for 'pure' scientific evidence. Moreover, from the perspective of scientific research, the central prerequisite for any viable research programme was the ability to direct attention in order to get one's research and opinions across, with the result that media formed the key channel for persuasive scientific language regarding BSE, instead of the established governance structures (Foreman 1994: 21).

The intimate and long-standing connection between science and politics has been particularly pronounced when, on the one hand, a lack of clear scientific advice and knowledge concerning some politically acute and reactive issue has left room for the need to clarify political viewpoints on scientific ambiguity. On the other hand, the generation of novel scientific evidence can result in the dramatic re-contextualization of political drama. This influence of new discoveries and evidence was clearly demonstrated by the fact that the BSE drama was propelled into existence by detailed scientific research. Whereas the history of international health cooperation clearly demonstrates the ease with which political considerations can take advantage of scientific disarray and competing theories, the initial accent of the BSE drama illustrated the sporadic, but still substantial, force of scientific evidence over politics.

Scientific studies had begun to proliferate in late 1995 and early 1996 demonstrating that BSE in cows was a likely cause of an emerging human variant of CJD. Most of these studies were dismissed by the UK government as dubious scaremongering.[16] However, a scientific study by the UK Government Surveillance Unit specializing in CJD clearly showed that BSE had been the source in at least some cases of human CJD. Thus, the scientific community had managed to mould the context in which British–European policy was going to be played out for several months, indicating a shift in the focus of European policy away from the usual discourses endogenous to politics, which took into account public health considerations.

The emergence of scientific evidence on BSE and its possible link with CJD not only shrank the space left for political manoeuvring along the accustomed routes but, more importantly, gave increasing political influence to various consumer and health-related groups. As it soon became evident that conclusive scientific proof could not be achieved without extensive and time-consuming research,[17] calls for immediate action based on the worst-case scenario gathered momentum in the EC, its member-states, and especially the UK. The discourse that pressed for immediate action consisted of a wide spectrum of different views united by the idea that a major health disaster might be imminent if drastic actions were not taken to alter the prevailing food production practices—for example, the cannibalistic practice of feeding bovine bone meal to cows—which, according to these perspectives, had produced the disease in the first place. In other words, the central argument behind the concerned and critical attitude had to do with motivating people for necessary change and with pointing at the imminent catastrophe stemming from the perversity of modern lifestyles.[18] In the BSE case, the conscientious discourse—that is, the discourse produced by many advocacy, consumer rights and public health groups—proceeded by expressing strong concern over existing food-processing methods and intensive farming practices based on the maximization of profit, instead of a respect for the 'natural' way of doing things (Baker and Ridley 1996: 242). The public health tone of the initial BSE peaking trajectory had not so much to do with scientific attitude and evidence than with a mixture of science, fear, anxiety, and concern, which yielded compatible and accordant political decisions. Thus, the scientific and quasi-scientific arguments—trying to establish causal explanations for natural phenomena—were momentarily blended with critical and normative points of view—emphasizing the corruptness of secretive state-centred politics that had led to unnatural means of taking advantage of nature—to produce the distinctive sense that something special was taking place. By focusing attention on the tradition of secretive, non-transparent, and deceptive state practices in public health, various normative discourses turned the traditional 'better safe than sorry' type of thinking inherent in the public health paradigm into primary focus (Slack 1991: 119).

The normative emphasis was initially shared by much of the European media. The public discourse highlighted images of people digesting beef that had been 'unnaturally' produced. The emphasis was on deeply embodied visuals. As such, these discourses turned the attention away from the inconclusive scientific studies and from the bickering between the different governance bodies. BSE turned into an embodied metaphor expressing in a highly emotional way many of the anxieties people felt at the time. Politics, human relationship with nature, and industrial food production were seen in one fevering scenario of huge potential risks and vulnerabilities.

From the perspective of the normative BSE discourse, the natural realm, unaffected by modern artificial practices, is in a state of natural order and equilibrium. Not surprisingly then, the root cause of emerging disasters and eruptive calamities is often seen as lying in the destabilizing effects of human unnatural actions. The revenge of the rainforest argumentation prevailed in the public arenas around Europe. These discourses disregarded the possibility of accidental mutations and natural transformation as a plausible cause for the emergence of new diseases. The suggestion was clear: it is not the external reality that is chaotic, it is the social reality in which we live that is unnatural, hedonistic, and, ultimately, self-destructive and prone to produce 'Frankensteinian' outcomes. Regardless of their diverse missions and reasons, various conscientious groups proceeded by perceiving the UK and Europe as fundamentally flawed, driven by special interest lobbies, and incapable of addressing crucial questions satisfactorily. This resulted in pressure to take political action. The sentiment grew that any action was better than no action. At the societal level, 'political' decisions were mobilized outside and beyond state-sanctioned channels, for example, in the form of consumer politics. The strength of various consumer and animal rights movements played to diverse transnational reactions that also manifested in financial market reactions. The myriad actors involved relied on informal networks that cut across international borders. Consequently, these actors were able to spread their message and influence people at the grassroots level, which could not be totally governed by states or international institutions. However, to continue to affect complex international politics for long periods of time, the societal level and transnational actors would have required politically sustainable coherence and a power base. The coherence of the message disappeared as the scientific evidence, and actual happenings discounted the idea of an acute public health emergency, and the power base vanished as the political trajectory turned to a vast reservoir of nationalistic sentiments and tendencies for their source of legitimacy. In this way, the British media, for example, started to appeal to enemy images that framed the various European governments as hungry to infringe upon British rights. The underlying complexity of the technical and medical knowledge led first to uncertainties and then to stronger assertions of state interest.[19] The EU governance was mocked as incoherent and incompetent in ways that had been used before and have been used since. As the UK was seen in the British public's eyes as a victim of the European overreaction, the underlying disease anxieties were channelled, internationalized, to outside antagonistic actors. The disease itself was less actual in this reframing whereas the continental infringement on British affairs was seen as the actual driver of the dynamic. As we saw in the case of Haiti, internationalization of an epidemic to outside foreign and infringing elements can be seen as one key dynamic when the epidemic burden is geographically uneven in a way that coincides with political borders.

The Waning Trajectory of the BSE Drama

After the initial push that set the BSE drama into motion, the focus started to shift from a tempo set and driven by public health considerations to one that was less coherent and more ambiguous as the political characteristics began to take hold and no new scientific information further clarifying the issue was immediately forthcoming. The partial admission by the UK government that some of the information it had earlier called ridiculous and outrageous scaremongering was correct after all questioned the legitimacy of its stance on BSE. However, the ambiguity of the scientific evidence and the contentious nature of the rivalling theories about what caused BSE and CJD started to give way to political manoeuvring around the issue. Because it was caused by an unconventional type of disease agent—a prion—it was difficult to discuss BSE in a popularized epidemiological context, and consequently, the scientific evidence allowed for both public misrepresentation and misinterpretation (Baker and Ridley 1996: 242). Instead of the science fiction-like prion hypothesis, the most embodied modality of the BSE saga was the link between the sick, jerking cows, and hamburger meat. The initial alarm caused by the pronouncement of a possible link between BSE and CJD also subsided as soon as it became evident that there were not going to be a large number of deaths in a short period of time because of the disease. The public health emergency concerns started to evaporate. Under these conditions, the political debate shifted away from implementing radical changes to taking into account the economic and national repercussions, domestic concerns, and international interests, alongside the public health and consumer rights viewpoints.

The science-based public health language was attention catching but also ambiguous and required interpretation. In other words, the question of who was the legitimate interpreter and representative of the scientific 'knowledge' became extremely important. The legitimacy of public health language has been reinforced by the much-publicized advances made in the field of disease causation and spread and in the eradication of many global diseases during the twentieth century. The tension that has traditionally existed between scientific research and politics seems to have been resolved in favour of the latter as a result of the triumphs of medicine and science against such formidable diseases as plague, cholera, and yellow fever. The scientific expertise and community have started to provide the anchoring discourse for health-related international governance. If this is absent, the lack of an authoritative scientific opinion allows governments to use trade, economics, and politics-related considerations to guide their decision-making on international health. That said, importantly in the BSE context, the 1980s and 1990s witnessed the emergence of new health hazards such as Ebola, HIV, and AIDS and the re-emergence of old lethal diseases such as tuberculosis (Altenstetter 1994: 416). The growing alarm and the associated popular anxiety have led to the perception that public health expertise cannot always handle emerging health hazards. The world is too technically complex and scientifically uncertain. This, in turn, has resulted in more leeway for political concerns in formulating public health policies. Such politicization has been reinforced by the emerging of more ideological, norma-tive, and ethical controversies in dealing with national, regional, and global public health issues.

In the BSE context, the ability to achieve political aims was therefore closely connected to the ability to speak in the name of science. Not surprisingly then, the initial BSE drama heavily emphasized the legitimacy of science and medi-cine over and above mere politics, which meant that to get the acceptance and backing needed for effective policy-making, governmental actions on international health could not be openly based on narrow or conventional conceptualizations of national self-interest. Attempts by the political players of the BSE games to speak in the name of science were present throughout the episode. The crux of the argument was clear and meant to downplay the scepticism that the government had interfered with expert knowledge and that the UK's policies were not based on sound and independent scientific advice. The same substantive stance was ech-oed by the European Council, which, on the conclusion of its 21–22 June 1996 meeting, stated: 'Such decisions will be taken only and exclusively on the basis of public health and objective scientific criteria and of the judgement of the Com-mission, in accordance with the existing procedure, that these criteria have been satisfied'. The council indicated that there was no politics involved, only science in its management of the affair. However, as all the parties involved knew, the focus and legitimacy of the scientific advice were starting to be increasingly blurred as the scenario developed. This was caused mostly by the natural time delay in the scientific community coming up with a consensus view on the basic nature and causation of the disease. Realization of this left room for political manoeuvring— other, more narrowly political arguments took the leading role, although not one of outright dominance at first.

By the time the UK introduced its policy of non-cooperation with the other EU member-states and the common institutions, the initial persuasiveness and attention-catching nature of the public health perspective had lost much of its ability to lead the discussion. As the shock and awe receded to the background, political controversies occupied the foreground in the discussion and in the decision-making processes. Furthermore, the emphasis shifted increasingly towards calming and soothing actions. Thus, the need to present the reassuring appearance of BSE being under control was a very prominent feature. Because it had become evident by the middle of March 1996 that the BSE matter could not be kept out of public scrutiny, the emphasis shifted to controlling and minimizing the economic and political implications of the situation by appearing vigilant and thorough. After some initial wavering, the language shifted markedly towards emphasizing control of public health risks rather than stressing the centrality of economic disturbances. However, the political management of the public appearance of the disease was still close to the surface. Although the EU discourse increasingly took on a public health facade, the position of this stance in the overall trajectory of the BSE drama resulted in it becoming more and more political as other actors began to adopt such co-optive 'scientific' standpoints. The BSE drama that was initially set in motion by non-governmental actors began to shift and spread in its scope as it was no longer supported by shocking new scientific discoveries or alarming news of rising or projected death rates.

In the context of the gradual waning of the BSE plays of morality and legitimacy, the identification of the UK as the source of BSE and its negative ramifications led to counter-narratives and arguments. These mainly British discourses emphasized that BSE was a European, rather than a solely British, problem. As far as the UK was concerned, the ban on its beef and beef products on the grounds that they might pose a hypothetical risk to human health was scientifically unfounded and, therefore, politically motivated.

The main justification for using the 'BSE as a Europe-wide problem' argument was that it reasoned against the justification and legitimacy of the EU's measures against the UK.[20] It was a political antidote to the European suggestion that BSE was a 'British disease'. The stances started to harden, and appeals to national sentiments started to appear as is apparent from newspaper headlines such as 'Major Goes to War' after the 21 May 1996 speech by British Prime Minister John Major, in which he announced the policy on non-cooperation: 'Madam Speaker, important national interests for Britain are involved in this matter. I cannot tolerate these interests being brushed aside by some of our European partners with no reasonable grounds to do so'. Major announced that the UK would veto key EU decisions, halt progress on the Intergovernmental Conference, and disrupt the approaching European summit.

By ceasing to cooperate with EU decision-making, the UK highlighted the sense of urgency and alarm it felt over the beef ban and the fact that the BSE drama had deviated alarmingly from being based on and guided by public health alone. In the same vein, it was argued by the UK that it had already implemented

BSE control measures that went far beyond the measures taken in other EU member-states:

> We have explained very clearly the extent of the measures we have taken—going well beyond those in many other Member States of the European Union—to ensure the safety of British beef and beef products.
>
> *(Statement by Prime Minister John Major in the House of Commons, 21 May 1996)*

Thus, the situation in which the UK was the sole target of BSE eradication was considered intolerable by the British government: the localization and nationalization of the issue as British was seen as distinctively and publicly pointing to British actions as reckless, ill-advised, and showing bad political judgement. As a result, the legitimacy of the British government was seen as suffering both domestically and internationally since it was perceived as being unable to contain the disease, which seemed to be well in control elsewhere. Furthermore, it soon became evident that the crisis was not going to be treated as a common European problem as the British might have hoped, but as a primarily British predicament. The UK's assertive disruptive actions changed the emergency into one of contestation between the UK and the continental member-states.

The 'taming' of the BSE emergency scenario to fit the interests of one's own nation signified the receding coherence. To break out of the unfavourable position in which the UK found itself, more crafty arguments were needed than a mere appeal to European mutuality and goodwill. The characteristic thrust of such arguments brought about appeals to national sentiments as is apparent from newspaper headlines such as 'Major Goes to War', which used the older language of enmities and co-opted nationalistic sentiments. By stopping its cooperation in EU decision-making, the UK highlighted the sense of urgency and alarm it felt over the beef ban and the fact that the BSE play was no longer based on and guided solely by science. The continuing public health narratives on both sides acquired a form that was increasingly decided upon by the craft and skill used in proceeding with international contestation.

Concerns over the danger BSE posed to public health and the sustainability of a risk-free environment were tangible at the beginning of the BSE affair. Not surprisingly, the pivotal question revolved round the measurability of the risks involved. In other words, how should the real risks be measured, were there any objective criteria for measuring health risks, what were the issues involved besides the immediate public health concerns, and how to best evaluate and balance all the issues that were at stake? Two themes emerged to occupy the central ground. First, the normal or usual state of affairs is that the management of diseases as a compartmentalized area of cooperation is left to presumably politically disinterested scientists and bureaucrats. From this perspective, the BSE crisis involved a breakdown of the boundary between politics and health as a functional area of cooperation. Second, the emergence of BSE in the public consciousness did not only bring about the politicization of international health cooperation, it also resulted in public health rhetoric saturating the political space. Thus, the nature of the BSE drama was embodied in discourses that did not only extend political intrigues to international health issues but distinctively produced arguments that were a unique mix of politics and science pertinent to the fleeting dynamics of the BSE trajectory.

The new combination of political and scientific characteristics culminated in an emphasis on normalcy, in the return of the usual wheeling and dealing in politics. The extraordinary sense of doing the right thing from the perspective of safeguarding public health changed into normalizing and situation downplaying language. The aim was to find a way out, to restore a commonsensical situation where the ban on British beef and the UK's disruption of European decision-making could be brought to an end.

The UK government's initial response had desperately tried to neutralize, normalize, and contain a situation that had the potential of getting completely out of hand. The assurances concerning the safety of and control over the situation, which appealed to the ordinary definition of the term 'safety', highlighted the desirability of stability in the face of the extraordinary BSE situation. Normalcy was given a practical content by associating it with the restorative measures that the UK government had already taken. Thus, normalcy was made dependent on the precautions taken against the extraordinary and unlikely health threat. The British hopes that things would soon return to 'normalcy' were soon dashed. The emphasis shifted to different co-options of scientific research. The UK government considered that its stance was a scientifically proven one. There were no longer any appeals to the solidarity of the European governments or attempts to convince them. John Major's government began strongly pushing its case that the European institutions had overreacted. During the final phase of the BSE drama, there was a search for solutions to the crisis that allowed each side to claim that they had not backed down. The search for the face-saving option also allowed all the parties involved to claim that their decisions were based on the best possible scientific evidence.

The BSE as an epidemic emergency scenario came to an end in the summer of 1996. At the Florence summit at the end of June 1996, the whole affair was 'resolved' by making it synonymous with a difficult but politically inert disease that could be managed by functional expertise through non-political means. After Florence, BSE no longer played a part in European international relations. The political language used by the UK government just before the Florence meeting, highlighting the national interests at stake due to the perceived unjustifiable actions by the EC and other member-states, was not in stark contrast with the way in which the matter was eventually dissolved by the language games of 'scientific and objective criteria', 'exclusively on the basis of public health', and 'scientists giving a clean bill of health'. The BSE language, which emphasized the UK's national interests, was actually quite compatible with insulating the whole BSE matter from politics and, incidentally, from the public visibility brought to it by high politics. The prominence of normal political language at the expense of science-dictated 'normalcy' was instrumental in pushing BSE out of the international scene and into a politically indistinct technical realm.

The British BSE narrative changed the balance between the attributes of the 'scientific' and the 'political'. In other words, the forces that were unleashed from political control at the beginning of the BSE crisis did not only instantiate themselves in public health concerns but also entailed the recontextualization of public health as a political phenomenon. During the first phase of the BSE drama, the scientific evidence concerning the possible link between BSE and CJD was later denounced by the UK as mere hysteria and, consequently, political actions and consumer reactions based on that evidence were defined as unjust, undeserved and not based on accurate science. In the second phase of the transformation, the policy decisions and the consumer reactions that were first denounced as uncontrollable outbursts of irrational fear and emotion were balanced against the British national interests at stake. Not surprisingly, what was considered hysteria and irrationality did not fare well with political interests. The scientific evidence that was considered unjustifiable from the point of view of national interests was downplayed. The final phase evolved from the fight over the science of BSE into the decision to lay the issue to rest.

For the EU, the supposedly obvious reaction to the publication of new scientific findings in the UK was to halt sales of British beef products as a precautionary measure. The measures that were considered entirely justifiable included actions with a significant impact on the political and economic interests of the UK. In other words, what had to be done and implemented seemed to flow naturally out of what was proper to the exceptional circumstances of a public health emergency. The spectrum of alternatives was, in other words, considerably reduced and condensed, with the result that only one interpretation of what should be done seemed prudent enough to calm public concern and market reactions. Under these unusual conditions, the heavy emphasis on the scientific approach seemed to offer a legitimate, stabilizing, and calming solution compatible with the essence of the BSE drama because, after all, it was scientific findings that had brought about the crisis in the first place.

It can be argued that the EU turned very inconclusive scientific evidence into an objective standard of safety by banning British beef, thereby setting into motion many of the interpretative dynamics that were distinctive of the BSE crisis. The best scientific evidence, which, in this case, meant the only evidence at hand, became a tool for minimizing the risk to public health. Moreover, the EU's language games proceeded along the logic that the smaller the perception of risk to public safety, the more fleeting the ramifications of the whole affair for the efficiency and stability of the Common Market. The phrases, 'all necessary measures', 'best available scientific evidence', and 'to minimize any potential risk', all were now being used. They determined and defined the nature of what could be done and on what evidence. Moreover, because the best evidence at the time was hopelessly inconclusive, the appropriate measures could not be too detailed and specific but had to be aimed at eliminating unknown risks. Thus, regardless of the sense of direction inherent in the initial BSE drama, it resulted in rather sweeping measures that, once in place, redefined the contextual meaning of the subsequent actions.

The surprise and novelty of the situation began to wear off, with the result that the course of action that was initially considered quite appropriate in the extraordinary situation turned into something that needed to be defended and justified. Suddenly, the 'natural' meaning of the BSE crisis became an increasing object of attention and revision. In the end, the 'overriding objective' had changed from a willingness to implement 'all necessary measures' to eliminate any potential public health risk to the fulfilment of 'necessary conditions' so that the export ban could eventually be lifted. Furthermore, the necessary conditions for the lifting of the ban no longer conveyed a sense of naturalness immediately self-evident to political decision makers but referred the whole matter to 'scientific and technical advice' and to 'public health and objective scientific criteria'. The last phase of the BSE order contained a sense of normalcy that indicated that additional pressures such as the necessities inherent in devastating epidemic diseases were no longer significant.

The eradication of BSE, which was taken as the fundamental goal, was defined as a matter of restoring confidence in European beef. However, the whole argument was somewhat self-referential and circular. In other words, the actions aimed at eradication were framed primarily as confidence restoring and only secondarily as geared to fighting the disease as an epidemic entity. Thus, the EU was soon engaged in eradicating a baffling disease by means that were aimed at the alarming loss of consumer confidence. However, as consumer confidence started to pick up, the distinctive measures imposed on the UK remained because of the original reason, the BSE–CJD link. Despite the fact that the number of BSE cases continued to rise during 1996, the demand for beef and beef products rose significantly. In this environment, the original BSE impetus lost its steam. The measures taken against the disease and to calm the markets were now mainly left over from the earlier more pressing political atmosphere. The power of the scientific standpoint to define and point to some logical solution to the BSE problem vanished as the primary actors of the BSE drama began to interpret science, rather than have the scientific standpoint interpreted to them by the expert community.

The Legacy of the BSE Drama

The BSE morality drama acted as an evolving guide to respectable behaviour. The EU's cordoning actions were initially considered inevitable even by the UK government. The apparent political victory achieved by the EU institutions on the BSE issue blended in with other happenings at the time so that the upper hand and initiative gained by the supranational EU was history before it had ever really been gained. The initial positions taken up by each side, which were made more distinct by the proximity of each to the BSE issue, were no longer valid when the focus of politics shifted elsewhere. The agreement reached at the Florence Council meeting on 21–22 June 1996, signalling the disappearance of BSE from the European international scene, was something of an anti-climax to the whole affair, which had been prepared for a more poignant resolution of the hyperbolic public health crisis. At the beginning of the BSE crisis, the general mood was one of a sense of alarm and emergency, which seemed to point at an imminent public health disaster. The awaited disaster failed to materialize in that the whole affair produced only contestation between the players, which found its clearest expression in the UK's non-cooperation policy vis-à-vis all EU decision-making. This policy seemed to make things hang in the balance, causing the initial anxiety over the looming public health crisis to recede into the background. However, the political contestation itself failed to produce anything significant as the attention shifted away from BSE politics to other more usual political issues.

Diseases are reflective of the underlying form of the political community. In this respect, BSE was caused as much by the political situation of the spring of 1996 as it was by the physical disease agent, the prion. This disease morality play had supranational and transnational protagonists. The legitimacy of consumer and public right groups grew after the BSE crisis as did the legitimacy of the European public health authorities. The crisis shaped the underpinnings of the European political space and left a legacy. Sensitivity to health scares has grown after 1996. The associated morality plays provided a recognizable form for political contestation, which has more lately surfaced in relation to food toxins, genetically manipulated food, and several different threatening diseases. The sick, jerking, stumbling cows of the UK provided the basic form for an important European morality play. The most lasting legacy of the BSE drama was the way in which the issues ebbed and waned in a matter of months. This same fleeting trajectory has been evident in later pandemic scares such as SARS and avian flu. The BSE crisis demonstrated how a pandemic drama can become part of high politics. However, it also pointed out the fleeting nature of such dramas. Second, the analysis of the BSE scare exemplified a situation in which the attribution of a disease to one state can lead to an interstate contestation. Third, the BSE drama highlighted the role of a myriad other international, supranational, and transnational actors in a public health spectacle.

Notes

1 The 'root' causes of most violent epidemics can be traced to the multilevel political structures and dynamics that provide the macro-level context for the disease-causing agents (e.g. Fassin 2007; Farmer 2004; Joralemon 1997).
2 MINUSTAH had a very diverse staff that originated from 22 countries. They were deployed in contingents based on country of origin to various geographical areas in Haiti. The more than 400 Nepalese troops sent to Haiti were stationed in three locations. One of them was the camp in Mirebalais. The troops were rotated every 6 months.
3 Already in 2011, Piarroux et al. (2011: 1165) had concluded that the symptomatic cases occurred inside the MINUSTAH camp. Thus, they directly challenged the official UN statements.
4 For resistance against this form of global governance, see, for example, Feldman (2008).
5 One such message was taped by the US ambassador to Haiti, Raymond Joseph: 'Listen, don't rush on boats to leave the country. If you do that, we'll all have even worse problems. Because I'll be honest with you: If you think you will reach the US and all the

doors will be wide open to you, that's not at all the case. And they will intercept you right on the water and send you back home where you came from' (NYT 2010).

6 The colonial project got much of its substance from racial and evolutionary 'scientific' doctrines. This enabled the discourse that the West was not in Africa to conquer, but to help (Brantlinger 1985: 167–8): 'Ostensibly removed from the realm of land and politics, colonization viewed through the lens of salutary medical aid was made to seem essentially humanitarian' (Kelm 1998: 101).

7 At this junction, there would have been alternative lines of inquiry based on Foucauldian or Deleuzian perspectives. This alternative would speak directly to Foucault's (2007) concepts presented in his 'Security, Territory, Population' lectures. On infectious diseases and biopolitics, see, for example, Elbe (2005).

8 Similarly, the disease at first did not spread to the neighbouring Dominican Republic, which led to the stigmatization of the Haitians there.

9 For example, HIV and AIDS were territorialized into Africa, racialized into Afro-American communities, and sexualized into gay communities. SARS was nationalized into China, and BSE was contained in the UK. Avian flu was localized into Indonesia, Turkey, and much of Asia. Swine flu became a Mexican disease.

10 Similarly, it may be further argued that the public meaning of suffering from AIDS changed the expressive pain behaviour of those who had HIV and AIDS. Their suffering was stigmatized and used for political purposes. The fact that the suffering became more 'silent' was in itself a politicosomatic phenomenon influencing the way people suffered, the way the disease spread, the policies for its management, and the politics of it.

11 On the relationship between international relations, political power, and pandemics, see, for example, Yanzhong (2004) and Price-Smith (2009).

12 On 19 March 1997, British Prime Minister John Major denied the link between BSE and CJD.

13 The necessity of a sense of rhythm in wise politics is most prominently demonstrated in Machiavelli. Success in political games depends on the ability to act at the right time, which is facilitated by prudent understanding of the moment's requirements and by a sense of political rhythm.

14 The UK's attempt to restrain and subdue the measures unleashed by the EU ban on British beef by blocking the EU's decision-making offers a case in point of an innovative venture of giving a new appearance to an acute problem in order to enable international actors to better manage the situation.

15 The public health model concentrates on a problem-solving perspective that is mainly medical in character. First, the problem is defined, and then the procedures that have worked previously in similar situations are vigorously and painstakingly applied. The emphasis is not on the other, more social, and political aspects of the disease such as economic welfare, trade, and poverty, which are considered important, but secondary to the main objective of controlling the outbreak.

16 In a letter to the mother of a CJD victim on 19 March 1997, British Prime Minister John Major maintained that no link existed between BSE and CJD.

17 Baker and Ridley (1996: 239–40) report on the difficulty of arriving at conclusive scientific evidence: 'A major problem in studying prion diseases results from the long-time course over which these diseases develop. Although the incubation period may be as short as a few months in some mouse and hamster adapted scrapie models, in large animals, the incubation period in acquired cases ranges from two to several years, depending on the route of contamination, and in acquired cases in humans (e.g. iatrogenic cases and kuru), it ranges from two to 30 years. This makes the collection of epidemiological data, the identification of causative events, and experimental transmission studies (other than in rodents) very difficult.'

18 The following example from Newsweek (22 May 1995: 19) might shed some light on these language games: 'Until recently, most experts thought of new viral diseases as accidents of genetic mutation. But of late, they have become less fearful of random genetic change—and more terrified by the effects of human social change.'

19 See, for example, Haas (1992: 1).
20 The scientific side of the British argument proceeded by denying the possibility of maternal transmission of BSE and CJD, which would justify the wholesale slaughter of the offspring of affected animals. In the case of older animals, it was argued that no slaughter programme was likely to have any effect because 'it is impossible to target with any accuracy cattle that may be incubating BSE, and killing all 11 million cattle in the UK in less than the three-four years (by which time the epidemic will be virtually over) is not practicable' (Baker and Ridley 1996: 242).

8

BEYOND PANDEMIC SECURITY

In Chapter 2, I reviewed the nexus between plague and power through its prototypical containment drama depictions in works of art. I used classical paintings as well as the cover art of Hobbes' *Leviathan* to exemplify the historical depth of the imageries relating to this often-forgotten yet still deeply felt nexus between human bodies and plague of the global reaches. Similar to war, plague has had a significant impact on how external, international, and global environments have been imagined because they come into our bodies and immediately connect us to others—centres to peripheries in many senses. The imaginaries of one's body's and community's position in the wider world are acutely important for today's global political and economic order. The point has been that diseases characterize yet also distort of the maps, and global political maps add to crystallizing the projected meanings of diseases. They are politically processed to mean something through the process of nationalizing and localizing them or their origin to somewhere and through internationalizing them to be the fault of global governance institutions or the global order itself by ethnicizing, racializing, or sexualizing a disease to originate from certain practices, habits, groups, and cultures. COVID-19 offers a good example of a disease that has been processed thus: it has been made to fit existing national, regional, and global patterns of enmity, and these enmities have given content to expressed disease language, which has been turned into potent omens of misgovernance and a vicious global order, and it has singled out the bad sinful habits and the groups of people exhibiting such habits. They are also made to fit the blame and status games; they become issues of (de)legitimacy, prestige, and power. They generally lower the levels of trust between and within societies/states and, thereby, catalyze expressions of mistrust such as unrest, repression, and war.

The use of art to make a point is itself an often-used epistemological tool that relies on the value and position of art in our society. Art is seen as deeply revelatory. It seems persuasive to argue through highly regarded art. I am basically claiming that the polito-somatic nexus makes sense and has a refined form since it has been depicted in works of

DOI: 10.4324/9781003169147-8

high culture for hundreds of years. This acknowledgement and recognition also offers a bridgehead for going beyond the claims of plagues and power having a rarefied higher pattern or intellectual form. Is it really so? Are we spellbound into repetition of a cycle of pandemic drama because of the often pre-cognitive patterns of politosomatics?

Going beyond global public health's proto-theoretical form involves recovering and acknowledging the deeply embodied substance of health worries as parts of differently lived lives, instead of pandemic security and scenarios of situated global practices. What do people actually do and need to do in the global space, and how is health compromised while doing this? Fittingly, in his *Art as Experience*, John Dewey (1980: 7) wants to remove art from the high pedestal on which it has been placed and reposition it in the stream of everyday life, as a part of the 'significant life of an organized community'. According to Dewey, art punctuates and accents the 'emotions and ideas that are associated with the chief institutions of social life'. In this way, Dewey intends to recover 'the continuity of aesthetic experience with normal processes of living' (1980: 10). Through this move, he also redefines the term 'art'. Art is part of everybody's life and, as a practice, in everyone's possession. The value of this repositioning is due to the practical worth of doing so: through everyday art, anybody can beautify, refine, and expand their everyday experiences. Similarly, going beyond public health involves the rediscovery of global health as a modality and function of everyday life. There should not be anything lofty about managing the flow of people's lives—it should not be placed on a high pedestal where it becomes a part, for example, of geopolitical blame and status games. Health should be a practical everyday issue rather than being a part of identity politics stemming from the politosomatic pandemic security scenarios. Scenarios of pandemic security easily lead into extraneous combinations where a sudden local outbreak in Wuhan becomes an issue of high political importance instead of being managed as what it is: a chain of infections that needs to be stopped as soon as possible in order to guarantee the basic foundations of global life. When a disease, as Susan Sontag pointed out, begins to embody epochal worries and fears, it turns into something which cannot be approached solely on the basis of key practical expertise and which thus cannot be contained because it connects with such potent underlying patterns of enmity. COVID-19 illustrates well this tendency of refining a disease into a mega-security issue. From the very beginning, it was part of state and geopolitical security to such an extent that it became impossible to uncover its actual point of origin. COVID-19 was turned into a mythological creature, and, as such, it contains fears from bodily infection all the way to the sustainability of the global order and the decline and fall of the great powers. It becomes so lofty of a syndrome that it is impossible to contain because the cascading effects spread from the practical level in different ontological directions. Much harm can emanate even from a relatively small outbreak, such as the cholera in Haiti, and can have long-lasting harmful implications because its origin cannot be acknowledged because of reasons of legitimacy, prestige, and legal litigation. In his memoir, the UN general secretary of the time, Ban Ki-moon, laments the enduring effects of the cholera—in the form of general mistrust of the UN—in Haiti: 'The cholera epidemic continues to poison the Haitian people's relationship with the United Nations' (Ban Ki-moon 2021: 226). However, the issue's lofty complexities prevented him from clearly expressing the likelihood that the disease was brought to Haiti by UN peacekeepers. Things remain stuck. These stubborn and difficult-to-manage complexities result from the politosomatic relationship, which, if unacknowledged and mismanaged, can catapult the pandemic situation from a local outbreak into an enduring syndrome that keeps on having negative effects at many levels.

The key paradox is that if the historically well-established linkages between plagues and people are bypassed, the expertise-based management of infectious diseases will continue to be hampered by politicizations of diseases. This has been, I am afraid, made even more likely by the emergence and spread of COVID-19. However, if the combinatorial patterns are taken into account from the very beginning, they can be better identified and contained. The aim is to empower, to gain from the increased self-awareness about the forms that give rise to so much anxiety as people's lives become increasingly intertwined with the mobilities of global life. Such de-mythologizing and de-glorifying of the hyperbolic descriptor of 'pandemics' allows for a re-examination of many lived life anxieties that go into the building of such lofty complexities of enmity and fear. Going beyond these can result in disentangling the often unrecognized complexities that are lumped together under the term 'pandemic'. This disentanglement aims at showing the complex web of life that makes pandemics ideally comprehensible signifiers of 'fatal blows' pertinent to our times.

Dewey's point encourages rediscovery. It is a means to an end, an end that is ultimately just and fair democracy. By bringing pandemics into the everyday life context, they can start to function in a more transformative way. The transformative element, for Dewey, is one of recombination. It extends and reshuffles existing cultural connections, acts as a catalyst in thinking beyond the taken for granted, offers new insights, and broadens the potential for new meanings (Goldblatt 2006: 17). Such a transformational process highlights the ability of innovative imageries to refine people's thinking and open their minds to new and alternative connections and combinations as well as to disentangle existing complexities that seem too complicated and mythological to serve any meaningful purpose (e.g. Dewey 1980: 131). My intention is that in this manner, through the mapping out of the disease-related cultural form's inherent imageries, new ways of rediscovering the more encompassing entanglements of 'pandemics' be opened up in order to facilitate a transformative and empowering going beyond mere activity. For now, it seems that when people hear the descriptor, 'pandemic outbreak', they stop thinking and get stuck in the ritualistic behavioural patterns of a pandemic emergency that has so long roots that people do not have ownership over them. They remain largely proto-theoretical and pre-cognitive meaning that we are likely to repeat them. They are so engrossed in signifiers such as 'fatal blow' and 'contagion' that they are no longer cognizant of the fundamental role that pandemics play and could play in their wider scenarios of situated life. This book has made an attempt to describe historical patterns and rediscover historical roots so as to allow for the recognition of what goes into the construction of the ideally comprehensive but, at a closer look, difficult-to-describe phenomenon of pandemics.

To help us on, Dewey's work on art seems to suggest a refined memory—a residue of experience—that can be used in the 'magical' re-attachment of feeling, value, and meaning to a new circumstance in ordinary life. The excitable memory cues provide a vehicle for rendering new events 'poignant and momentous'. This transformative and democratic rediscovery of every person as an artist appears to fit well into the scheme of things in experimental and even serendipitous trying out of one's wider surroundings. Pandemics can turn from detached signifiers of doom into sources of insights into how we feel and sense our surroundings and into how we might change them. Dewey's (1980: 122) notion that the transformative function of imageries provides 'knowledge of something else' seems to find its place in the tradition of innovative memory, in which memories are not only about the past but a vehicle for 'remembering' something anew. Thus, it is possible to find justification for the Deweyan combinatory plays that rely on such rediscovery and the gaining of insights by experimentally trying out different combinations of images and thereby forming new imageries. This type of 'combinatorics' refers to the possibility of transformative remembering of the possibilities of richer and more democratic lives. Pandemics might at first seem to contain too much forceful, violent, and brute factuality to allow for playing and tinkering around. However, as I have tried to show in this work, pandemics are already as they stand works of power, knowledge, and culture. Our conceptions of them are rich, and they contain much historical experimentalism and 'transformativity'. This part should be repossessed as the pandemic cultural form is one of the foremost ways of feeling, sensing, and knowing about our global surroundings.

From the perspective of Deweyan transformative combinatorics, the act of seeing new connections allows for the recognition of knowledge of the 'what if' type. The ability of this type of knowledge to convey new types of certainty derives from the intensity of the accompanying experience. When the intensity reaches a high point, the term 'revelatory' seems appropriate. Such moments when hitherto unattained possibilities are 'acknowledged' contain a guiding tendency whereby people act 'in deference to' what they have acknowledged (Dewey 1958: 144). These poignant and momentous revelatory moments carry with them a particular sense of certainty about what is taking place. This sense of reality can be seen as a function of being engrossed with events in a particular way. Interpreted thus, the sense of reality becomes a quality attached to circumstances; certain ways of being engrossed with events produce a sense that the situation is especially real and true. It is significant that Erving Goffman (1974: 2), the developer of frame analysis, located himself in the tradition of Dewey and ultimately William James and followed James' modus operandi expressed in the question, 'Under what circumstances do we think things are real?' The emergent moment may reveal something as real—an infectious disease as an ideally comprehensive entity. For example, the revelatory moments of pandemics rely on specific circumstances and situational characteristics to carry meaning and start to be revelatory. COVID-19 contains intense and irresistible cascades ripping through and across the globality. The avian flu pandemic scare in 2004 needed many conceptual innovations and reconfigurations, such as mutability and crossing the interspecies boundary, to become engrossing. It also needed the sudden and striking precedent of SARS in 2003 to catapult it into prominence. The engrossing images of dead birds and animals being culled seemed to carry with them a profound message about the meaning of the times and what should be done, but only as a function of the right circumstances, combinations, and confluences. Gaining awareness of these situational characteristics and entanglements can open up ways of understanding the roughness of pandemics in a more innovative and even transformative way. We need to understand the enmities and fears that are projected onto a pandemic and that are the materials of which pandemics are constructed, in addition to the disease agents and disease causation. Better knowledge of the factors coming into play from this politosomatic relationship would allow for better management of disease as a physical entity as well as for containment of its immediate cascading effects.

Furthermore, Dewey's thought, in connection with Goffman and James, points to the non-cognitive emphasis in general pragmatist thought. It is possible to contextualize Dewey's ideas about extending and transforming meaning with the Jamesian emphasis that religious-like experiences have a fundamental role in the way meaning and certainty are apprehended. James highlights the role of non-cognitively gained preconceptual revelations over empirically verified objectivity. He seems to suggest that the broad aspect of experience is fuelled by pre-cognitively gained disclosures and schemes (James 1985: 352). This suggests that the grounding of everyday experience is not abstract and intellectual but proto-theoretical, pre-cognitive, emotional, and quasi-religious (James 1985: 397).[1] The important point here is that the revelatory way of gaining 'knowledge' is not based on occasions of reasoned choice but on moments of believing, learning, experiencing, growing up, inheriting, and accepting. This type of knowledge requires constant reminding and reminders, a role that striking and engrossing events such as pandemic outbreaks can play. We could rediscover pandemics as something other than sublime and almost mythological events and fatal blows. Rediscovering pandemics—that is, going beyond them—can involve democratization of the underlying historically deep memories, which are often used for purposes that are anything but democratic.

Ludwig Wittgenstein's emphasis on reminders provides one further element to the current pandemic-related combinatorics. More precisely, his later philosophy may be used to shed some light upon the degrees of freedom in the underlying combinatorics. Discernible wholes of language, in the Wittgensteinian sense of language games, do not come together in some strictly formal way (Wittgenstein 1968: 108).[2] Wittgenstein uses the term 'family resemblance' to bring forth the elusive and indeterminate character of language use (Wittgenstein 1968: 23, 67). He continuously points out the dangers of an omnipresent and more imprisoning use of language games. He sees that language games—that is, scenarios of situated knowledge—can and often do 'conjure up' fairly determinate senses that go beyond mere family resemblance (Wittgenstein 1968: 426–8). On the one hand, thus, language games can be used in an imprisoning way of conveying how things must be. On the other hand, language offers a highly desirable way of showing, demonstrating, and teaching how things could be. In the second sense, the means of social activity can be used to bind actions and things loosely and innovatively together, whereby the game brings up whole patterns of similarity and dissimilarity: 'The language games are rather set up as objects of comparison which are meant to throw light on the facts of our language by way not only of similarities, but also of dissimilarities' (Wittgenstein 1968: 130). Besides this character of language games, they have a more dogmatic use, which can 'hold us captive' (Wittgenstein 1968: 115). The 'picture' invoked by a language game holds people captive, and they 'cannot get outside of it' for it lies in their language, and language seems to repeat it to them 'inexorably' (Wittgenstein 1968: 105). 'Pandemic' can be used as>>> an example of something captivating instead of offering points of contrasts and patterns of dissimilarity. Reminding, in this Wittgensteinian sense, refers to the activity of offering objects of comparison meant to awaken those captivated by imprisoning and determinate lumps of knowledge/authority. This understanding of 'going beyond' offers a way to 'unfreeze' the consolidated memory systems. The Wittgensteinian continuum between 'showing how things can be' and 'demonstrating how they must be' offers a clue to the political use of image combinations that comprise modern ideas about pandemics. My efforts in this book have been concentrated on reminding readers of a whole gamut of interrelationships between pandemics and their somatic and political surroundings. In a nutshell, the very idea of politosomatics is connected with getting us unstuck from our compelling and imprisoning pandemic imageries so that we are not held captive by them and so that they are no longer able to repeat themselves on us inexorably. However, this cannot be achieved without first, as I have done in this book, reading the wider historical patterns that have formed between plagues and people. What repeats inexorably needs to be recognized and acknowledged first in order to become aware of their status and dynamics.

The democratization of pandemics aims at making its connections with the daily lives of people and their political contexts more evident. The pandemic-related public health discourse often relies on an opposite movement: making pandemics more insular and more of a field of expert knowledge and less of an issue of people and their politics. Further light can be shed on the relatively undemocratic field of pandemics through Susan Sontag's masterful account of the disease metaphors of bodily illnesses. In her pioneering *Illness as a Metaphor* (2001), Sontag ponders over the cultural history of the different conditions of being ill in Western societies. Distinct diseases have highly readable social meanings, with long and mutating historical roots. The most horrid and culturally memorable of these diseases involve the regressive bodily processes of decomposition. They are readable not only in a cognitive way but also in more embodied ways. These killer diseases have their own temporal tempos. Time becomes of essence as there is a rush to find a cure. This temporization changes the situation of ethics as long-term deliberation becomes a vice and hectic rush prevails as a virtue. The tempo of events becomes accentuated by the perceived progress of the disease as it spreads across and deeper into people and their communities. Besides bringing its own time and its corresponding ethics, a disease emergency contains its own affective regime. Fear and anxiety saturate the air. The dimension of power changes as well. The authorities that are recognized and the knowledge that is acknowledged come to be seen from the perspective of their ability to provide a sense of relief from the pain. The communities themselves change as more and more people become inhabitants of what Sontag calls 'the kingdom of the sick'. This medically maintained domain inhabited by sick people was a deeply personal focus for Sontag. Illness was more than a metaphor for her. She survived two cancers but died after a long and painful illness when a third cancer claimed her. Her knowledge of the isolating conditions in the kingdom of the sick is deeply embodied. The ways in which the disease decomposed her body is closely mirrored in the way she was stripped away from her usual social relationships and in the way she became de-individualized in the medical machinery in the frantic search for a cure. As a template for a community, the 'hospital' provides for quite a different set of rights and responsibilities for its citizens than the communal metaphor of a 'polis'—a deeply autocratic, instead of democratic, polity.

This brings to my mind a child's drawing I saw while I was working as a good governance expert in an EU–India programme in 2004–06 meant to educate the media on HIV and AIDS. The drawing carried the caption: 'This man is being chased by HIV and HIV is trying to stab him with the dagger of sadness and loneliness!'[3] The captivating and mentally disempowering quality of the signifier 'pandemic' has much to do with this basic observation.

Although the desirable going beyond would involve recognition that diseases are always political, the modern global health governance language often treats perceived health issues in terms of the so-called functions rather than in terms of territorial entities such as states. The functionalist perspective involves a conceptual move away from the relevance of possible specific territorial concerns and people's embeddedness in their specific geographical contours. The conceptual move contrasts with the territorial approach, which puts the emphasis on political markers of discontinuity, on the other signifiers of political separation: while borders disjoin the political powers by attaching them to a plurality of territories, it conjoins the map into one whole consisting of similar homogenous territorial entities. In offering a substantive alternative to traditional politics, the (neo)functionalist approach treats the possible adversarial power relations between political entities as an obstacle to rational decision-making. Functionalism imagines the relationship between a rational planning approach and a traditional political perspective as potentially at odds: power is connected to politicization and seen as having a negative impact on rational problem-solving in various functional areas of cooperation. The functional ideal, according to which efficiency and accountability are connected with proven technical expertise, is prone to distil what is considered to be undue politicization out of the functional fields of cooperation. A corresponding measure of efficiency starts from the idea that the most commonsensical thing to do is to entrust the matter to experts with scientifically grounded practical know-how. However, although this idea sounds compelling and rational, it erases as unnecessary the very thing that almost always happens in a pandemic situation as the disease becomes a part of a wider complex where politics and power play a vital role. The functionalist approach insufficient if the power politics of pandemics is ignored as irrational and unneeded. What is required, instead, is to see how power politics finds its way into pandemic scenarios.

To understand the radical nature of functionalism, one needs to appreciate the way in which it defines 'a function'. The roots of the concept draw from the perception that human needs can be ordered hierarchically. The most basic human needs form the basis of what is meant by functions. These basic needs, such as food and health, highlight the importance placed on the material and natural needs of human beings as biological organisms. From this perspective, it may be argued that the function of human health comprises a distinct area similar to the material needs of food and sustenance. The idea is that the more basic the need, the more clearly it should be beyond politics and politicization. The argument is that people's basic physical, social, material, and mental wants and needs have to replace divided and narrow political considerations in the interest of building more prosperous and peaceful polities.

Because of the desire to keep disease out of politics, it is useful to further examine the interface between traditional politics and modern functionalist practice. It is clear that politics has a positive role to play even from the functionalist perspective. The positive role of politics consists of arguments, disagreements, and debates that do not disturb rational expertise. Politics, in this respect, consists of the capability and willingness to act to establish and maintain the separation of politics in a more negative sense and the function of public health. For example, the willingness to invest in global vaccination programmes reflects the positive role that politics can play in order to enable experts to do their work. Politicians can allocate the necessary resources for functional areas and to experts. Such positive politics establishes and maintains the institutional framework for any effective functional expertise. Besides being connected with important institutional arrangements, public health work involves a more mundane, yet equally necessary, role for politics—one has to choose the personnel to work in the functional field, allocate money for the building of offices and laboratories, finance large-scale inspection programmes, and so on. Often, this seems rather clear-cut and straightforward, but, as the controversies over stem cell research illustrate, there is no guarantee that these decisions can be left to the public health experts themselves. As long as the justifications and reasons are based on common rational interest, this role of politics is not seen as harmful even when it results in low levels of disagreement so long as they do not result in the paralysis of expertise. The politics internal to a functional field is perceived in a similar way. Experts can argue over the best course of action in maintaining public health. Even though the public perception is usually one of there being only a single best course of action, there usually exist multiple ways in which a problem can be solved. The belief is that this type of expert 'politics' is instrumental and even necessary for the advancement of right and effective programmes. Scientific debates, disagreements, and compromises are not in themselves seen as political in the negative sense of the word. From the functionalist perspective, negative politics, therefore, involves failure to control a disease because the protective barriers and borders between functions and politics are dangerously crossed. What this means is that negative politics is in many respects synonymous with diseases themselves as when Chinese secrecy was seen as a factor in the initial spread of SARS and COVID-19. The controlling of diseases and maintaining of public health has a lot to do with the ability to keep negative politics out of the functional field so that it cannot 'pollute' common interests. In this context, it should be noted that attempts to ignore, bypass, and deny politics lead easily into technocratic naivety as the way in which a particular perception of a disease influences a whole gamut of responses ranging from people's reactions to the way in which governments and institutions continuously reassess their situation awareness.

Even a cursory look at the COVID-19 outbreak, to cite just one pandemic example, reveals that different actors have their own at least partly incompatible goals, and it also illuminates how the politics of health will defy any attempts to differentiate between positive and negative forms of politicization. The key point of contention is the origin of the disease. However, it remains doubtful that it will be conclusively resolved. While the origin is being disputed and becoming part of power political games, the mutating disease itself becomes more mysterious. Nobody knows for sure where it came from and in what direction its variants are developing. Similarly, the global vaccination effort had a slow start as developed nations were quick to herd the vaccines for their own use. A sense of global injustice prevailed, and this is going to be one of the lingering consequences of COVID-19. Main issues and side challenges are mushrooming in ways that are uncontained and cannot be resolved by the functional approach alone.

The public health framework has gained some independence from the state system, and it has the proven ability to capture people's sympathies, which cannot be tapped in their totality by a state-centric world view. At the mythological level, the transnational spirit of public health has some protagonist figures that draw identification, respect, and a sense of awe. These figures inspire and embody to a degree the otherwise technocratic, abstract character of global public health. In moving beyond, the protagonists and their imageries provide clues to how global public health can be independently embodied. Usually, these protagonist heroes suffer adverse circumstances while they carry on with the healing activity and reform mission. These heroic figures are humanitarian because of the pain they endure for the sake of helping others. However, they are figures that can at times represent the nodal point between the individual's and humanity's embodiments relatively unmediated by national hagiographies and narratives. The present-day gallery of such figures include, in addition to the aid workers in distant places, doctors who break government codes of secrecy and scientists who try to develop new cures. It is at this level that the cosmopolitan framings of global public health can find their heroic embodiments and offer some substantive alternative to the traditional political embodiments. The gallery of heroic inventors—such as Koch and Pasteur—can become articulated as a gallery of human progress in general, instead of national manifest destiny. However, in today's highly polarized and power political climate, the protagonists for humanity are also usually contested and controversial figures. For example, the key figures that played leading roles in the US pandemic control institutions were dragged into deep politicization in the context of the 2020 US presidential elections.

Thus, there are some notable hero figures in pandemic spectacles. The heroism of unselfish other-interested health-care workers and the diligent hard work of the officials of the various public health agencies are often noted in pandemic narratives. These figures are made to stand out above the political realm in a pantheon reserved for the heroes and martyrs of humanity. The hagiography of humanity, as defined in the public health discourse, includes some exceptional people who died fighting pandemics and whose memory is commemorated in many places—in the media, on the internet, and in journals—that are receptive to the idea of a humanity that transcends national states. One such notable figure was that of Dr Carlo Urbani who died fighting SARS. The eulogy for Urbani carried in the *New England Journal of Medicine* (Reilley *et al.* 2003: 1951) of 15 May 2003 is telling. It makes a revealing statement: 'In some ways, the SARS outbreak in Hanoi is a story of what can go right, of public health's coming before politics'. Similarly, in January 2020, Chinese doctor Li Wenliang became a hero when he alerted others on the uncontained SARS-like outbreak. He was admonished for making 'false' statements by the Chinese authorities and died of COVID-19 in early February 2020. These examples reveal the difficulties faced by the transnational community and its protagonists in the face of complex physical and political events.

Public health is taken as a higher-order realm that should at least in emergency situations prevail over political considerations. The eulogy for Urbani continues by pointing out the importance and also the risks involved in being part of the first line of defence in public health:

> First-line health-care providers quickly alerted the WHO of an atypical pneumonia. Dr Urbani recognized the severity of the public health threat. Immediately, the WHO requested an emergency meeting on Sunday, March 9, with the Vice Minister of Health of Vietnam. Dr Urbani's temperament and intuition and the strong trust he had built with Vietnamese authorities were critical at this juncture. The four-hour discussion led the government to take the extraordinary steps of quarantining the Vietnam French Hospital, introducing new infection-control procedures in other hospitals, and issuing an international appeal for expert assistance. Additional specialists from the WHO and the Centers for Disease Control and Prevention (CDC) arrived on the scene, and Médecins sans Frontières (MSF, or Doctors without Borders) responded with staff members as well as infection-control suits and kits that were previously stocked for outbreaks of Ebola virus.

The personal efforts of Urbani are seen as instrumental in the efforts of various public health agencies to realize the grave nature of the situation and in getting the political officials in Vietnam to allow for the introduction of public health-driven policies. The eulogy ends by stressing the pride that the medical community feels in the heroic deeds of Urbani:

> [I]t is clear that Dr Urbani's decisive and determined intervention has bought precious time and saved lives. We remember Dr Urbani with a mixture of pride in his selfless devotion to medicine and unspeakable grief about the void his departure has left in the hearts of his colleagues around the world.

Public health embraces a form of humanity-based political theology. The corresponding heroes' gallery and hagiography can provide clues to the particular ways in which the pandemic narrative proceeds. These prototypical figures empower individuals and organizations that are seen fighting the pestilence in ways that give them political clout and agency. However, despite these progressive heroes and functionalist ideology, the power of the public health narratives still captures our attention and holds us captive to the state-centric figure galleries and political theologies.

Thus, it is difficult to conceive of pandemic scares' public health dramas without taking into account the traditional value placed on the dramas of 'containment' and on the efforts 'to contain'. Cultural geographer Yi-Fu Tuan, in his book, *Landscapes of Fear* (1979: 6), argues that much of human activity is directed at constructing material and conceptual technologies to secure human existence free from what he calls chaos: 'In a sense, every human construction whether mental or material is a component in a landscape of fear because it exists to contain chaos'. This is especially pertinent to the conceptual configurations of political theory and international thought. Both can be seen as traditions that aim to contain the effects of insecurity, anarchy, and injustice in and between polities. Thucydides saw politics as an activity aimed at maintaining and, if possible, expanding the most human of spaces, political space, against the mechanistic ideas of necessity and absence of alternatives—the 'might is right' type of thinking—and against the accidental qualities of complex human-to-human or human-to-nature relationships—for example, passions of the moment. He saw war and plague as factors that constricted the political space to the point of hysteria, factionalism, and lack of deliberation. Defined from this perspective, politics turns into a supportive construction aiming at the creation of healthy political communities. Thucydides seems to suggest how shared memories and the shared beliefs embedded in them contribute to the emergence of a consensual communal realm of persuasibility (Cogan 1980: 168). This resource is seen as vital for governability because any significant splits in communal together-mindedness may lead to the possibility of potentially disastrous whimsical and erratic actions. From this classical perspective, it can be stated that political rhetoric and deliberation are seen as being based on the existence and on the continuous rediscovery of the area of together-mindedness: The mission of political rhetoric is not to persuade but to rediscover and reinvent the underlying persuasive element (Entralgo 1970: 177). Communal together-mindedness can be seen as a playground of alikeness and contrast in a way that leads to likeliness and predictability when it comes to the future course of the community. This classical background may be seen as foregrounding the more modern ideas concerning building containment-oriented frameworks that constrain the perceived sources of erratic, accidental, and chaotic actions and events. However, these classical ideals place much emphasis on the need to safeguard the realm of political deliberation against haste and hyperbole.

Throughout this book, I have highlighted how the modern public health frame's manifest technocratic and expert-centric modalities are easily overshadowed by the cryptic language and practices of the considerably older discourse of intertwined plagues and power. One of the most prominent reasons why the explicitly medical and epidemiological language of the contemporary global health community inevitably borrows from these older signifiers is the basic reality that its disease language is fully embodied with complex appealing polysemy. The centuries of interaction between diseases and politics have produced a mutually resonating object world that enables discussing political processes as disease-like processes and discussing physical diseases in terms of hostile enemies against whom it is possible to wage wars. Because abstract knowledge of global public health cannot resonate with such historically embedded meanings, it is bound to resort to using quasi-political language. This public health language insinuates, suggests and says indirectly things that are pertinent to the lives of people in their political embeddings. Let us consider an obvious example of this need to embody and anchor the abstract medical realms. This context is made apparent by descriptions of how the human immunity system functions:

> White blood cells are responsible for protecting the body from invasion by foreign substances such as bacteria and viruses. The majority of white blood cells are produced in the bone marrow, where they outnumber red blood cells by 2 to 1. However, in the bloodstream, there are about 600 red blood cells for every white blood cell. There are several types of white blood cells. Granulocytes and macrophages protect against infection by surrounding and destroying invading bacteria and viruses, and lymphocytes aid in the immune defence. Granulocytes are prepared by apheresis or by centrifugation of whole blood. They are transfused within 24 hours after collection and are used for infections that are unresponsive to antibiotic therapy.

This prototypic account, which imagines a system of human immunological defence against 'invading' disease agents, is from the webpage of the American Red Cross.[4] The language of political enmity makes the internal workings of human physiology more tangible by comparing it to the military response against an invading foreign army. Furthermore, the workings of the human body are understood to be relating to a system in which the 'reds' are the nutrient-carrying workers defended by the guardian 'whites'. The respective roles of the whites and reds are given meanings that remind us of the societal roles of owners and labourers during the time when white blood cells were first discovered and described at the turn of the twentieth century. From this perspective, the accounts of human immunology draw from conservative political visions of ideal harmony. These accounts turn the descriptions of the hard-to-understand invisible world into stimulating and easy-to-grasp imageries. One should note that the borrowings from the world of politics into the world of immunology are not merely descriptive. Some of the ideological content of the political world also gets transferred into the world inside the human bloodstream. Organized and systematized knowledge/power configurations access the world of expert and scientific knowledge. A representative quote from a scientific journal further underscores this tendency:

> An academic domain is established when the knowledge within is systematized. We have acquired knowledge by conquering the evils that have attacked and threatened humankind. In the case of germs, humans identified them and invented methods to control them. But more importantly, the experiences of fighting against various diseases were collected and systematized into the academic field of bacteriology. The knowledge systematized into an academic field can never be lost through the generations, and it can be readily utilized by anyone thereafter.
>
> *(Yoshikawa 1999: 1)*

The notion of scientific progress often narrates itself in terms of an increasingly successful and carefully planned and executed military campaign. The demonstration of the authority of scientific knowledge draws from a theatre of proof whereby expert knowledge authority is revealed rather than cognitively and intellectually proven. Such revelatory demonstrations would be harder to come by without the existence of the plague and power template.

Similarly, accounts of pandemic challenges share the same dramaturgy as the defence of the contemporary world order against its visions of enemies in the so-called rogue elements that are 'spreading' through failed and failing polities. This dramaturgy is as ancient as it is embodied. For example, Hippocrates' medical models were embodied in the narrative form that Thucydides utilized in his *History of the Peloponnesian War*, and Hippocrates can be argued to have borrowed from the political theories of his own time. From this perspective, it is not surprising that this shared cultural form is omnipresent in contemporary pandemic imageries and in their interpretations by political authorities. Let's consider another example of the ideological underpinnings of the plague to power nexus: the PEPFAR in the US aimed to alleviate the plight of those suffering from HIV and AIDS in Africa. Africa, as the world's perceived periphery, became a signifier of the dismal state of affairs and a bad omen of things to come in the 1990s. This connection made the pestilences in the hierarchical world order's periphery hyperbolic and anticipated.

With increasing and accelerated global connectedness, the periphery is no longer a place only for demonstrating Western goodness through acts of charity, healing, and humanitarianism. The periphery's conditions, disorders, and diseases have been worried about and turned into prognoses for the future. Deriving from this perspective, there was a lot of prestige to be derived from 'curative' and containing actions in Africa. Former US President George W. Bush used the Lazarus miracle allegory of Christianity to point out how PEPFAR, an American initiative, could bring the African people back from certain death in his speech on Africa and AIDS on 29 April 2003. His explicit reference was to the new HIV and AIDS policies of the US, which 'gave hope' to the otherwise doomed people of Africa:

> There are only two possible responses to suffering on this scale. We can turn our eyes away in resignation and despair, or we can take decisive, historic action to turn the tide against this disease and give hope of life to millions who need our help now. The United States of America chooses the path of action and the path of hope.

In the same speech, Bush drew an explicit connection between the high political agenda and AIDS:

> We believe that everyone has a right to liberty, including the people of Afghanistan and Iraq. We believe that everyone has a right to life, including the children in the cities and villages of Africa and the Caribbean.

The Lazarus allegory refers to such concrete instances of helping to save people as well as the more abstract ability to set people free from oppression and death. However, the Lazarus allegory also has the effect of designating the US as an almost sacred community—that of the helper and the healer. In the context of the African HIV and AIDS disaster, Bush assumes the high role of a sacred benefactor. While highlighting the near messianic role of the sole superpower in the world today, he points out the moral roots of HIV and AIDS in Africa: the lack of the right types of values and social practices, rather than the rampant social exclusion, marginalization, and economic destitution of sub-Saharan Africa.[5] The Bush administration's eagerness to concentrate on the ABC (abstinence, be faithful, and correct and consistent condom use) approach to HIV and AIDS revealed the promotion of 'right' morals as the proper method of fighting the spread of the syndrome. What the US administration was spreading was not medical know-how, but the values it thought were the proper bases of a sustainable way of life.[6] It also gave a prominent role to the various faith-based organizations fighting HIV and AIDS. The story of Lazarus is one of conversion and production of belief. Akin to this, the Bush administration's policy on HIV and AIDS in Africa, through its emphasis on the role of abstinence and marital fidelity, designated the moral community that Africa should join in order to fight HIV and AIDS successfully. This example indicates how

HIV/AIDS was translated into an eradication programme in Africa. It needed to be made societally and ideologically understandable. Even any seemingly expert-driven programme has to be based on consensus over the underlying values and over what constitutes a proper programme in the first place.

The points which are taken by relevant actors as persuasive and based on which some knowledge becomes acknowledged are also the starting points of the eradication and containment policies of international functional organizations such as the WHO. The larger context of arriving at such consensus is moulded by the overall contemporaneous processes. The values and ideologies inherent in the zeitgeist inevitably spill over onto the global public health efforts because, in the absence of addressing these processes, any talk about pandemics would not be coherent or persuasive. Pandemics as frames are extremely real. However, this sense of realness does not necessarily have to do with our perception of them as being factual in the sense of our ideas of them corresponding with the state of affairs in the physical world. Some have claimed that pandemics are not such a hyperbolic threat as they are made out to be:

> [The pandemic worst-case scenario] makes good press copy, attracts TV cameras, and raises grant funding. Are influenza pandemics likely? Possibly, except for the preposterous mortality rate that has been proposed. Inevitable? No, not with global warming and increasing humidity, improved animal husbandry, better epizootic control, and improving vaccines. This does not have the inevitability of shifting tectonic plates or volcanic eruptions. Pandemics, if they occur, will be primarily from respiratory tract pathogens capable of airborne spread. They can be quickly blunted by vaccines, if administrative problems associated with their production, distribution, and administration are promptly addressed and adequately funded.
>
> *(Kilbourne 2009: 218)*

The threat posed by pandemics appears persuasive and factual because the pandemic frame and cultural form fits well with other ideas of threat that are pertinent. Different worst-case scenarios lend mutual support to each other. Pandemics are believable because they allow for the articulation and addressing of more generalized fears and anxieties. They provide a speculative locus for envisioning 'better' global societies that are 'prepared' and 'resilient'.

Thus, it is possible to see how ideologies play a role in public health efforts and how public health promotes political visions to defeat dystopian pandemic threats. The threat posed by pandemic diseases is accented and hyperbolized partly because it is 'the standard operating procedure' in the present global polity, which faces many anxieties connected with the global lowering of borders. However, as has been pointed out through this book, there is nothing inherently new or surprising in this. Diseases have always allowed for the effective articulation of political dystopias. They have always been played up if knowledge about them has not been able to be played down and suppressed. Diseases are relevant as one of the foremost grounds of political imageries and loci of the normative shoulds and should-nots. However, pandemic imageries' political uses have been altered recently due to the processes of globalization. The global lowering of boundaries and barriers has created a more interconnected world. Although this process is generally seen as a preferred change, much hesitation and worry remain. Pandemic speculation provides a high reading on the Richter scale of global fears. At the same time, much of the overall substance remains shared. Pandemics rehearse the prominent themes when it sees threats arising from the failed and failing places of the world. The good practice stories concerning mutating disease elements that penetrate borders resonate well with the ontological imageries of the geopolitics of our times and make ideally comprehensible the dangers of a seamless global order and point to the need to create as yet an elusive resilient global order. The ideal comprehensibility of pandemics comes with a political message—they do political work and mobilize resources for this purpose.

Thus, it is possible to redefine pandemics differently from how they are usually used in speculative scenarios about the 'coming plague'. Talk about pandemics represents a re-examination of contemporary ways of articulating pain and also of the ways in which pains and fears of pandemics articulate the modern global experience. People's everyday beliefs, values, and practices concerning different scenarios of pain and suffering contain an important power-political modality. The fears and pains involved in one of the most global ways of suffering—pandemics—give deeply sensible coherence to the ways of feeling globality and flows of power in the global space. Pandemics arouse fear of immediate danger for the people living in the Global North, yet they also narrate stories of the obvious health disparities between the Global North and South. The globally constituted existence exerts considerable influence on individual-level suffering and anxieties and opens new avenues of sensing and feeling global worries in bodily ways. The social construction of pandemics registers the many fears and anxieties felt by the perceived distortions and transgressions of the contemporary world. Because of this, pandemics can also be reframed to embody the complexities entailed in ethical subjectivity and right actions. This realization that pandemics are political and embodied may allow for their repossession to be parts of lived life in an empowering and democratic way. They are not hyperbolic and sublime; in fact, people's fears of them are anything but lofty and mythological.

Notes

1 See also Wittgenstein (1968: 378).
2 A language game ties words together with simple actions and things: '[T]he term, "language game", is meant to bring into prominence the fact that the speaking of language is part of an activity or of a form of life' (Wittgenstein 1968: 34).
3 Jain and Jain (2005).
4 www.redcrossalabama.org/all.htm. Accessed 10 April 2009.

5 The root causes of most violent epidemics can be traced to the multilevel political structures and dynamics which provide the macro-level context for the disease-causing agents
(Fassin 2007; Farmer 2004; Joralemon 1997).

6 Western public health discourse appears to use the tropes of 'lifestyle' and way of life'
to articulate the broader, more encompassing normative vision that accounts for social,
economic, and political structures (Tesh 1988: 99).

REFERENCES

Aaltola, Mika (1999) 'International epidemics: A short expedition to places inhabited by states and mad cows', *Medicine, Conflict and Survival*, 15(3): 235–54.

———— (2005) 'The international airport: The hub-and-spoke pedagogy of the American empire', *Global Networks*, 5(3): 261–78.

———— (2008) *Sowing the Seeds of Sacred: Political Religion of Contemporary World Order and American Era*, Leiden: Brill.

———— (2009) *Western Spectacles of Governance and the Emergence of Humanitarian World Order*, London: Palgrave Macmillan.

———— (2012a) *Understanding the Politics of Pandemic Scares: An Introduction to Global Politosomatics*, London: Routledge.

———— (2012b) 'Contagious insecurity: War, SARS and global air mobility', *Contemporary Politics*, 18(1): 53–70.

———— (2020) *Democratic Vulnerability and Autocratic Meddling: The 'Thucydidean Brink' in Regressive Geopolitical Competition*, London: Palgrave Macmillan.

Aaltola, Mika, Ketola, Johanna, Peltonen, Aada and Vaakanainen, Karoliina (2021) 'An abrupt awakening to the realities of a pandemic: Learning lessons from the onset of Covid-19 in the EU and Finland', FIIA Briefing Paper 112. Online. Available HTTP: < https://www.fiia.fi/en/publication/an-abrupt-awakening-to-the-realities-of-a-pandemic> (accessed 3 March 2021).

Abbate, C. (2016) ' "Higher" and "lower" political animals: A critical analysis of Aristotle's account of the political animal', *Journal of Animal Ethics*, 6(1): 54–66.

Agamben, G. (1998) *Homo Sacer: Sovereign Power and Bare Life*, Stanford: Stanford University Press.

Alaszewski, A. (2021) *COVID-19 and Risk: Policy Making in a Global Pandemic*, Bristol: Bristol University Press.

Ali, A., Chen, Y., Johnson, J. *et al.* (2011) 'Recent clonal origin of cholera in Haiti', *Emerging Infectious Diseases*, 17(4): 699–701.

Ali, S.H. and Keil, R. (2006) 'Multiculturalism, racism and infectious disease in the global city: The experience of the 2003 SARS outbreak in Toronto', *Topia*, 16: 23–49.

Allard, James and Martin, Mathew (2009) *Staging Pain 1580–1800*, London: Ashgate.

Allison, Graham (2017) *Destined for War: Can America and China Escape Thucydides's Trap?* New York: Houghton Mifflin Harcourt.

Altenstetter, C. (1994) 'European Union response to AIDS/HIV and policy networks in the ore-Maastricht era', *Journal of European Public Policy*, 1–3: 413–40.

Alteri, C., Cento, V., Piralla, A. *et al.* (2021) 'Genomic epidemiology of SARS-CoV-2 reveals multiple lineages and early spread of SARS-CoV-2 infections in Lombardy, Italy', *Nature Communications*, 12, article no. 434. https://doi.org/10.1038/s41467-020-20688-x.

Amnesty International (2021) 'Amnesty international report 2020/21', Online. Available HTTP: < https://www.amnesty.org/download/Documents/POL1032022021ENGLISH.PDF> (accessed 23 March 2021).

Anderlini, Jamil (2020) 'Xi Jinping faces China's Chernobyl moment', *Financial Times*, 10 February. Online. Available HTTP: < https://www.ft.com/content/6f7fdbae-4b3b-11ea-95a0-43d18ec715f5>

Andersen, K.G., Rambaut, A., Lipkin, W.I. *et al.* (2020) 'The proximal origin of SARS-CoV-2', *Nature Medicine*, 26: 450–2.

Andrus, J.K., Aguilera, X., Oliva, O. *et al.* (2010) 'Global health security and the international health regulations', *BMC Public Health*, 10(S2).

Annas, G. (1999) 'The impact of health policies on human rights_ AIDS and TB control', in J. Mann, M. Grodin, S. Griskin and G. Annas (eds), *Health and Human Rights: A Reader*, London: Routledge.

Appian (2000) *Wars of the Romans in Iberia*, J. Richardson (ed), Liverpool: Liverpool University Press.

Baccini, L., Brodeur, A. and Weymouth, S. (2021) 'The COVID-19 pandemic and the 2020 US presidential election', *Journal of Population Economics*, 34: 739–67.

Baker, H. and Ridley, R. (1996) 'What went wrong in BSE? From prion disease to public disaster', *Brain Research Bulletin*, 40(4): 237–44.

Barbarossa, C. (2018) 'Consumer reactions to food safety scandals: A research model and moderating effects', in A. Gray and R. Hinch (eds), *A Handbook of Food Crime: Immoral and Illegal Practices in the Food Industry and What to Do about Them*, Bristol: Bristol University Press.

Barnes, B. (1995) *The Elements of Social Theory*, London: UCL Press.

Barr, Robert (1962) 'The two cities in Saint Augustine', *Laval théologique et philosophique*, 18(2): 211–29.

Barr, Stephen (1964) *Experiments in Topology*, New York: Thomas Y. Crowell Co.

Barsalou, L.W. (1999) 'Perceptual symbol systems', *Behavioral and Brain Science*, 22(4): 577–660.

Bartelson, Jens (1998) 'Second natures: Is the state identical with itself?', *European Journal of International Relations*, 4(3): 295–326.

Barthes, R. (1980) *Mythologies*, New York: Hill and Wang.

Benini, Aldo and Bradford, Janet (1995) 'Ebola strikes the global village: The virus, the media, the organized response'. Online. Available HTTP: <http://adder.colorado.edu/~hazctr/benini.htm>.

Bever, Edward (2000) 'Witchcraft fears and psychosocial factors in disease', *Journal of Interdisciplinary History*, xxx(4): 573–90.

Biden, J.R. (2021) 'Remarks by President Biden on the American jobs plan', 31 March. Online. Available HTTP: <www.whitehouse.gov/briefing-room/speeches-remarks/2021/03/31/remarks-by-president-biden-on-the-american-jobs-plan/> (accessed 3 May 2021).

Bloomberg (2020) 'The Coronavirus may be "disease X" health experts warned about', 22 February. Online. Available HTTP: < https://www.bloombergquint.com/business/coronavirus-may-be-the-disease-x-health-agency-warned-about> (accessed 12 December 2021).

Bolder, Patrick (2020) *COVID-19 and World Peace: An Overture to a New Era or Business as Usual?* Hague: Hague Centre for Strategic Studies.

Bollyky, Thomas J. (2021) 'A year out: Addressing international impacts of the COVID-19 pandemic', Council on Foreign Relations. Online. Available HTTP: <www.cfr.org/report/year-out-addressing-international-impacts-covid-19-pandemic> (accessed 3 May 2021).

Boroditsky, L. (2000) 'Metaphoric stucturing: Understanding time through spatial metaphors', *Cognition*, 75: 1–28.

Bowen, J. and Laroe, C. (2006) 'Airline networks and the international diffusion of severe acute respiratory syndrome (SARS)', *The Geographical Journal*, 172(2): 130–44.

Brantlinger, Patrick (1985) 'Victorians and Africans: The genealogy of the myth of the dark continent', *Critical Inquiry*, 12(1): 166–203.

Bronfen, Elisabeth (1998) *The Knotted Subject: Hysteria and Its Discontents*, Princeton, NJ: Princeton University Press.

Brown, C. (1987) 'Thucydides, Hobbes, and the derivation of anarchy', *History of Political Thought*, 8(1): 33–62.

Brown, Peter (1965) 'Saint Augustine', in Beryl Smalley (ed), *Trends in Medieval Political Thought*, Oxford: Blackwell.

Brown, Peter (1980) *The Cult of the Saints: Its Rise and Function in Latin Christianity*, Chicago, IL: University of Chicago Press.

Brunt, P. (1967) 'Thucydides and human irrationality', *Classical Review,* 17(3): 278–80.

Bryant, R.C. (2021) 'Localism', in *Governance for a Higgledy-Piggledy Planet: Crafting a Balance Between Local Autonomy and External Openness*, Washington, DC: Brookings Institution Press.

Burns, B., Busby, C. and Sawchuk, K. (1999) *When Pain Strikes*, Minneapolis, MN: University of Minnesota Press.

Byerly, C. (2010) 'The U.S. military and the influenza pandemic of 1918–1919', *Public Health Reports*, 125(3): 82–91.

Caballero, M. (2005) 'SARS in Asia: Crisis, vulnerabilities and regional responses', *Asian Survey,* 45(3): 475–95.

CANSO (2015) 'Seamless ATM workshop'. Online. Available HTTP: <www.canso.org/sites/default/files/03%20-%20Airport%20Role%20in%20Support%20of%20Seamless%20Sky%20-%20Mr%20SL%20Wong,%20ACI.pdf>.

Caporaso, J.A. (1997) 'Across the great divide: Integrating comparative and international politics', *International Studies Quarterly*, 41(4): 563–92.

Carlowe, Jo (2010) 'Coming to Haiti's aid', *Nursing Standard*, 25(14): 19–22.

Carmichael, Ann G. (1986) *Plague and the Poor in Rennaissance Florence*, Cambridge: Cambridge University Press.

Carver, C.S. (1998) 'Resilience and thriving: Issues, models, and linkages', *Journal of Social Issues*, 54(2): 245–66.

Castelli, C. (2008) 'Obama adviser urges public-private teaming to tackle bioterror', *Inside the Pentagon*, 24(43): 3–4.

Catanach, I. (2001) 'The "globalization" of disease? India and the plague', *Journal of World History*, 12(1): 131–53.

CDC (2020) 'CDC advises travelers to avoid all nonessential travel to China', 28 January. Online. Available HTTP: <www.cdc.gov/media/releases/2020/s0128-travelers-avoid-china.html> (accessed 3 May 2021).

Chapman, C.R. and Wyckoff, Margo (1981) 'The problem of pain: A psychobiological approach', in S. Haynes and L. Gannon (eds), *Psychosomatic Disorders: A Psychophysiological Approach to Etiology and Treatment*, New York: Praeger.

Cheng-Chia, Tung and Yang, Allan (2020) 'How China is remaking the UN in its own image', *The Diplomat*. Online. Available HTTP: <https://thediplomat.com/2020/04/how-china-is-remaking-the-un-in-its-own-image/> (accessed 3 May 2021).

Child, R. (2014) 'Two models of the global order', *Public Affairs Quarterly*, 28(3): 197–214.

Chiu, Remi (2017) *Plague and Muci in the Renaissance*, Cambridge: Cambridge University Press.

Cioffi, Frank (2010) 'Overviews: What are they of and what are they for?', in W. Day and V. Krebs (eds), *Seeing Wittgenstein Anew*, Cambridge: Cambridge University Press.

Cipolla, C. (1979) *Faith, Reason, and the Plague: A Tuscan Story of the Seventeeth Century*, Brighton: The Harvest Press Ltd.

Cipolla, C. (1981) *Fighting Plague in Seventeeth-Century Italy*, Madison: University of Wisconsin Press.

Clark, C., Foster, E. and Hallett, J. (eds) (2015) *Kinesis: The Ancient Depiction of Gesture, Motion, and Emotion*, Ann Arbor: University of Michigan Press.

Clark, Candace (1987) 'Sympathy biography and sympathy marginb,' *American Journal of Sociology*, 83: 290–321.

Clark, Ian (1989) *The Hierarchy of States: Reform and Resistance in the International Order*, Cambridge: Cambridge University Press.

Cliff, A., Smallman-Raynor, M., Haggett, P., Stoup, D. and Thacker, S. (2009) *Infectious Diseases: Emergence and Re-Emergence: A Geographical Analysis*, Oxford: Oxford University Press.

Cogan, Marc (1980) *The Human Thing*, Chicago, IL: University of Chicago Press.

Collinge, J. (2012) 'The risk of prion zoonoses', *Science*, 335(6067): 411–13.

COM (2005) *On Strengthening Coordination on Generic Preparedness Planning for Public Health Emergencies at EU Level*, Brussells: Commission of the European Communities.

Connor, Walter Robert (1984) *Thucydides*, London: Princeton University Press.

Cooke, Jennifer (2009) *Legacies of Plague in Literature, Theory and Film*, London: Palgrave-Macmillan.

Craik, E.M. (2001) 'Thucydides on the plague: Physiology of flux and fixation', *Classical Quarterly*, 51(1): 102–8.

Crang, M. (2002) 'Between places: Producing hubs, flows and networks', *Environment and Planning A*, 34: 569–74.

Cravioto, A., Lanata, C.F. and Lantagne, D.S. (2011) 'Final report of the independent panel of experts on the cholera outbreak in Haiti'. Online. Available HTTP: <https://static1.squarespace.com/static/54694fa6e4b0eaec4530f99d/t/54d75728e4b05ca7b54f2292/1423398696771/UN+Report+on+Haitian+cholera+epidemic.pdf> (accessed 3 May 2021).

Crawford, D. (2007) *Deadly Companion: How Microbes Shape Our History*, Oxford: Oxford University Press.

Crawford, Neta (2000) 'The passion of world politics: Propositions on emotion and emotional relationships', *International Security*, 24(4): 116–56.

Crosse, M. and Gootnick, D. (2007) *Influenza Pandemic: Efforts under Way to Address Constraints on Using Ativirals and Vaccines to Forestall a Pandemic*, Darby: Diane Publishing Co.

Curtin, Philip D. (1964) *The Image of Africa: British Ideas and Action, 1780–1850,* Madison: University of Wisconsin Press.

Daddow, O. (2012) 'The UK media and "Europe": From permissive consensus to destructive dissent', *International Affairs (Royal Institute of International Affairs 1944–),* 88(6): 1219–36.

Dahlberg, Charles (1988) *The Literature of Unlikeness,* London: University Press of New England.

Daileda, D.A. (2008) 'America on the move', in N. Solomon and R. Ivey (eds), *Architecture: Celebrating the Past, Designing the Future,* New York: Visual Reference Publications.

Dalby, Simon (1996) 'The environment as geopolitical threat: Readind Robert Kaplan's *coming anarchy'*, *Ecumene,* 3(4): 472–96.

D'Andrade, R.G. (1987) 'A folk model of the mind', in D. Holland and N. Quinn (eds), *Cultural Models in Language and Thought,* Cambridge: Cambridge University Press.

Darwin, Charles (1859) *Origin of Species,* Lomdon: Murray.

Dassel, Kurt and Reinhardt, Eric (1999) 'Domestic strife and the initiation of violence at home and abroad', *American Journal of Political Sciences,* 43(1): 56–85.

Delaporte, F. (1986) *Disease and Civilization: The Cholera in Paris, 1932,* London: The MIT Press.

Desmond, W. (2006) 'Lessons of fear: A reading of Thucydides', *Classical Philology,* 101(4): 359–79.

Deudney, D. (2008) *Bounding Power: Republican Security Theory from the Polis to the Global Village,* Princeton: Princeton University Press.

Dewey, John (1958) *Experience and Nature,* New York: Dover.

——— (1980) *Art as Experience,* New York: Perigee.

Diamond, Jared (1997) *Guns, Germs, and Steel: The Fates of Human Societies,* New York: W. W. Norton & Company.

Dillon, Michael and Reid, Julian (2000) 'Global governance, liberal peace and complex emergency', *Alternatives,* 25(1): 117–43.

DiMaggio, P. (2002) 'Why cognitive (and cultural) sociology needs cognitive psychology', in K. Cerulo (ed), *Culture in Mind: Toward a Sociology of Culture and Cognition,* New York: Routledge.

Dionysius of Halicarnassus (1940) *Antiquitates Romanae,* Cambridge: Harvard University Press.

The Diplomat (2020) 'Wuhan Coronavirus: China plays the blame game', 27 January. Online. Available HTTP: < https://thediplomat.com/2020/01/wuhan-coronavirus-china-plays-the-blame-game/> (accessed 30 January 2020).

Dodge, Martin, and Kitchin, Rob (2004) 'Flying through code/space: The real virtuality of air travel', *Environment and Planning A,* 36(2): 195–211.

Dols, Michael (1974) 'The comparative communal responses to the Black death in Muslim and Christian societies', *Viator—Medieval and Renaissance Studies,* 5: 269–88.

Donelan, Michael (1978) 'The political theorists and international theory', in M. Donelan (ed), *The Reason of States: A Study in International Political Theory,* London: George Allen & Unwin.

Donelly, J. (1986) 'International human rights: A regime analysis', *International Organization,* 40(3): 599–639.

Donini, A. (2010) 'The far side: The meta functions of humanitarianism in a globalized world', *Disasters,* 34: 220–37.

Dowell, Scott and Braden, Christopher (2011) 'Implications of the introduction of cholera to Haiti', *Emerging Infectious Diseases,* 17(7): 1299–300.

Dowsett, G. (2003) 'HIV/AIDS and homophobia: Subtle hatreds, severe consequences and the question of origins', *Culture, Health & Sexuality,* 5(2): 121–36.

Duffield, M. (1998) 'NGO relief in war zones: Toward an analysis of the new aid paradigm', in T. G. Weiss (ed), *Beyond UN Subcontracting*, London: Macmillan.

Durkheim, Emile (1965) *The Elementary Forms of the Religious Life*, New York: Free Press.

Dutta, Arin (2008) *The Effectiveness of Policies to Control a Human Influenza Pandemic: A Literature Review*, Washington, DC: The World Bank Development Research Group Pwerty Team.

Eckert, E. (2000) 'The retreat of plague from Central Europe, 1640–1720: A geomedical approach', *Bulletin of the History of Medicine*, 74(1): 1–28.

Ehrenberg, Victor (1960) *The Greek State*, Oxford: Blackwell.

Elbe, Stefan (2006) 'AIDS, security, biopolitics', *International Relations*, 19(4): 403–19.

——— (2011) 'Pandemics on the radar screen: Health security, infectious disease and the medicalisation of insecurity', *Political Studies*, 59(4): 848–66.

Ellis, C. (2002) 'Shattered lives: Making sense of September 11th and its aftermath', *Journal of Contemporary Ethnography*, 31: 375–410.

Ellis, J.R. (1991) 'The structure and argument of Thucydides' archaeology', *Classical Antiquity*, 10(2): 344–76.

Ellis, R. (2001) *Vertical Margins: Mountaineering and the Landscape of Neoimperialism*, Madison: University of Wisconsin Press.

Entralgo, Lain (1970) *The Therapy of the Word in Classical Antiquity*, New Haven: Yale University Press.

Eurosurveillance (2006) 'Early containment strategy: A protocol to contain pandemic influenza when it first emerges globally', *Eurosurveillance*, 11: 13.

Evans, Richard (1992) 'Ëpidemics and revolutions: Cholera in nineteenth-century Europe', in T. Ranger and P. Slack (eds), *Epidemics and Ideas: Essays on the Historical Perception of Pestilence,* Cambridege: Cambridge University Press.

Evenett, S., Hoekman, B., Rocha, N. *et al.* (2020) 'The COVID-19 vaccine production club: Will value chains temper nationalism?' Policy Research Working Paper no. 9565, World Bank, Washington, DC. Online. Available HTTP: <https://openknowledge.worldbank.org/handle/10986/35244> (accessed 3 May 2021).

Falk, Francesca (2011) 'Hobbes' Leviathan un die aus dem Blick gefallenen Schnabelmasken', *Leviathan*, 39(2): 247–66.

Farkas, J. and Schou, J. (2020) *Post-truth, fake news and Democracy. Mapping the politics of falsehood.* New York: Routledge.

Farmer, Paul (2004) Pathologies of Power: Health, Human Rights, and the New War on the Poor, Berkley, CA: University of California Press.

Farmer, Paul (2006) *AIDS and Accusation: Haiti and Geography of Blame*, Berkeley, CA: University of California Press.

Fassin, Dider (2007) *When Bodies Remember: Experience and Politics of AIDS in South Africa*, Berkeley, CA: University of California Press.

Feldman, Ilana (2008) 'Refusing invisibility: Documentation and memorialization in Palestinian refugee claims', *Journal of Refugee Studies*, 21(4): 498–516.

Felter, C., Bussemaker, N., Persaud, S. and Speier, M. (2021) *A Guide to Global COVID-19 Vaccine Efforts*, Washington, DC: Council on Foreign Relations.

Ferguson, J. (1990) *The Anti-Politics Machine: Development, Depoliticization and Bureaucratic Power in Lesotho*, Cambridge: Cambridge University Press.

Ferguson, J. and Lohmann, L. (2016) 'The anti-politics machine: "Development" and bureaucratic power in Lesotho', in N. Haenn, R. Wilk and A. Harnish (eds), *The Environment in Anthropology: A Reader in Ecology, Culture, and Sustainable Living*, 2nd edition, New York: New York University Press.

Ferhani, Adam and Rushton, Simon (2020) 'The international health regulations, COVID-19, and bordering practices: Who gets in, what gets out, and who gets rescued?', *Contemporary Security Policy*, 41(3): 458–77.

Fidler, D.P. (2004) *SARS, Governance and the Globalization of Disease*, London: Palgrave Macmillan.

Fidler, D.P. and Gostin, L.O. (2008) *Biosecurity in the Global Age: Biological Weapons, Public Health and the Rule of Law*, Stanford: Stanford University Press.

Fiering, Norman (1976) 'Irresistible compassion: An aspect of eighteeth-century sympathy and humanitarianism', *Journal of the History of Ideas*, 37(2): 195–218.

The *Financial Times* (2020) 'Coronavirus is speeding up the decoupling of the global economies', 23 February. Online. Available HTTP: <www.ft.com/content/5cfea02e-549f-11ea-90ad-25e377c0ee1f>.

Fine, G. and Manning, P. (2003) 'Erving Goffman', in G. Ritzer (ed), *The Blackwell Companion to Major Contemporary Social Theorists, Part II,* London: Blackwell.

Finkelstein, S. and Curdt-Christiansen, C.M. (2003) 'ICAO's anti-SARS airport activities', *Aviation Space Environment Medicine*, 74(11): 1207–8.

Fiott, Daniel. and Zeiss, Marco (2021) 'The EU and Covid-19', in *Yearbook of European Security*, Paris: European Union Institute for Security Studies (EUISS).

Foreman, C. (1994) *Plagues, Products and Politics: Emergent Public Health Hazards and National Policymaking*, Washington, DC: The Brookings Institution.

Foster, E. (2009) 'The rhetoric of materials: Thucydides and Lucretius', *The American Journal of Philology*, 130(3): 367–99.

Foucault, M. (2007) *Security, Territory, Population*, London: Palgrave Macmillan.

Franko, G.F. (2009) 'Epidamnus, Thucydides, and "the comedy of errors"', *International Journal of the Classical Tradition*, 16(2): 234–40.

Freedom House (2019) 'Freedom in the world: Democracy in retreat', https://freedomhouse.org/report/freedom-world/2019/democracy-retreat (accessed 12 January 2022).

Frerichs, R.R. (2016) 'Inquiry', in *Deadly River: Cholera and Cover-Up in Post-Earthquake Haiti*, Ithaca: Cornell University Press.

Garrett, Laurie (1994) *The Coming Plague: Newly Emerging Diseases in a World Out of Balance*, New York: Farar, Straus and Giroux.

Gelpi, C. (1997) 'Democratic diversion: Governmental structure and externalization of domestic conflict', *Journal of Conflict Resolution*, 41(2): 255–82.

Ginzburg, Carlo (1990) 'Killing a Chinese mandarin: The moral implications of distance,' *Critical Inquiry*, 21(1): 46–60.

Glover, Jonathan (2000) *Humanity: A Moral History of the Twentieth Century*, New Haven: Yale University Press.

Goffman, Erving (1974) *Frame Analysis*, New York: Harper.

—— (1997) *Goffman Reader*, London: Blackwell.

Goldblatt, P. (2006) 'How John Dewey's theories underpin art and art education', *Education and Culture*, 22(1): 17–34.

Goldstein, P. (1985) 'The drugs-violence nexus: A tripartite framework', *Journal of Drug Issues*, 15: 493–506.

Gonos, George (1997) '"Situations" versus #frame": The "interactionist" and "structuralist" analyses of everyday life,' *American Sociological Review*, 42(6): 854–67.

Goodman, R. (2006) 'Humanitarian intervention and pretexts for war', *The American Journal of International Law*, 100(1): 107–41.

Gostin, L. (2014) 'Global polio eradication: Espionage, disinformation, and the politics of vaccination', *The Milbank Quarterly*, 92(3): 413–17.

Greenwood, E. (2020) 'Thucydides in times of trouble', in M. O'Rourke (ed), *A World Out of Reach: Dispatches from Life under Lockdown*, New Haven/London: Yale University Press.

The Guardian (2021) 'Influencers say Russia-linked PR agency asked them to disparage Pfizer vaccine', 25 May. Online. Available HTTP: < https://www.theguardian.com/media/2021/may/25/influencers-say-russia-linked-pr-agency-asked-them-to-disparage-pfizer-vaccine> (accessed 26 May 2021).

Guittet, E. (2017) 'Unpacking the new mobilities paradigm: Lessons for critical security studies?' in M. Leese and S. Wittendorp (eds), *Security/Mobility: Politics of Movement*, Manchester: Manchester University Press.

Gulland, A. (2012) 'Polio vaccination worker is shot and killed in Pakistan', *BMJ: British Medical Journal*, 345(7867): 6.

Gwyn, R. (1999) ' "Killer bugs," "silly burgers" and "politically correct pals": Competing discourses in health scare reporting', *Health*, 3(3): 335–46.

Gyu, Lee Dong (2021) 'The belt and road initiative after COVID: The rise of health and digital silk roads', Issue Brief, The Asan Institute for Policy Studies. Online. Available HTTP: <http://en.asaninst.org/contents/the-belt-and-road-initiative-after-covid-the-rise-of-health-and-digital-silk-roads/> (accessed 3 May 2021).

Haas, P. (1992) 'Introduction: Epistemic communities and international policy coordination', *International Organization*, 46(1): 1–35.

Hafner, M., Yerushalmi, E., Fays, C. *et al.* (2020) *COVID-19 and the Cost of Vaccine Nationalism*, Santa Monica, CA: RAND Corporation.

Hamamoto, Darrell Y. (2002) 'Empire of death: Militarized society and the rise of serial killing and mass murder', *New Political Science*, 24(1): 105–20.

Hamilton, Daniel (2004) 'Reconciling November 9 and September 11', in C. Balis and S. Serfaty (eds), *Visions of America and Europe: September 11, Iraq, and Transatlantic Relations*, Washington, DC: Center for Strategic & International Studies.

Hamilton, L.C. and Hamilton, J.D. (1983) 'Dynamics of terrorism', *International Studies Quarterly*, 27(1): 39–54.

Hardt-Mautner, G. (1995) ' "How does one become a good European?": The British press and European integration', *Discourse & Society*, 6(2): 177–205.

Hardt, M. and Negri, Antonio (2001) *Empire*, Cambridge: Harvard University Press.

Harle, V. (2000) *The Enemy with a Thousand Faces: The Tradition of the Other in Western Political Thought and History*, London: Praeger Publishers.

Harper, Kyle (2017) 'The old age of the world', in *The Fate of Rome: Climate, Disease, and the End of an Empire*, Princeton: Princeton University Press.

Harrison, Mark (1996) 'The tender frame of man: Disease, climate and racial difference in India and the West Indies, 1760–1860', *Bulletin of the History of Medicine*, 70(1): 68–93.

Hazdra, R.J. (2001) *Air Mobility the Key to the United States National Security Strategy*, Alabama: Air University Press.

Health Canada (2003) 'Learning from SARS: Renewal of public health in Canada', in *A Report of the National Advisory Committee on SARS and Public Health*, Ottawa: Health Canada.

Henson, Jayne R. and Olson, Loreen N. (2010) 'The monster within: How male serial killers discursively manage their stigmatized identities', *Communication Quarterly*, 58(3): 341–64.

Herdt, Gilbert (1992) *Gay Culture in America*, Boston: Beacon Press.

Hermann, R. and Fischerkeller, M. (1993) 'Beyond the enemy image and spiral model: Cognitive-strategic research after the cold war', *International Organization*, 49(3): 415–50.

Heymann, D. and Rodier, G. (2004) 'SARS: A global response to an international threat', *The Brown Journal of World Affairs*, 10(2): 185–97.

Hitzer, Bettina and Leon-Sanz, Pilar (2016) 'The feeling body and its diseases: How cancer went psychosomatic in twentieth-century Germany', *Osiris*, 31(1): 67–93.

Hobbes, Thomas (1982) *Leviathan*, New York: Penguin.

Holden, Robert (1986) 'The contagiousness of aircraft hijacking', *The American Journal of Sociology*, 91(4): 874–904.

Hollingsworth, T., Ferguson, N. and Anderson, R. (2007) 'Frequent travelers and rate of spread of epidemics', *Emerging Infectious Diseases*, 13(9): 1288–94.

Honingsbaum, Mark (2013) 'Regulating the 1918–19 pandemic: Flu, stoicism and the Northcliffe Press', *Medical History*, 57(2): 165–85.

Horden, Peregrine (1992) 'Disease, dragons and saints: The management of epidemics in the Dark Ages', in T. Ranger and P. Slack (eds), *Epidemics and Ideas: Essays on the Historical Perception of Pestilence*, Cambridge: Cambridge University Press.

Houston, A. (2017) 'UNstoppable: How advocates persevered in the fight for justice for Haitian cholera victims', *Health and Human Rights*, 19(1): 299–303.

Hoy, S. and Nuget, W. (1989) 'Public health or protectionism? The German-American pork war', *Bulletin of the History of Medicine*, 62: 45–52.

Huang, C., Wang, Y., Li, X. *et al.* (2020) 'Clinical features of patients infected with 2019 novel coronavirus in Wuhan, China', *The Lancet*, 395(10223): 497–506. Online. Available HTTP: <https://doi.org/10.1016/S0140-6736(20)30183-5> (accessed 3 May 2021).

Hufnagel, L., Brockmann, D. and Geisel, T. (2004) 'Forecast and control of epidemics in a globalized world', *Proceedings of the National Academy of Sciences*, 101: 15124–9.

Huntington, Samuel (1965) 'Political development and political decay', *World Politics*, 17(3): 386–430.

——— (1997) 'The erosion of American national interest', *Foreign Affairs*, 76(5): 28–49.

——— (2004) 'Hispanic challenge', *Foreign Policy*, March–April: 30–45.

——— (2005) *Who Are We? The Challenge to America's National Identity*, New York: Simon & Schuster.

Hutchison, Emma (2018) 'Emotions, bodies, and the un/making of international relations', *Millennium: Journal of International Studies*, 47(2): 284–98.

IATA (2005) 'Comments of international air transport association (IATA) on draft international health regulation'. Online. Available HTTP: <http://158.232.12.119/ihr/revisionprocess/iatacomments.pdf> (accessed).

ICAO (2011) 'Proposal to provide a framework for the next steps in establishment of Asian skies—seamless ATM in Asia/Pacific', Asia/Pacific Seamless ATM Symposium, Bangkok. Online. Available HTTP: <www.icao.int/APAC/Meetings/2011_Seamless_ATM/IATA%20Speech%20SEAMLESS%20ATM%20ASIAN%20SKIES%20-%20%20NETWORK%20MANAGEMENT.pdf> (accessed 3 May 2021).

ICAO (2019) 'Implementation of a seamless sky', 22nd Meeting of the AFI Planning and Implementation Regional Group. Online. Available HTTP: <www.icao.int/WACAF/Documents/APIRG/APIRG%2022/WPs%20-%20FINAL%20ENG/WP%2049%20%20-%20Implementation%20of%20Seamless%20Sky.pdf> (accessed 3 May 2021).

Ignatow, Gabriel (2007) 'Theories of embodied knowledge: New directions for cultural and cognitive sociology', *Journal for the Theory of Social Behaviour*, 37(2): 115–35.

Ikenberry, G.J. (2009) 'Liberal internationalism 3.0: America and the dilemmas of liberal world order', *Perspectives on Politics*, 7(1): 71–87.

The Independent Panel for Pandemic Preparedness and Response (2021) 'COVID-19: make it the last pandemic'. Online. Available HTTP: < https://theindependentpanel. org/wp-content/uploads/2021/05/COVID-19-Make-it-the-Last-Pandemic_final.pdf> (accessed 14 May 2021).

Jain, M. and Jain, S. (2005) *HIV/AIDS Media Manual India 2005*, New Delhi: The Thomson Foundation.

James, S. and Prilleltensky, I. (2002) 'Cultural diversity and mental health: Towards integrative practice', *Clinical Psychology Review*, 22(8): 1133–5.

James, William (1985) *Varieties of Religious Experience*, London: Penguin Classics.

Jasanoff, S. (1997) 'Civilization and madness: The great BSE scare of 1996', *Public Understanding of Science*, 6(3): 221–32.

Jasper, James M. (1998) 'The emotions of protest: Affective and reavtive emotions in and around social movements', *Sociological Forum*, 13(3): 397–424.

Johnson, Chalmers (2000) *Blowback: The Costs and Consequences of the American Empire*, New York: Henry Holt & Co.

Joralemon, S. (1997) 'Civilization and madness: The great BSE scare of 1996', *Public Understanding of Science*, 6(3): 221–32.

Jouanna, Jacques (2012) *Greek Medicine from Hippocrates to Galen*, Leiden: Brill.

Jung, Carl G. (1973) *On the Psychology of the Trickster-Figure: Four Archetypes*, Princeton: Princeton University Press.

Kalimtzis, Kostas (2000) *Aristotle on Political Enmity and Disease: An Inquiry into Stasis*, Albany: State University of New York Press.

Kaplan, Robert (1994) 'The coming anarchy', *The Atlantic Monthly*, 272(2): 44–76.

Kelm, Mary-Ellen (1998) *Colonizing Bodies: Aboriginal Health and Healing in British Columbia, 1900–50*, Vancouver: University of British Columbia Press.

Kemper, T.D. (1981) 'Social constructionist and positivist approaches to the sociology of emotions', *The American Journal of Sociology*, 87: 337–62.

—— (1987) 'How many emotions are there? Wedding the social and the autonomic components', *The American Journal of Sociology*, 93(2): 263–89.

—— (1991) 'Predicting emotions from social relations', *Social Psychology Quarterly*, 54: 330–42.

Kennan, George (1946) 'George Kennan's "long telegram", history and public policy program digital archive, national archives and records administration, department of state records'. Online. Available HTTP: <http://digitalarchive.wilsoncenter.org/document/ 116178> (accessed 23 December 2021).

Kilbourne, Edwin (2009) 'Plagues and pandemics: Past, present, and future', in N. Bostrom and M. Cirkovic (eds), *Global Catastrophic Risks*, Oxford: Oxford University Press.

Kilwein, J.H. (1995) 'Some historical comments on quarantine: Part one', *Journal of Clinical Pharmacy and Therapeutics*, 20: 185–7.

Ki-moon, Ban (2021) *Resolved: Uniting Nations in a Divided World' Review: Child of War to Man of Peace*, New York: Columbia University Press.

Kiple, K. (2001) 'Response to Sheldon Watts', *Journal of Social History*, 34(4): 975–6.

Kishi, R., Pavlik, M. and Jones, S. (2021) *Armed Conflict Location & Event Data Project*, Washington, DC: ACLED.

Kleinman, A. (1986) *Social Origins of Distress and Disease: Depression, Neurasthenia and Pain in Modern China*, New Haven: Yale University Press.

Kleinman, A. and Becker, A. (1998) 'Sociosomatics: The contribution of anthropology to psychosomatics', *Psychosomatic Medicine*, 60: 389–93.

Knox, H., O'Doherty, D., Vurdubakis, T. and Westrup, C. (2007) 'Rites of passage: Organization as an excess of floes', *Scandinavian Journal of Management*, 23: 265–84.

Koslowski, Rey and Kratochwil, Friedrich (1994) 'Understanding change in international politics: The Soviet empire's demise and the international system', *International Organization*, 48(2): 215–47.

Lakoff, G. and Kovecses, Z. (1987) 'The cognitive model of anger inherent in American English', in D. Holland and N. Quinn (eds), *Cultural Models in Language and Thought*, Cambridge: Cambridge University Press.

The Lancet (2010) 'As cholera returns to Haiti, blame is unhelpful', *The Lancet Infectious Diseases*, 10(12): 813.

Larrey, J.D. (1831) *Mémoire sur le cholera-morbus*, Paris: 27–33, quoted in F. Delaporte (1986) *Disease and Civilization*, London: The MIT Press.

Larson, B., Nerlich, B. and Wallis, P. (2005) 'Metaphors and biorisks: The war on infectious diseases and invasive species', *Science Communication*, 26(3): 243–68.

Latour, Bruno (1988, 1993) *The Pasteurization of France*, Cambridge: Harvard University Press.

Lebow, Richard (1981) *Between Peace and War*, Baltimore: Johns Hopkins University Press.

Lee, Debbie (1998) 'Yellow fever and the slave trade: Coleridge's *the Rime of the Ancient Mariner*', *ELH*, 65(3): 675–700.

Leng, Russell (1993) *Interstate Crisis Behavior, 1816–1980: Realism versus Reciprocity*, Cambridge: Cambridge University Press.

—— (2000) *Bargaining and Learning in Recurring Crises: The Soviet-Americal, Egyptian-Isreali, and Indo-Pakistani Rivalries*, Ann Arbor: University of Michigan Press.

Levy, Jack (1988) 'Domestic politics and war', *Journal of Interdiciplinary History*, 38(4): 653–73.

Lewis, H. (1971) *Shame and Guilt in Neurosis,* New York: International Universities Press.

Li, Richard P.Y. and Thompson, William R. (1975) 'The "coup contagion" hypothesis', *The Journal of Conflict Resolution*, 18(1): 63–88.

Lindenbaum, Shirley (2001) 'Kuru, prions, and human affairs: Thinking about epidemics', *Annual Review of Anthropology*, 30: 363–85.

Linn, J. (2018) Recent Threats to Multilateralism. *Global Journal of Emerging Market Economies*, 9(1–3), 86–113.

Longrigg, James (1992) 'Epidemics, ideas, and classical Athenian society', in T. Ranger and P. Slack (eds), *Epidemics and Ideas: Essay on the Historical Perception of Pestilence*, Cambridge: Cambridge University Press.

Loosemore, M., Raftery, J., Reilly, C. and Higgon, D. (2006) *Risk Management in Projects*, London: Routledge.

Louis, Marieke and Maertens, Lucile (2021) *Why International Organizations Hate Politics—Depoliticizing the World*, London: Routledge.

Luckhurst, Roger (2020) 'The Chinese virus', Critical Quarterly, 62(4): 54–62.

Lundborg, T. and Vaughan-Williams, N. (2011) 'Resilience, critical infrastructure, and molecular security: The excess of "life" in biopolitics', *International Political Sociology*, 5(4): 367–83.

Lutz, Catherine A. and Abu-Lughod, Lila (eds) (1990) *Language and the Politics of Emotion*, London: Cambridge University Press.

Mahy, B. and Brown, C. (2000) 'Emerging zoonoses: Crossing the species barrier', *Revue scientifique et technique*, 19(1): 33–40.

Maizland, Lindsay (2020) *How Countries Are Holding Elections During the COVID-19 Pandemic*, New York: Council on Foreign Relations.

Malkki, Liisa (1996) 'Speechless emissaries: Refugees, humanitarianism, and dehistoricization', *Cultural Anthropology*, 11(3): 377–404.

Malkki, Liisa (2002) 'News from nowhere: Mass displacement and globalized "problems of organization"', *Ethnography*, 3(3): 351–60.

Manicas, Peter (1982) 'War, stasis, and Greek thought,' *Comparative Studies in Society and History*, 24(4): 673–88.

Marlin-Bennett, Renee (2013) 'Embodied information, knowing bodies, and power', *Millennium: Journal of International Studies*, 41(3): 601–22.

Marshall-Cornwall (1967) J. *Napoleon as Military Commander*, Princeton: Van Nostrand.

Martini, M., Gazzaniga, V., Bragazzi, N. and Barberis, I. (2019) 'The Spanish influenza pandemic: A lesson from history 100 years after 1918', *Journal of Preventive Medicine and Hygiene*, 60(1).

Mayer, Arno J. (1969) 'Internal causes and purposes of war in Europe: A research assigment', *The Journal of Modern History*, 41(3): 291–303.

McCormick, Michael (2003) 'Rats, communications, and plague: Toward an ecological history', *Journal of Interdisciplinary History*, 34(1): 1–25.

McKinley, Jr, James C. (2010) 'Homeless Haitians told not to flee to U.S.', *The New York Times*, 18 January. Online. Available HTTP: <www.nytimes.com/2010/01/19/us/19refugee.html> (accessed 1 January 2021).

McNeill, William (1976) *Plagues and People,* Garden City, NY: Anchor Press/Doupleday.

Meisel, M. (2016) 'War', in *Chaos Imagined: Literature, Art, Science*, New York/Chichester: Columbia University Press.

Mellish, T., Luzmore, N. and Shahbaz, A. (2020) 'Why were the UK and USA unprepared for the COVID-19 pandemic? The systemic weaknesses of neoliberalism: A comparison between the UK, USA, Germany, and South Korea', *Journal of Global Faultlines*, 7(1): 9–45.

Ministry of Foreign Affairs of the People's Republic of China (2020) 'Foreign ministry spokesperson Hua Chunying's daily briefing online on February 3, 2020'. Online. Available HTTP: <www.fmprc.gov.cn/mfa_eng/xwfw_665399/s2510_665401/2511_665403/t1739548.shtml> (accessed 3 May 2021).

Minow, Martha (2002) *Breaking the Cycle of Hatred: Memory, Law, and Repair*, Princeton, NJ: Princeton University Press.

Mitchell, Melanie (2009) *Complexity: A Guided Tour*, Oxford: Oxford University Press.

Mojola, S. (2017) 'AIDS in Africa: Progress and obstacles', *Current History*, 116(790): 170–5.

Monoson, S.S. and Loriaux, M. (1998) 'The illusion of power and the distribution of moral norms: Thucydides? Critique of Periclean policy', *American Political Science Review*, 92(2): 285–97.

Monten, J. (2006) 'Thucydides and modern realism', *International Studies Quarterly*, 50(1): 3–25.

Mordechai, Lee, Eisenberg, Merle, Newfield, Timothy P. *et al.* (2019) 'The justinianic plague: An inconsequential pandemic?', *Proceedings of the National Academy of Sciences of the United States of America*, 116(51): 25546–54.

Morgenthau, Hans (1955) *Politics Among Nations: The Struggle for Power and Peace*, New York: Alfred Knopf.

Most, Ben and Starr, Harvey (1980) 'Diffusion, reinforcement, geopolitics, and the spread of war', *American Journal of Political Science*, 74(4): 932–46.

Mykhalovskiy, E. and Weir, L. (2006) 'The global public health intelligence network and early warning outbreak detection: A Canadian contribution to global public health', *Canadian Journal of Public Health*, 97(1): 42–4.

Nelkin, D. and Gilman, S. (1991) 'Placing blame for devastating disease', in A. Mack (ed), *In Time of Plague: The History and Social Consequences of Lethal Epidemic Disease,* New York: New York University Press.

Nerlich, Brigitte (2007) 'Media, metaphors and modelling: How the UK newspapers reported the epidemiological modelling controversy during the 2001 foot and mouth outbreak', *Science, Technology & Human Values,* 32(4): 432–57.

Noun, A. and Chyba, C. (2008) 'Biotechnology and biosecurity', in N. Bostrom and M. Cirkovic (eds), *Global Catastrophic Risk*, Oxford: Oxford University Press.

NSS (2010) 'US national security strategy', May. Online. Available HTTP: <https://obamawhitehouse.archives.gov/sites/default/files/rss_viewer/national_security_strategy.pdf> (accessed 1 January 2021).

NSS (2015) 'US national security strategy', February. Online. Available HTTP: <https://obamawhitehouse.archives.gov/sites/default/files/docs/2015_national_security_strategy_2.pdf> (accessed 1 January 2021).

NSS (2017) 'US national security strategy', December. Online. Available HTTP: <https://trumpwhitehouse.archives.gov/wp-content/uploads/2017/12/NSS-Final-12-18-2017–0905.pdf> (accessed 1 January 2021).

NYT (2020a) 'China grapples with mystery pneumonia-like illness – Beijing is racing to identify a new illness that has sickened 59 people as it tries to calm a nervous public', 6 January. Online. Available HTTP: <https://www.nytimes.com/2020/01/06/world/asia/china-SARS-pneumonialike.html> (accessed 1 January 2021).

NYT (2020b) 'The test a deadly coronavirus outbreak poses to China's leadership', 21 January. Online. Available HTTP: < https://www.nytimes.com/2020/01/21/world/asia/china-coronavirus-wuhan.html>. (Accessed 1 January 2021).

OHCHR (2016) 'Statement by Professor Philip Alston, special rapporteur on extreme poverty and human rights UN responsibility for the introduction of cholera into Haiti on 25 October 2016', UN Human Rights Office of the High Commissioner. Online. Available HTTP: <www.ohchr.org/EN/NewsEvents/Pages/DisplayNews.aspx?NewsID=20794&LangID=E> (accessed 3 May 2021).

Orwin, C. (1988) 'Stasis and plague: Thucydides on the dissolution of society', *Journal of Politics*, 50(4): 831–47.

Padmawati, Siwi and Nichter, Mark (2008) 'Community response to avian flu in Central Java, Indonesia', *Anthropology & Medicine*, 15(1): 31–51.

Palmer, R. (1982) 'Fighting the plague in seventeenth-century Italy', *Sociology of Health and Illness,* 4(3): 358–9.

Panisset, Ulysses (2000) *International Health Statecraft: Foreign Policy and Public Health in Peru's Cholera Epidemic,* Lanham: University Press of America.

Parish, Steven (2008) *Subjectivity and Suffering in American Culture: Possible Selves*, London: Palgrave-Macmillan.

Patterson, K. and Pyle, G. (1991) 'The geography and mortality of the 1918 influenza pandemic', *Bulletin of the History of Medicine*, 65(1): 4–21.

Peer, A. (2015) 'Julius Caesar and the Roman *stasis*', *Hermathena*, 199: 71–92.

Perry, G. (2002) 'Huntington and his critics: The West and Islam', *Arab Studies Quarterly*, 24(1): 31–48.

Petit-Goâve, Carrefour, Canapé Vert, Léogane and Haitian Red Cross Psychological Support Programme (2010) 'Cholera outbreak: Note on community beliefs, feelings and perceptions'. Online. Available HTTP: <http://haiti.humanitarianresponse.info/LinkClick.aspx?link=HRC+PSP+-+Cholera+beliefs+and+perceptions.pdf&tabid=77&mid=860&language=en-US> (accessed 10 April 2010).

Piarroux, R., Barrais, R., Faucher, B. *et al.* (2011) 'Understanding the cholera epidemic, Haiti', *Emerging Infectious Diseases*, 17(7): 1161–8.

Pijpers, R. (2006) ' "Help! The poles are coming": Narrating a contemporary moral panic', *Geografiska Annaler, Series B, Human Geography*, 88(1): 91–103.

Pillinger, Mara (2020) 'Virus travel bans are inevitable but ineffective', *Foreign Policy*, 20 February. Online. Available HTTP: <https://foreignpolicy.com/2020/02/23/virus-travel-bans-are-inevitable-but-ineffective/> (accessed 1 May 2020).

Plutarch (2010) *Select Lives by Plutarch, viz. Pericles, Pelopidas, Aristides, Philopœmen, Lysander, Cimon, Nicias, Agesilaus, Alexander the Great,* Oxford: Gale ECCO.

Poole, Thomas (2020) 'Leviathan in lockdown', *LRB,* 1 May. Online. Available HTTP: <https://www.lrb.co.uk/blog/2020/may/leviathan-in-lockdown> (accessed 3 May 2021).

Posner, Richard (2004) *Catastrophe: Risk and Response,* Oxford: Oxford University Press.

Price-Smith, Andrew (2009) *Contagion and Chaos: Disease, Ecology, and National Security in the Era of Globalization,* Cambridge: The MIT Press.

Princen, Sebastiaan (2007) 'Advocacy coalitions and the internationalization of public health policies', *Journal of Public Policy,* 27(1): 13–33.

Pullan, Brian (1992) 'Plagues and perception of the poor in early modern Italy', in T. Ranger and P. Slack (eds), *Epidemics and Ideas: Essays on the Historical Perception of Pestilence,* Cambridge: Cambridge University Press.

Pyle, Kenneth (2007) *Japan Rising: The Resurgence of Japanese Power and Purpose,* New York: Public Affairs.

Ramadan, A. (2013) 'Spatialising the refugee camp', *Transactions of the Institute of British Geographers,* 38(1): 65–77.

Rao, Mohan (1992) 'Of cholera and post-modern world', *Economic and Political Weekly,* 27(24): 1792.

Rasmussen, A.L. (2021) 'On the origins of SARS-CoV-2', *Nature Medicine,* 27(9). https://doi.org/10.1038/s41591-020-01205-5.

Reicher, S., Cassidy, C., Wolpert, I., Hopkins, N. and Levine, M. (2006) 'Saying Bulgaria's Jews: An analysis of social identity and the mobilization of social solidarity', *European Journal of Social Psychology,* 36: 49–72.

Reilley, B., Van Herp, M., Sermand, D. and Dentico, N. (2003) 'SARS and Carlo Urbani', *New England Journal of Medicine,* 348: 1951–2.

Retzinger, S. (1991) *Violent Emotion: Shame and Rage in Marital Quarrels,* Newbury Park: Sage.

Robins, R.S. (1981) 'Disease, political events, and populations', in H. Rothschild and C. Chapman (eds), *Biocultural Aspects of Disease,* London: Academic Press.

Rogalin, C., Soboroff, S. and Lovaglia, M. (2007) 'Power, status, and affect control', *Sociological Focus,* 40(2): 202–20.

Rollet, V. (2014) 'Framing SARS and H5N1 as an issue of national security in Taiwan: Process, motivations and consequences', *Extrême-Orient Extrême-Occident,* 37: 141–70.

Rorty, Richard (1989) *Contingency, Irony and Solidarity,* Cambridge: Cambridge University Press.

Rosenthal, Elizabeth (2003) 'The SARS epidemic: The path; From China's provinces, a crafty germ breaks out', *The New York Times,* 27 April. Online. Available HTTP: <www.nytimes.com/2003/04/27/world/the-sars-epidemic-the-path-from-china-s-provinces-a-crafty-germ-breaks-out.html> (accessed 3 May 2021).

Rotberg, R. (2002) 'The new nature of nation-state failure', *The Washington Quarterly,* 25(3): 85–96.

Rozakou, K. (2012) 'The biopolitics of hospitality in Greece: Humanitarianism and the management of refugees', *American Ethnologist,* 39(3): 562–77.

Rudan I. (2020) 'A cascade of causes that led to the COVID-19 tragedy in Italy and in other European Union countries', *Journal of Global Health,* 10(1). https://doi.org/10.7189/jogh-10-010335.

Rudd, K. (2015) 'The great guessing game: America, China, and the future of the global order', *Horizons: Journal of International Relations and Sustainable Development,* 5: 32–49.

Rushton, Simon (2019) *Security and Public Health—Pandemics and Politics in the Contemporary World*, Cambridge: Polity Press.

Russell, Timothy W., Wu, Joseph T., Clifford, Sam *et al.* (2021) 'Effect of internationally imported cases on internal spread of COVID-19: A mathematical modelling study', *Lancet Public Health*, 6. Online. Available HTTP: <www.thelancet.com/action/showPdf?pii=S2468-2667%2820%2930263-2> (accessed 5 May 2021).

Saab, Bilal Y. (2016) *After Hub-and-Spoke: US Hegemony in a New Gulf Security Order*, Washington, DC: Atlantic Council. Online. Available HTTP: < https://www.atlanticcouncil.org/wp-content/uploads/2016/04/Hub_and_Spoke_0414_web.pdf> (accessed 1 April 2021).

Salter, Mark (2008) 'Introduction', in M. Salter (ed), *Politics at the Airport*, Minneapolis: University of Minnesota Press.

Scarry, Elaine (1987) *The Body in Pain: The Making and Unmaking of the World*, New York: Oxford University Press.

Scheff, Thomas (1993) *Bloody Revenge*, Boulder: Westview.

Schepin, O. and Yermakov, W. (1991) *International Quarantine*, Madison: International University Press, Inc.

Schlosser, J. (2012) '"Hope, danger's comforter": Thucydides, hope, politics', *The Journal of Politics*, 75(1): 169–82.

Schraff, D. (2020) 'Political trust during the Covid-19 pandemic: Rally around the flag or lockdown effects?', *European Journal of Political Research*. Online. Available HTTP: < https://ejpr.onlinelibrary.wiley.com/doi/epdf/10.1111/1475-6765.12425> (accessed 1 December 2020).

Shaoul, J. (1997) 'Mad cow disease: The meat industry is out of control', *Ecologist,* 27(5): 182–7.

Sharat, G.L. (1995) 'Geopolitics of communicable diseases: Plague in Surat, 1994', *Economic and Political Weekly*, 30(46): 2912–14.

Shen, J. (2021) 'What roles do population and migration flows play in the spatial diffusion of COVID-19 from Wuhan City to provincial regions in China?', *China Review*, 21(3): 189–220.

Siddiqi, Javed (1995) *World Health and World Politics: The World Health Organization and the UN System*, Columbia: University of South Caroline Press.

Skillen, James (2001) *Putting the Focus in Context: Comments on President Bush's September 20 Address*, Washington. Online. Available HTTP: <https://web.archive.org/web/2009*/http://www.cpjustice.org/node/593> (accessed 10 December 2021).

Skinner, Q. (1988) 'A reply to my critics', in J. Tally (ed), *Meaning and Context*, London: Polity.

Skultety, Steven C. (2009) 'Delimiting Aristotle's conception of stasis in the politics', *Phronesis*, 54(4–5): 346–70.

Slack, Paul (1991) 'Responses to plague in early modern Europe: The implication of public health', in A. Mack (ed), *In Time of Plague: The History and Social Consequences of Lethal Epidemic Disease*, New York: New York University Press.

Slim, Hugo (2001) 'Violence and humanitarianism', *Security Dialogue*, 32(3): 325–39.

Slomp, G. (1990) 'Hobbes, Thucydides and the three greatest things', *History of Political Thought*, 11(4): 565–86.

Smith, Alastair (1998) 'International crises and domestic politics', *The American Political Science Review*, 92(3): 623–38.

Smith, Karen (2005) 'The outsiders: The European neighborhood policy', *International Affairs*, 81(4): 757–73.

Snowden, F.M. (2019, 2020) *Epidemics and Society: From the Black Death to the Present*, New Haven: Yale University Press.

Sontag, Susan (1978) 'Disease as political metaphor', *The New York Review of Books*, 23 February. Online. Available HTTP: < www.nybooks.com/articles/1978/02/23/disease-as-political-metaphor/> (accessed 10 December 2021).

Sontag, Susan (1988) *AIDS and Its Metaphors*, New York: Farrar, Straus and Giroux.

——— (2001) *Illness as Metaphor and AIDS and Its Metaphors*, New York: Picador.

Sowerby, R. (1998) 'Thomas Hobbes's translation of Thucydides', *Translation and Literature*, 7(2): 147–69.

Spilerman, S. (1970) 'The causes of racial disturbances: A comparison of alternative explanations', *American Sociological Review*, 35: 627–9.

Spitzer, Leo (1947) 'Ragamuffin, ragman, rimarole and rogue', *Modern Language Notes*, 62(2): 85–93.

Stahl, Hans-Peter (1966) *Die Stellung des Menschen im Geschichtichen Prozess*, Munich: Beck.

St John, R., King, A., de Jong, D., Bodie-Collins, M., Squires, S. and Tam, T. (2005) 'Border screening for SARS', *Emerging Infectious Diseases,* 11(1): 6–10.

Symonds, R. and Carder, M. (1973) *The United Nations and the Popuation Question 1945–70*, New York: McGraw-Hill.

Tesh, Sylvia (1988) *Hiden arguments: Political ideology and Disease Prevention Policy*, Piscataway: Rutgers University Press.

Thomas, E., Zhang, A. and Wallis, J. (2020) *Viral Videos: Covid-19, China and Inauthentic Influence on Facebook*, Sydney: Australian Strategic Policy Institute.

Thomas, N. (2006) 'The regionalization of avian influenza in East Asia: Responding to the next pandemic', *Asian Survey*, 46(6): 917–36.

Thucydides (1959) *The Peloponnesian War: The Thomas Hobbes Translation*, David Grene (ed), Ann Arbor: University of Michigan Press.

Torgman, A. (2012) 'Haiti: A failed state? Democratic process and OAS intervention', *The University of Miami Inter-American Law Review*, 44(1): 113–37.

Troy, K. (1996) 'The plague that wasn't', *Newsweek*, 9 December: 18.

Truex, Rory (2020) 'China's chernobyl never seems to arise', *The Atlantic*, 17 February. Online. Available HTTP: < https://www.theatlantic.com/ideas/archive/2020/02/cor onavirus-wont-be-chinas-chernobyl/606673/> (accessed 12 December 2021).

Tuan, Y. (1995) 'Island selves: Human disconnectedness in a world of interdependence', *Geographical Review*, 85(2): 229–39. https://doi.org/10.2307/216065.

Tuan, Yi-Fu (1979) *Landscapes of Fear*, New York: Pantheon Books.

Tuite, A., Tien, J., Eisenberg, M. *et al.* (2011) 'Cholera epidemic in Haiti, 2010: Using a transmission model to explain spatial spread of disease and identify optimal control interventions', *Annals of Internal Medicine*, 154: 593–601.

Turner, V. (1957) *Schism and Continuity in an African Society*, Manchester: Manchester University Press.

Ungar, Sheldon (1998) 'Hot crises and media reassurance: A comparison of emerging diseases and Ebola Zaire', *British Journal of Sociology*, 49(1): 36–56.

United Nations Secretary-General (2016) 'Statement attributable to the spokesman for the secretary-general on Haiti'. Online. Available HTTP: <www.un.org/sg/en/content/ sg/statement/2016-08-19/statement-attributable-spokesman-secretary-general-haiti> (accessed 11 October 2018).

Urry, J. (2009) 'Aeromobilities and the Global', in S. Cwerner, S. Kesselring and J. Urry (eds), *Aeromobilities*, London: Routledge.

The Wall Street Journal (2020) 'Beijing Faults U.S. Stance on coronavirus', 6 February. Online. Available HTTP: <www.wsj.com/articles/beijing-faults-u-s-stance-on-corona virus-11581014266> (accessed 28 May 2020).

Wardrip, Noah (1996) 'Writing Networks: New Media, Potential Literature'. *Leonardo*, 29(5): 355–373.

Watts, S. (2001) 'Yellow fever immunities in West Africa and the Americas in the age of slavery and beyond: A reapprisal', *Journal of Social History*, 34(4): 969–74.

Weiss, Meira (1997) 'Signifying the pandemics: Metaphors of AIDS, cancer and heart disease', *Medical Anthropology Quarterly*, 11(4): 456–76.

Wen, Y. (2021) 'Branding and legitimation: China's party diplomacy amid the COVID-19 pandemic', *China Review*, 21(1): 55–90.

Wenham, Clare (2019) 'The oversecuritization of global health: Changing the terms of debate', *International Affairs*, 95(5): 1093–110.

Westlake, M. (2020) 'Conclusions: Chronicle of a Brexit foretold?' in *Slipping Loose: The UK's Long Drift Away from the European Union*, Newcastle upon Tyne: Agenda Publishing.

White House (2003a) 'O'Neil, Fauci discuss president's AIDS initiatives', 3 May.

——— (2003b) 'Joint statement between the United States of America and Singapore', 6 May. Online. Available HTTP: <https://georgewbush-whitehouse.archives.gov/news/releases/2003/05/20030506-12.html> (accessed 3 May 2021).

——— (2004) 'Fact sheet: President bush signs biodefense for the 21st century', 28 April. Online. Available HTTP: <https://fas.org/irp/offdocs/nspd/biodef.html> (accessed 3 May 2021).

——— (2005) 'National strategy for pandemic influenza', 1 November. Online. Available HTTP: <https://georgewbush-whitehouse.archives.gov/homeland/pandemic-influenza.html> (accessed 31 December 2021).

——— (2021) 'Quad leaders' joint statement: "The spirit of the Quad"', 12 March. Online. Available HTTP: <www.whitehouse.gov/briefing-room/statements-releases/2021/03/12/quad-leaders-joint-statement-the-spirit-of-the-quad/> (accessed 18 March 2021).

WHO (2003) 'Consensus document on the epidemiology of severe acute respiratory syndrome (SARS)'. Online. Available HTTP: < https://www.who.int/csr/sars/en/WHO-consensus.pdf> (accessed 23 March 2021).

——— (2005) 'Revision of the international health regulations'. Online. Available HTTP: <www.who.int/csr/ihr/WHA58-en.pdf> (accessed 5 May 2021).

——— (2005, 2016) *International Health Regulations*, 3rd edition. Online. Available HTTP: <https://apps.who.int/iris/bitstream/handle/10665/246107/9789241580496-eng.pdf;jsessionid=EEC296B19D29D4FC23DAB8E4F19369F9?sequence=1> (accessed 5 May 2021).

——— (2006a) *WHO Pandemic Influenza Draft Protocol for Rapid Response and Containment Updated Draft 30 May 2006*, Geneva: World Health Organization.

——— (2006b) *SARS: How a Global Epidemic Was Stopped*, Geneva: WHO Press.

——— (2007a) *The World Health Report 2007: A Safer Future – Global Public Health Security in the 21st Century*, Geneva: World Health Organization.

——— (2007b) *WHO Interim Protocol: Rapib Operations to Contain the Initial Emergence of Pandemic Influenza*, Geneva: World Health Organization.

——— (2015) 'Blueprint for R&D preparedness and respose to public health emergencies due to highly infectious pathogents'. Online. Available HTTP: < https://www.who.int/docs/default-source/blue-print/blueprint-for-r-d-preparedness-and-response-meeting-report.pdf?sfvrsn=156d23be_2> (accessed 12 December 2021).

——— (2018) 'Prioritizing diseases for research and development in emergency contexts'. Online. Available HTTP: < https://www.who.int/activities/prioritizing-diseases-for-research-and-development-in-emergency-contexts> (accessed 12 December 2021).

——— (2020a) 'WHO advice for international travel and trade in relation to the outbreak of pneumonia caused by a new coronavirus in China', 10 January. Online. Available HTTP: <www.who.int/news-room/articles-detail/who-advice-for-international-travel-and-

trade-in-relation-to-the-outbreak-of-pneumonia-caused-by-a-new-coronavirus-in-china> (accessed 5 May 2021).

———— (2020b) 'Updated WHO advice for international traffic in relation to the outbreak of the novel coronavirus 2019-nCoV', 24 January. Online. Available HTTP: <www.who.int/news-room/articles-detail/updated-who-advice-for-international-traffic-in-relation-to-the-outbreak-of-the-novel-coronavirus-2019-ncov-24-jan/>(accessed5May 2021).

———— (2020c) 'Updated WHO advice for international traffic in relation to the outbreak of the novel coronavirus 2019-nCoV', 27 January. Online. Available HTTP: <www.who.int/news-room/articles-detail/updated-who-advice-for-international-traffic-in-relation-to-the-outbreak-of-the-novel-coronavirus-2019-ncov> (accessed 5 May 2021).

———— (2020d) 'Updated WHO recommendations for international traffic in relation to COVID-19 outbreak', 29 February. Online. Available HTTP: <www.who.int/news-room/articles-detail/updated-who-recommendations-for-international-traffic-in-rela tion-to-covid-19-outbreak> (accessed 5 May 2021).

———— (2021a) 'WHO-convened global study of origins of SARS-CoV-2: China part'. Online. Available HTTP: <www.who.int/docs/default-source/coronaviruse/final-joint-report_origins-studies-6-april-201.pdf?sfvrsn=4f5e5196_1&download=true> (accessed 5 May 2021).

———— (2021b) 'WHO calls for further studies, data on origin of SARS-CoV-2 virus, reiterates that all hypotheses remain open'. Online. Available HTTP: <www.who.int/news/item/30-03-2021-who-calls-for-further-studies-data-on-origin-of-sars-cov-2-virus-reiterates-that-all-hypotheses-remain-open> (accessed 5 May 2021).

Willer, David, Lovaglia, Michael and Markovsky, Barry (1997) 'Power and influence: A theoretical bridge', *Social Forces*, 76(2): 571–603.

Wittgenstein, L. (1968) *Philosophical Investigations*, Oxford: Basil Blackwell.

———— (1980) *Culture and Value*, Chicago: University of Chicago Press.

Woodward, Bob (2010) *Obama's Wars*, New York: Simon & Schuster.

Yanzhong, Huang (2004) 'The SARS epidemic and its aftermath in China: A political perspective', in S. Knobler *et al.* (eds), *Learning from SARS: Preparing for the Next Disease Outbreak*, Washington, DC: The National Academies Press.

Yoshikawa, Hiroyuki (1999) 'ICSU opening the door to the new millenium', *Science International Newsletter*, 71: 1–2.

Zacher, M. and Sutton, B. (1996) *Governing Global Networks: International Regimes and Communications*, Cambridge: Cambridge University Press.

Zaretsky, Robert (2020) 'When the plague came to Athens: For Thucydides, history was flux and humanity was constant', *Foreign Affairs*, 21 May. Online. Available HTTP: <www.foreignaffairs.com/articles/greece/2020-05-21/when-plague-came-athens> (accessed 21 November 2020).

Zartman, William (1995) 'Introduction', in W. Zartman (ed), *Collapsed States: The Disintegration and Restoration of Legitimate Authority*, SAIS African Studies Library, Boulder: L. Rienner Publishers.

Zerubavel, E. (1997) *Social Mindscapes: An Invitation to Cognitive Sociology*, Cambridge: Harvard University Press.

Zuckerman, A. (2004) 'Plague and contagionism in eighteenth-century England: The role of Richard Mead', *Bulletin of the History of Medicine*, 78(2): 273–308.

INDEX

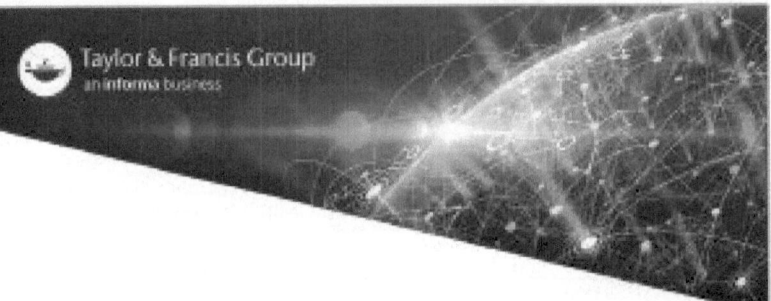
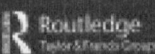
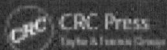